BASIC MATERNAL-
NEWBORN NURSING

BASIC MATERNAL-NEWBORN NURSING

FIFTH EDITION

Barbara G. Anderson
Pamela J. Shapiro

DELMAR PUBLISHERS INC. ®

NOTICE TO THE READER

Executive Editor: Leslie Boyer
Project Editor: Carol Micheli
Editing Manager: Barbara Christie
Production Coordinator: Linda Helfrich
Design Coordinator: Susan Mathews

For information, address Delmar Publishers Inc.
2 Computer Drive West, Box 15–015
Albany, New York 12212

10   9   8   7   6   5   4   3

Printed in the United States of America
Published simultaneously in Canada
by Nelson Canada,
A division of The Thomson Corporation

Library of Congress Cataloging-in-Publication Data

Anderson, Barbara G.
    Basic maternal-newborn nursing / Barbara G. Anderson,
Pamela J. Shapiro, 5th ed.
        p. cm.
        Rev. ed. of: Obstetrics for the nurse / Barbara G. Anderson,
Pamela J. Shapiro, 4th ed. c1984.
        Bibliography: p.
        Includes index.
        1. Obstetrical nursing. I. Shapiro, Pamela J.
II. Anderson, Barbara G. Obstetrics for the nurse.
III. Title.
        [DNLM: 1. Obstetrical Nursing. WY 157 Ar4ro]
RG951.A52   1989   610.73'678—dc19   88-2039
ISBN: 0-8273-3373-0 (pbk.)
ISBN: 0-8273-3374-0 (instructor's guide)

CONTENTS

PREFACE

The fifth edition of *Basic Maternal-Newborn Nursing* (formerly *Obstetrics for the Nurse*) continues to place emphasis on the nursing process as an approach to family-centered maternity care. The text has been revised and updated to include the latest developments in the care of the child-bearing family. Information on cultural variances has been included in this edition. Also, information on bonding and attachment to the newborn has been expanded to enable the nursing student to more fully understand this important process.

In order to promote student understanding and continuity of patient care, the discussion of normal pregnancy and childbirth has been separated from the presentation of complications that can occur during pregnancy, labor, and delivery. Expanded sections on maternal-infant nutritional needs, breast-feeding, including a chart dealing with breastfeeding problems, fetal monitoring, non-stress tests and biophysical profiles, amniocentesis, ultrasonography, Doppler instrumentation, and alternative birthing centers contribute to the comprehensiveness of this text. Additional information on the nursing process and nursing care plans reflect current trends and updated approaches to patient care.

Information regarding gestational diabetes, screening for neural tube defects and chorionic villi sampling have been added to help the nursing student's understanding of the prenatal screening techniques now available. Detriments to fetal health including smoking, alcohol consumption, drugs, and environmental influences have been expanded. A more complete section has been added regarding sexually transmitted diseases, including AIDS. The CDC's recommendation for health care workers has been provided.

New illustrative material and charts demonstrating various positions for labor and delivery have been included to help orient the student to ways of enhancing the birthing process. A section on newborn evaluation has also been included.

In addition to these textual changes, the fifth edition of *Basic Maternal-Newborn Nursing* retains from previous editions the following learning/teaching aids:

- learning objectives that precede each chapter
- review questions at the end of each unit and self-evaluation tests at the end of each section which reflect the learning objectives and reinforce student comprehension and retention

- suggested activities at the end of each chapter that provide opportunities for further enrichment and application of knowledge
- extensive use of color illustrations and tables, providing visual-interest and promoting retention of information
- step-by-step procedural instructions for certain nursing techniques
- color highlighting of material or information that is of special significance to the nurse
- an expanded glossary and index for quick reference

The authors appreciate the in-depth reviews of the fifth edition by numerous maternity nursing instructors. We are gratified to know the text serves as an ideal resource for review in preparation for the nursing board exams as well as a basic introductory text to family-centered maternity care.

The Authors

The authors have had many years of experience in obstetrical nursing and are also co-authors of EMERGENCY CHILDBIRTH HANDBOOK. Barbara Anderson received her basic nursing education at St. Mary's Hospital in Waterbury, Connecticut and her B.S. degree from Chaminade University in Honolulu, Hawaii. She is currently retired as administrator of Kaiser Moanalua Medical Center in Honolulu, Hawaii.

Pamela Shapiro received her B.S.N. from California State University in 1970. She has worked as a public health nurse and has also had experience in psychosocial counseling in a rehabilitation center. She received additional training in 1975 from ICEA to prepare expectant couples for childbirth and early parenting. She has taught Lamaze technique and parenting classes for twelve years. Recently Ms. Shapiro completed an OB-GYN Nurse Practitioner program through California State University, San Jose. She is currently practicing as a women's health care nurse practitioner in a private physician's office in Kirkland, Washington.

Reviewers for the Fifth Edition

Pauline Goss, Riverside Community College, Riverside, California
Lois Butts, Del Mar College, Corpus Christie, Texas
Nancy DiDona, Elizabeth Seton College, Yonkers, New York
Helen M. Binda, Orleans Niagara BOCES, Sanborn, New York
Adeline M. Hardin, Former Instructor, St. Paul Technical Institute, Mesa, Arizona
Darlene Ross, St. Paul Technical Institute, St. Paul, Minnesota

SECTION 1

The Beginning of Life

UNIT 1

THE HISTORY OF MATERNAL-INFANT NURSING

OBJECTIVES

After studying this unit, the student should be able to:

- Identify noteworthy midwives.
- State the training given to midwives.
- List factors that have influenced changing trends in obstetrics.
- Identify legislation affecting midwives.
- Explain the role of the obstetrical nurse and the obstetrical technician.
- Describe current trends in obstetrical nursing.

From the earliest recorded time and in every culture women have attended other women in childbirth. As late as the eighteenth century, care of the pregnant woman was considered beneath the dignity of the physician. Men were summoned only in complicated and neglected cases.

MIDWIVES AND MIDWIFERY

In the fifth century B.C. the first formal training for midwives was instituted by Hippocrates. However, for several centuries thereafter efforts toward education were ineffectual. Basic obstetrical knowledge for midwives was contained in two books: one published in 1513 by a surgeon named Rodien, the other written by Jacob Rueff in 1554. Self-taught or instructed by older midwives, most midwives remained ignorant of the simple principles of obstetrics.

A few European midwives of the seventeenth and eighteenth centuries, by contrast, achieved wide renown for their skill, writing and devotion. Loyse Boursier (1563-1636) was a midwife to the French court and royal family for twenty-seven years. Elizabeth Nihell (1723-?) was a famous English midwife who wrote *A Treatise on the Art of Midwifery* in 1760. During the seventeenth century, physicians still did not participate in either a normal or abnormal

1

delivery. Their role was limited to writing prescriptions for drugs that a midwife wished to administer.

The first known instance of midwifery in the United States occurred in 1621 when Mrs. Bridget Lee Fuller, with knowledge acquired from practical experience, helped in a delivery on the Mayflower.

Anne Hutchinson, America's best remembered midwife, was of invaluable service in the mid-seventeenth century. In addition to her involvement as a midwife she was also active in religious work. In 1637 she was condemned in Boston for her interpretations of the Bible. She was accused of witchcraft after she helped Jane Hawkins deliver a monsterlike baby. Anne Hutchinson was massacred by Indians in the late summer of 1643. The Hutchinson River Parkway near New York City was named after this notable midwife.

Midwifery gradually became an accepted practice. Testimony of midwives became acceptable when questions of pregnancy or paternity arose. In the 1660s midwives were paid a salary of 100 guilders per year for attending the poor.

Throughout the eighteenth and nineteenth centuries most labors were still attended by midwives although the role of the physician was gradually increasing. Some midwives were called granny midwives or granny women; these women were untrained, often illiterate, and superstitious. Most were foreign-born or Black and served in cities of the Northeast or on plantations of the South. The inept practices of the granny midwives were reflected in the maternal and infant mortality statistics and the countless cases of gonorrheal ophthalmia resulting in blindness of the newborn.

Regulation of Standards

By the sixteenth century, rules and regulations were being drawn up in many countries in order to improve the work of the midwives. In the seventeenth century, many cities required prospective midwives to work under a recognized and experienced midwife before being allowed to practice.

Legal regulation of midwifery standards began earlier in Western Europe than in America. The first formal edicts governing obstetric practice were so general that they were virtually without effect. New York's ordinance of July 16, 1716 was more specific but dealt mainly with the midwife's ethical conduct and ignored her professional qualifications.

During the nineteenth century, medical licensure came under state control but there was little regulation. A significant beginning toward effective regulation came in 1907 with the enactment of the State Midwifery law which transferred control of midwives in New York City to the city's board of health. The city's midwives were now required to register annually, to demonstrate their ability to read and write, to be of good moral character, and to have attended a minimum of twenty cases of labor under the supervision of a licensed and registered physician. Enforcement of this law, however, was difficult and many women continued to practice midwifery without sanction.

In 1910 about 50 percent of all births in the United States were reported by midwives. However, a commissioned study made by New York State revealed that midwifery practices in the state were essentially medieval and very different from European midwifery. This study resulted in the tightening of existing legislation. A new institution was created with licensing and supervision. This eventually led to the establishment of the Bellevue School of Midwives. In the early 1900s, it was the midwife's duty to assist in labor and delivery and to keep the household running normally. The midwife's training consisted of at least six months to a year of instruction on pregnancy, asepsis, care during labor, and care of mother and child after delivery. Above all, the midwife was taught to recognize any condition that indicated a doctor was needed.

Revival of Midwifery

A commendable revival of educating midwives has taken place in the United States. Since 1915, the Maternity Center Association in New York City has been teaching midwifery. Also, training has taken place in several obstetrical centers such as Yale and Johns Hopkins Medical Center. Moreover home deliveries, which had become obsolete, began to increase. A revival of lay midwifery in the United States began in the mid 1970s with the formation of several groups dedicated to the restoration of childbirth in the home. By the end of 1977, lay midwives were licensed in fourteen states, mostly in the South.

Even though the number of home births have increased, the American College of Nurse Midwives considers the hospital or maternity home to be the preferred site for childbirth. This is because these institutions can better provide for the physical welfare of both the mother and infant. The College encourages members of the obstetrics team to provide for the personal needs of the family by combining a family-centered atmosphere with the safety of readily available obstetrical care, including the services of a physician.

HOSPITAL BIRTHS

During the period from 1930 to 1960 the proportion of births in hospitals increased from 36.9 percent (1935) to 88 percent (1950) to 96 percent (1960). During this period the campaign to hospitalize birth was supported by obstetricians, public health officials, upper class women and insurance companies. In 1946 the Hill-

Burton Act provided funds for the construction of hospitals in rural areas creating the possibility of hospital birth for women which previously had no choice but to give birth at home.

In the 1930s when half the deliveries in the United States were carried out at home, the maternal mortality rate was 60 per 10,000 live births. In 1975 with over 99 percent of deliveries in hospitals, maternal mortality was less than 3 per 10,000 live births. This is not a coincidence.

In the past ten years, there has been a significant change in the hospital environment for obstetrical patients. There is a trend toward family-centered maternity units. Women enter the hospital to a nicely decorated, home-like room. They labor, deliver their babies, recover and remain in the same room throughout their hospital stay, figures 1-1, 1-2, and 1-3. This combines many of the benefits of a home delivery with the safety aspects of a hospital birth.

THE OBSTETRICAL NURSE

Special obstetric training for nurses began in the United States with the founding of maternity hospitals in the late nineteenth century and the

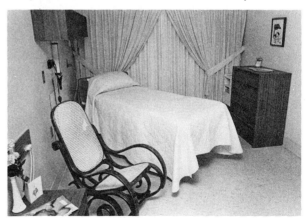

Figure 1-1
Home-like birthing room

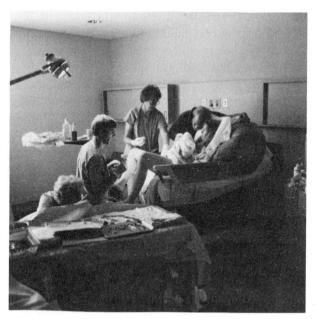

Figure 1-2

Teamwork in action

establishment of separate departments of obstetrics in general hospitals. Instruction in specific problems of pregnancy, labor and delivery became a standard part of the curriculum in nurses' training schools. As American medicine grew in complexity, nursing demanded greater skills. Maternity nurses known as Ob-Gyn nurse practitioners were trained to carry out many of the functions of the obstetric physician. These nurses (1) take the patient's history, (2) perform the physical examination, (3) make an obstetric evaluation, (4) manage and support the patient through labor up to the time of delivery, and (5) recognize obstetric complications.

The most significant source of support for the obstetrical nurse in the United States and Canada is the Nurses Association of the American College of Obstetricians and Gynecologists (NAACOG). The Association was formed in 1969 and is committed to the goal of improving the health

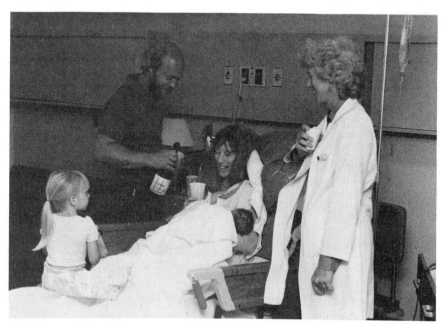

Figure 1-3

The expanding family gets acquainted.

of women and newborn babies. The NAACOG conducts educational programs in obstetric and gynecologic nursing and publishes the bimonthly *Journal of Obstetric, Gynecologic and Neonatal Nursing.*

To stimulate and recognize excellence in obstetric and gynecologic nursing, the Association has formed the NAACOG Certification Corporation. This Corporation has organized a voluntary joint certification program in maternal-gynecological-neonatal nursing in conjunction with the Division on Maternal and Child Health Nursing Practice of the American Nurses' Association. Examinations for certification were offered for the first time in 1976 to registered nurses who have been engaged in obstetric-gynecologic nursing for at least two consecutive years and who are currently devoting at least half of their practice time to patient care.

The Obstetrical Technician

The drastic shortage of nurses qualified to care for women during labor and delivery was apparent more than a decade ago. Analysis of the problem showed that an obstetrical technician could fill the need, just as the surgical technician fills a role in the operating room. In 1963, the first trained and qualified obstetrical technicians began to take over specific tasks in obstetrical units. With a basic understanding of the physiological principles relating to pregnancy and its termination, a technical knowledge of the process of normal labor, awareness of the symptoms of abnormal labor, and knowledge of procedures, an obstetrical technician fills a definite need in the health service field.

CONSUMER INFLUENCE

The practice of obstetrics has changed radically since 1920 with the introduction of blood transfusions, knowledge of the Rh factor, the advent of antibiotics, progress in anesthesiology, and other new knowledge. Since the 1960s, maternity care has rapidly improved not only because of advances in technology and better trained nurses, but also because of a continuing emphasis on educating consumers. This phenomenon has been very visible in the health field, particularly in the area of obstetrics.

The pregnant woman is involved in a natural process and does not have an illness or disease. However, prenatal health care is essential to prevent complications before they occur. With increased information and support from physicians and nurses, prepared childbirth classes, and an increasing abundance of literature for the expectant mother, women are finding they have more knowledge to actively take part in their own health care.

Consumers have already had a great effect on changing policies in obstetrics. Husbands now actively participate in labor and delivery and babies are allowed to stay with their mothers during the hospital stay (rooming-in) rather than being viewed behind glass in the nursery. Other medical practices such as positions for delivery (semi-sitting, squatting, or side-lying), enemas on admission and the availability of walking during labor have been influenced by the consumer.

Prepared childbirth classes have become a recommended choice by many expectant parents and allow the couple to participate more actively in the birth of their baby. Lamaze, Dick-Read and Bradley are the three best known methods of childbirth preparation. All use special breathing techniques and relaxation and all attempt to educate participants about the physiology of childbirth. The methods differ mainly in the specific breathing patterns and the specific comfort-producing behaviors taught to couples for use during labor. All prepared childbirth philosophies have the common goal of making the birth experience personally satisfying and safe.

Hospitals and personnel are attempting to meet the desires of consumers. Many hospitals today have birthing rooms with colorful wallpaper, curtains and dressers to create a more homelike atmosphere.

Variations of the birthing room concept are found across the country. Some are a compromise between traditional delivery rooms and alternative birth centers (ABC), which began to open between 1976 and 1982. Some hospitals use the Borning Bed that provides safe options for positioning of the mother.

The concept underlying birthing rooms is that of humanizing the birth experience and emphasizing the individual. Traditionally the mother has been moved to a postpartum unit after delivery. A single unit provides for labor, delivery, and recovery of the mother and baby. This minimizes nursing staff, and prevents disruption of the family unit during hospitalization. Advantages of a birthing room are:

1. The nursing staff no longer has to make the decision when to move the mother.
2. No second room needs to be set up.
3. Cost in staff, linen, and equipment is reduced.
4. Client satisfaction is increased.

ABCs have home-like accommodations including a crib for the newborn, private bathroom facilities, and lounge area. The philosophic difference between the ABC concept and a birthing room is screening criteria and should be limited to use by low-risk mothers. The concern of the nurse is to encourage couples to explore the birthing alternatives available to them in order that they can make a responsible informed decision.

SUGGESTED ACTIVITY

- Describe the setting and the style of care a patient might expect in a/an:
  a. hospital
  b. alternative birth center
  c. home birth with midwife

REVIEW

A. Multiple Choice. Select the best answer.

1. The first formal training for midwives was instituted in
    a. the 14th century
    c. the 17th century
    b. the 5th century B.C.
    d. the 19th century

2. The first known instance of midwifery in the United States occurred when
    a. Anne Hutchinson delivered a baby in New York City
    b. Bridget Lee Fuller helped in a delivery on the Mayflower
    c. Elizabeth Nihell wrote a book on midwifery
    d. Loyse Boursier came to the United States from France to practice midwifery

3. During the seventeenth century, the physician's role in obstetrics was to
   a. deliver the baby only
   b. attend the labor and delivery
   c. supervise the midwife
   d. write prescriptions for drugs that a midwife wished to administer

4. After 1935, the trend toward hospital births
   a. decreased the maternal mortality rate
   b. increased the infant mortality rate
   c. was limited only to upper class women
   d. all of these

5. The American College of Nurse Midwives recommends
   a. home deliveries
   b. strict laws governing midwives
   c. hospital or maternity home deliveries
   d. prohibiting the licensing of lay midwives

6. During 1935, hospital births in the United States occurred at the rate of
   a. 36.9 percent   c. 88 percent
   b. 50 percent   d. 96 percent

7. The Hill-Burton Act of 1946 provided for
   a. tuition for education of midwives
   b. better regulation and licensing of midwives
   c. construction of hospitals in rural areas
   d. training of the obstetrical technician

8. Factors that have influenced the changing trends in obstetrics since 1960 include
   a. advances in technology
   b. better trained nurses
   c. consumer education
   d. all of these

9. Midwife training in the early 1900s consisted of instruction in
   1. pregnancy and asepsis
   2. care during labor
   3. care of the mother and child after delivery
   4. recognizing conditions requiring a doctor
   a. 2 and 3
   b. 1, 2 and 3
   c. 4 only
   d. 1, 2, 3 and 4

10. Duties of the midwife included
    1. keeping the household running normally
    2. assisting in labor and delivery
    3. providing self-care instructions to the mother
    4. providing postnatal care for the newborn
       a. 1 and 2
       b. 2 only
       c. 1, 2 and 3
       d. 1, 2, 3 and 4

B. Match the term in column II to the correct statement in column I.

Column I	Column II
____ 1. homelike atmosphere where labor, delivery and recovery take place	a. Ob-Gyn nurse practitioner
____ 2. conducts educational programs in obstetric and gynecologic nursing	b. obstetrical technician
____ 3. babies stay with their mothers during the hospital stay	c. granny women
____ 4. carries out many of the functions of the obstetric physician	d. Anne Hutchinson
____ 5. transferred control of midwives in New York City to the board of health	e. Rodien
____ 6. untrained, illiterate, superstitious midwives	f. Dick-Read
____ 7. helps out in the obstetrical unit	g. Elizabeth Nihell
____ 8. wrote a basic obstetrics text in 1513	h. State Midwifery Law
____ 9. method of childbirth preparation	i. Maternity Center Association
____ 10. wrote *A Treatise on the Art of Midwifery*	j. Nurses Association of the American College of Obstetricians and Gynecologists
____ 11. notable American midwife of the seventeenth century	k. birthing room
____ 12. teaches midwifery	l. rooming-in

UNIT **2**

THE FEMALE REPRODUCTIVE SYSTEM

OBJECTIVES

After studying this unit, the student should be able to:

- State the primary functions of the female reproductive system.
- Identify the primary parts of the female reproductive system.
- Explain the functions of each of the primary parts of the female reproductive system.

*O*bstetrics is the branch of medical science which deals with childbirth and that which precedes and follows it. The nurse must acquire an understanding of the reproductive process in order to administer nursing care to the obstetric patient before and during childbirth. A knowledge of this process is also essential to caring for the mother and child following delivery.

Human life begins with the union of two cells: one from the female, called the ovum, and one from the male, called the sperm. This union of male and female cells, known as *fertilization* or *conception*, takes place within the female. She is responsible, both directly and indirectly, for the growth and development of the fertilized ovum which eventually results in the birth of a child. A beginning study should first examine the female reproductive system to discover how it is specially adapted for this purpose.

The female reproductive system has four basic functions:

- To produce ovarian hormones which are responsible for the female sex characteristics and reproductive functions.
- To produce the ovum and deliver it to the place where conception may take place.
- To nurture and sustain the developing fertilized ovum (product of conception) until birth.
- To accomplish delivery of the product of conception.

The female reproductive system includes the external genitals, internal organs, the breasts, pelvis, and related pelvic structures.

THE EXTERNAL GENITALS

The external genitals are those structures adjacent to but outside of the entrance to the vagina, figure 2-1. They protect the vagina and provide access for the male reproductive organ.

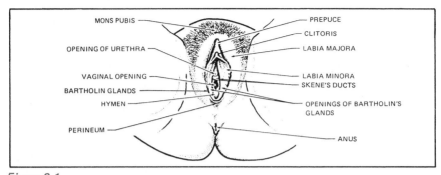

Figure 2-1

External genitalia

The Vulva

The *vulva* consists of two heavy lips called the *labia majora* and the external structures contained within them. The outside surface of the labia majora is composed of skin and fat and covered with pubic hair. The inner surface resembles mucous membrane. The labia extend from the *mons veneris*, a pad of fat covering the pubic area, to the perineum. The function of the labia majora is to cover and protect the vaginal entrance.

Inside the labia majora are two smaller lips called the *labia minora*. These thinner lips meet to form a partial hood called the *prepuce* which covers a tiny erectile structure, the *clitoris*. This is a small elongated mass of tissue, nerves, and muscle richly supplied with blood vessels and covered with mucous membrane. The clitoris is like the male organ, the penis, in that it is extremely sensitive and responds to sexual excitation. *Bartholin's glands* secrete a mucoid, lubricating substance during sexual intercourse. One gland is located on each side of the labia minora. Below the clitoris are two raised ridges with an opening between them; this is called the *urinary meatus* through which urine is voided.

Just below the meatus is a fold of mucous membrane called the *hymen* which protects the vaginal opening. The hymen partly (and occasionally completely) closes the outlet of the vagina.

Contrary to popular belief, rupture of the hymen is not necessarily an indication of the loss of virginity. It could occur from injury, surgery, use of tampons for menstruation, active sports, premarital examination, or sexual intercourse.

The Perineum

The area of skin, connective tissue, and muscle which lies between the vulva and the anus is known as the *perineum*. The muscle tissues affect the opening and closing of the vagina and the anus. The perineum stretches to accommodate delivery of the newborn. Injury to the perineum during birth may affect the support of the internal organs and bowel control.

The Anus

While not considered to be a part of the reproductive system, the anus is adjacent to the external reproductive organs. The *anus* lies below the perineum and is a deeply pigmented, puckered opening which serves as the outlet of the rectum. The anus is controlled by a circular muscle called the *anal sphincter*. This muscle controls the passage of feces and flatus. The mucous membrane of the rectum is very sensitive and easily injured. Because of its anatomical position, the rectum is sometimes used for examining procedures during pregnancy and labor.

INTERNAL ORGANS

The internal reproductive organs are those which lie within the pelvic cavity. They consist of the vagina, uterus, fallopian tubes, and ovaries. Also included are the supporting structures.

The Vagina

The vagina is a curved tubelike passage 8 to 12 centimeters long that leads from the vulva to the uterus. The lower portion of the cervix of the uterus protrudes into it. It is internally situated between the bladder and rectum. The vagina is made up of muscle and connective tissue and is capable of great distention during labor. It is lined with mucous membrane containing many folds called *rugae*. The secretion observed in the vagina is largely derived from the glands of the cervix. The vagina serves three important functions as a passage: (1) introduction of the penis and reception of *semen* (fluid in which sperm is carried), (2) discharge of menstrual flow and uterine secretions, and (3) delivery of the product of conception.

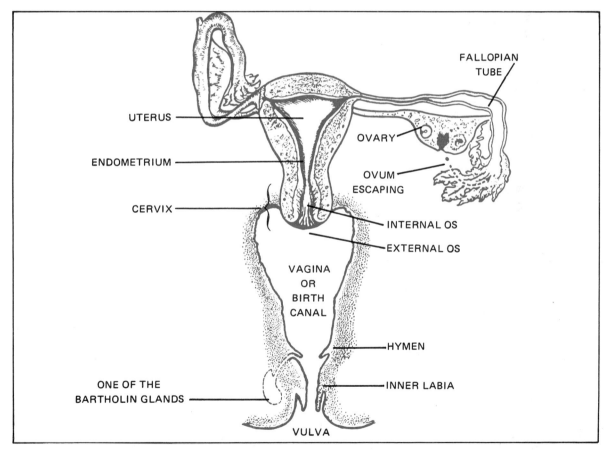

Figure 2-2

Internal female reproductive organs (Educational Department, Tampax, Inc., New York, NY)

The Uterus

The *uterus* is the organ which carries the fetus during pregnancy. It is a hollow, pear-shaped organ with thick muscular walls, and is 2 1/2 to 3 inches long and 3/4-inch thick. It occupies the middle of the pelvis between the bladder and the rectum and consists of the *fundus* (rounded top part), the *body* (middle part), and a narrow lower portion called the *cervix* (neck). The fundus and body make up the *corpus* of the uterus. The lining of the uterus is called the *endometrium.* The endometrium receives and nourishes the fertilized egg. During pregnancy, the uterus grows very soft and increases greatly in size to hold the growing fetus. By the end of pregnancy, the uterus becomes a thin, soft-walled muscular sac which yields to the movement of the fetus.

About half the length of the cervix projects into the vagina where the vaginal walls are attached to it. The cervix has a small round passageway called the cervical canal; the *internal os* of the canal opens into the uterus, and the *external os* opens into the vagina. Uterine secretions, the menstrual flow, the unfertilized ovum, the fetus during labor, and the *lochial discharge* (vaginal drainage during the six-week period following delivery) pass through the cervix to the vagina.

The Uterine Ligaments. The *broad ligaments* are two structures which extend from the side walls of the uterus to the pelvic walls. The ovaries and fallopian tubes are attached to these ligaments. The *round ligaments* of the uterus, attached to the side walls of the uterus, pass through the broad ligaments to reach the mons veneris. These ligaments help to support the pelvic organs. The *uterosacral ligaments* extend from the posterior cervical portion of the uterus to the sacrum and support the cervix.

The Fallopian Tubes

The two *fallopian tubes,* or *oviducts,* extend outward from the upper corners of the uterus to the abdominal cavity. They are about the diameter of a drinking straw and are largely muscular structures. The distal portion of the tube curves around the ovary in such a way that the fingerlike projections cup over the ovary but are not actually attached to it, figure 2-2. Their function is to carry the ovum along the canal by peristaltic action from the ovary to the uterus. Conception usually takes place in the outer third of the fallopian tube.

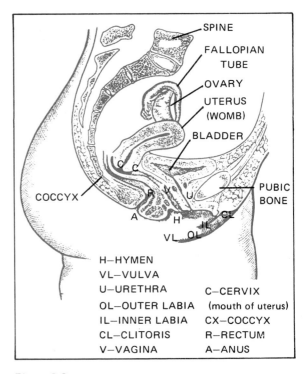

H—HYMEN
VL—VULVA
U—URETHRA
OL—OUTER LABIA   C—CERVIX
IL—INNER LABIA   (mouth of uterus)
CL—CLITORIS   CX—COCCYX
V—VAGINA   R—RECTUM
                  A—ANUS

Figure 2-3

Side view of the female pelvic organs (Educational Department, Tampax, Inc.)

The Ovaries

The two *ovaries* are also known as the sex glands of the female. In shape and size, they resemble an almond: hard, fibrous, silvery-white, and dimpled. Their functions are to mature and discharge ova and to produce hormones necessary to the process of reproduction. Several hundred thousand immature ova are present in the ovaries of the female at birth. At puberty, the ovaries systematically release one ovum at a time. The process continues until the time of menopause unless interrupted by pregnancy or the use of oral contraceptives. After menopause, the ovaries *atrophy* (decrease in size) and shrivel.

THE BREASTS

The breasts are considered to be accessory reproductive organs since they play an important part in pregnancy and lactation. They are located over the anterior part of the chest. The external breast is divided into three portions: (1) the soft area of skin, (2) the areola which surrounds the nipple and contains the glands of Montgomery, and (3) the nipple.

Internally, each breast is composed of 15 to 20 lobes containing glandular tissue (the mammary glands) and fat. The mammary glands are responsible for milk production (lactation). The lobes of each mammary gland consist of several lobules arranged in clusters around tiny ducts. These clusters are called *alveoli* and are lined with milk-producing cells called *acini.* As the ducts leading from the alveoli to the lobes and from the lobes approach the nipple, they are dilated to form little reservoirs in which milk is stored. The size of the breasts varies with the amount of fat deposited in them, but there is no relationship between size and the ability to pro-

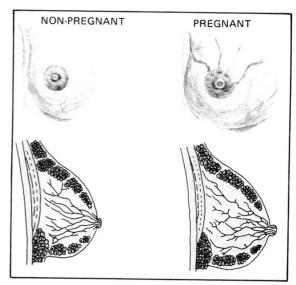

Figure 2-4

The mammary glands prepare the breasts for nursing the newborn. (Adapted from Nursing Education Aid, No. 10, Courtesy of Ross Laboratories)

duce milk. As pregnancy progresses, the breasts undergo physiological changes to make them ready for the demands of nursing the newborn infant.

THE PELVIS

The difference between the male and female pelvis is that the male pelvis is heavier, narrower, and deeper. A female pelvis can be *gynecoid* (typically womanlike) or *android* (manlike). The gynecoid pelvis is slightly heart-shaped and is the best shape for childbearing. The android pelvis is wedgeshaped and angular and is less suitable for childbearing.

The pelvis is formed by three innominate bones (the *ilium,* the *ischium* and the *pubis*), the sacrum, the coccyx and the ligaments

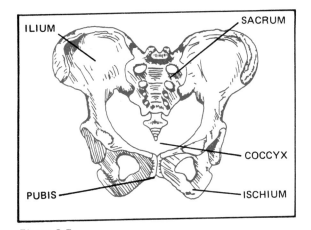

Figure 2-5

Structures of the pelvis

of the pelvis. The *coccyx* is a small, triangular bone made up of four vertebrae fused together, located at the end of the spine. It is connected to the sacrum by a hinge-type joint and forms part of the posterior boundary of the pelvis. The coccyx also helps support the pelvic floor.

The pelvis is further separated into the false pelvis and the true pelvis. The upper flaring part is termed the false pelvis. The false pelvis is seldom involved in the problems of labor. The true pelvis is the lower part of the pelvis. It forms the bony canal through which the baby must pass during delivery. The pelvic inlet, sometimes referred to as the pelvic brim, divides the false pelvis from the true pelvis.

The Pelvic Floor

All the organs in the pelvis are supported by *ligaments* and *fascias* which are made up of connective tissue, strands, bands, and layers. A powerful muscle called the levator ani reinforces

connecting them, figure 2-5. The innominate bones form the lateral and anterior boundaries of the pelvis. The *sacrum* is a large, wedge-shaped bone composed of five consolidated sacral vertebrae which forms the posterior wall

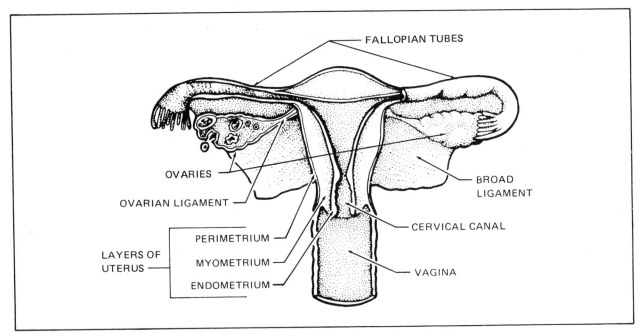

Figure 2-6

Uterus suspended by ligaments, round, broad and utero-sacral

the pelvic ligaments and fascias. The levator ani forms a "hammock" which extends from the side walls of the pelvis and meets in the middle line around the anus and vagina. The vagina, the rectum, the bladder, and the uterus are suspended by ligaments and fascias above the levator ani, figure 2–6.

The internal reproductive organs, which form a canal for the passage of the ovum and sperm, contain muscle and connective tissue completely lined with mucous membrane. They are partly covered by the peritoneum, a transparent membrane that lines the abdominal cavity. Characteristics of the mucous membrane vary according to the function required by the part. The membrane of the vulva is very sensitive; in the vagina it is rough and strong; the membrane lining the cervix and uterus is very vascular and strong. The epithelium is a layer of cells forming the surface layer of mucous membrane of the fallopian tubes and uterus. In the fallopian tubes, it is covered with microscopic "hairs" or cilia which, by their waving action, assist in transporting the ovum.

Related Structures of the Pelvis

Related pelvic structures are the ureters, bladder, urethra, and rectum. The *ureters* convey the urine from the kidneys to the bladder. The *bladder* lies behind the pubis and in front of the uterus. It is a storage space for urine. The *urethra* leads from the bladder to the opening in the vulva called the urinary meatus. Bladder distention delays the progress of labor.

The rectum is the terminal portion of the bowel. It opens externally to the anus and lies behind the uterus in the pelvic cavity.

SUGGESTED ACTIVITY

- Using a diagram of the female reproductive system, identify each part and explain its role in reproduction.

REVIEW

Multiple Choice. Select the best answer.

1. At the opening of the vagina is a fold of mucous membrane called the
   a. urinary meatus
   b. hymen
   c. clitoris
   d. corpus

2. Ova travel from the ovaries to the uterus through the
   a. internal os
   b. external os
   c. fallopian tubes
   d. fascia

3. The union of the sperm and ovum is called
   a. gestation
   b. conception
   c. fertilization
   d. conception or fertilization

4. The labia extends from the perineum to the
   a. clitoris
   b. vagina
   c. urinary meatus
   d. mons veneris

5. The lining of the uterus is called the
   - a. labia majora
   - b. endometrium
   - c. clitoris
   - d. cilia

6. The organ of sexual excitation in the female is the
   - a. cervix
   - b. vagina
   - c. clitoris
   - d. labia majora

7. The basic functions of the female reproductive system are to
   1. produce ovarian hormones which are responsible for the female sex characteristics and reproductive functions
   2. produce the ovum and deliver it to the place where conception may take place
   3. nurture and sustain the product of conception until birth
   4. accomplish delivery of the product of conception.
   - a. 1 and 4
   - b. 1 and 3
   - c. 2, 3 and 4
   - d. 1, 2, 3 and 4

8. The organs of the pelvis are supported by
   - a. fascia and ligaments
   - b. muscle
   - c. levator ani
   - d. cilia

9. The function of the ovaries is to
   - a. mature and discharge ova
   - b. produce hormones
   - c. neither of these
   - d. a and b

10. The part of the pelvis which is most involved with childbirth is the
    - a. coccyx
    - b. sacrum
    - c. true pelvis
    - d. false pelvis

11. The area of skin, connective tissue, and muscle between the vulva and anus is called the
    - a. perineum
    - b. urinary meatus
    - c. endometrium
    - d. fascia

12. Conception usually takes place in the
    - a. uterus
    - b. fallopian tube
    - c. ovary
    - d. cervix

13. The neck of the uterus is called the
    - a. vagina
    - b. perineum
    - c. cervix
    - d. labia majora

14. Located on each side of the labia minora and responsible for secreting a mucoid, lubricating substance during sexual intercourse are the
    - a. cilia
    - b. Bartholin's glands
    - c. fallopian tubes
    - d. hymen

UNIT 3

MENSTRUATION AND OVULATION

OBJECTIVES

After studying this unit, the student should be able to:

- State the physiological changes which take place in the female during adolescence and menopause.
- Explain the interrelated processes of menstruation and ovulation.
- State the reasons for female infertility.
- List the functions of estrogen, progesterone, FSH, and LH.

The female reproductive system undergoes great changes during the life cycle of the individual. Even before birth, the reproductive organs are undergoing growth and development as the fetus grows and develops. The reproductive organs generally reach maturity during puberty. *Puberty* is the period between the eleventh and sixteenth year during which the individual becomes capable of reproduction. In women, the production of a mature ovum (*ovulation*) usually occurs several months after the first menstrual period (*menarche*). During puberty, the size of the external and internal genitalia increases, pubic hair develops, and the breasts enlarge due, in most part, to the secretions of increasing amounts of the hormone, estrogen. The breasts contain mammary glands which are the milk secreting organs of the female. Although mammary glands are present in both sexes, they normally develop and function only in the female. At puberty, female breasts are influenced to develop by the hormones estrogen and progesterone. The childbearing years extend from the onset of ovulation to the menopause.

Menopause is the permanent physiological cessation of the menstrual flow. The ovaries atrophy as do the uterus, breasts, and external genitalia. Ovulation ceases and childbearing is no longer possible.

Menopause, sometimes referred to as the "change of life," is a normal physiological process and is not an illness. Like the menarche, the time it occurs varies with the individual. The menopause usually occurs between the ages of 45 and 50 in 50 percent of all females. Others may experience menopause prior to age 45 or after 50 years of age. Surgical removal of the ovaries also causes menopause. Between the ages of 35 and 55 years, there are approximately 10,000 ova remaining in the ovaries; more than 400,000 are present at birth.

The tendency to gain weight during menopause is common. Nervous disturbances, hot flashes, and sweating may occur due to the decreased level of sex hormones. The woman may show signs of anxiety and irritability during a two-to-five year period. Hormone treatment may be ordered by the physician to relieve these conditions. Hormone therapy, after a woman's system stops producing its own hormones, also decreases the risks of cardiovascular disease and osteoporosis.

OVULATION AND MENSTRUATION

The processes of ovulation and menstruation are interrelated. Ovulation is the process by which a mature ovum is released and the uterus is made ready to receive the fertilized ovum. *Menstruation* is the process of casting off the unnecessary uterine lining when conception does not occur after ovulation.

The hypothalamus, which is located at the base of the brain, releases gonadotropin-releasing hormones (GnRH) that stimulate the anterior lobe of the pituitary gland. These hormones control the ovarian function in the female. These hormones are the *follicle-stimulating hormone* (FSH) and the *luteinizing hormone* (LH).

The interior of the ovary is made up of connective tissue in which several hundred thousand microscopic structures known as *primordial follicles* are imbedded. During the pre-ovulatory phase of the menstrual cycle, the FSH causes several of these follicles to enlarge and migrate toward the surface of the ovary. Under the influence of FSH, one of these follicles develops into a *graafian follicle* (microscopic sac in which the ovum develops). The FSH acts with the LH to cause the developing follicle to secrete the hormone, estrogen, and causes the follicle to rupture in the process of ovulation. *Estrogen* is the hormone that stimulates the glands of the uterine lining (endometrium) to thicken. About 12 to 16 days after the beginning of the menstrual period, the ovum reaches maturity. A surge in the LH level causes the ovum to be expelled from the follicle.

When the ovum appears on the surface of the ovary, it is drawn into the fallopian tube by the

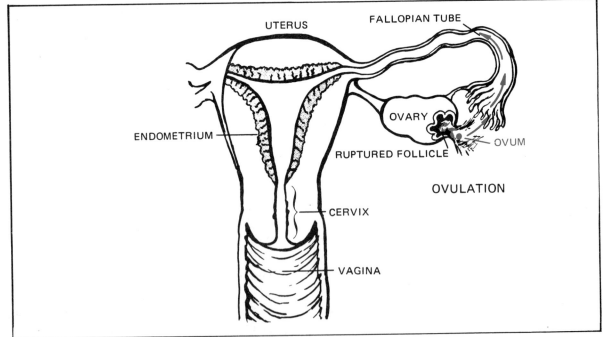

Figure 3-1

Ovulation: The release of the ovum from the follicle (Courtesy of DeLee's Obstetrics for Nurses, W.B. Saunders Co.)

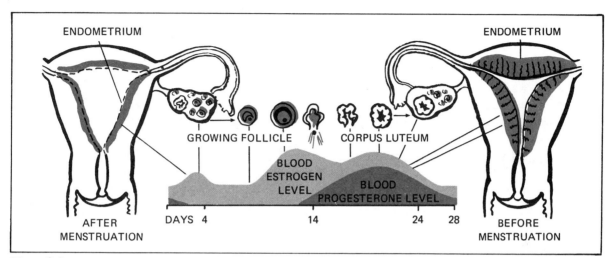

Figure 3-2

Hormones regulate the reproductive organs

cilia at the end of the tube, figure 3-1. The fallopian tube is lined with ciliated epithelium which propels the ovum along its route. After the follicle ruptures in ovulation, it develops into a structure known as the *corpus luteum* (sometimes called "yellow body" because of its yellow fatty substance). The LH stimulates the corpus luteum to secrete another hormone, *progesterone,* which increases the number and length of the blood vessels in the endometrium and causes uterine secretions. These changes prepare the uterus to receive the fertilized ovum. At this point, the uterine lining is engorged with blood and is thick and spongy. If conception does not occur, the corpus luteum disintegrates, the secretion of hormones decreases, and a portion of the endometrium is discharged through the vagina as the menstrual flow. The menstrual flow consists of mucous secretions, tissue fragments, and blood. After menstruation, the endometrium of the uterus is very thin.

If the ovum is fertilized, menstruation does not occur. After implantation, the fertilized ovum secretes a hormone called *human chorionic gonadotropin hormone* that enables the corpus luteum to continue to secrete progesterone during the first three months of pregnancy. After this period, the placenta assumes the secretion of progesterone.

The menstrual cycle begins with menstruation and is usually completed every 28 days. This approximate cycle, however, varies with the individual. The events which occur during the cycle are:

1. Menstruation lasts from three to seven days while the lining of the uterus is expelled. The discharge varies in amount from 30 to 200 milliliters.
2. Seven to ten days after menstruation, a period of repair is in progress. The estrogen hormone level is increasing and the lining of the uterus is thickening to prepare for an eventual pregnancy.
3. The next 12 to 14 days are known as the premenstrual period; the progesterone hormone level increases. Ovulation occurs around the first day of this period. It is during the premenstrual period that conception is most likely to occur.

The cycle begins again and continues at regular intervals except during pregnancy and after the menopause.

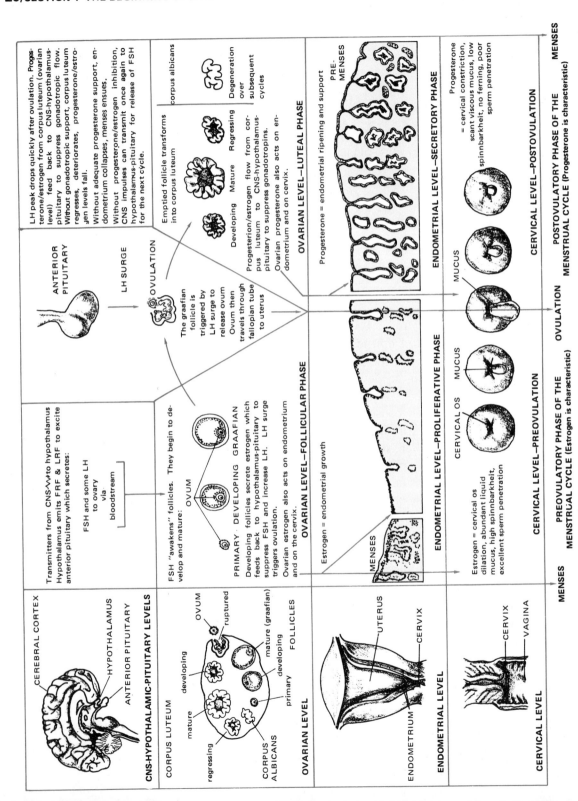

Figure 3-3

The normal menstrual cycle

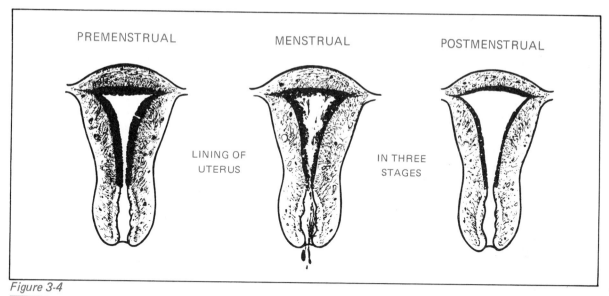

Figure 3-4

The uterus changes during the menstrual cycle (Courtesy of Educational Department, Tampax, Inc.)

ABNORMAL CONDITIONS RELATING TO MENSTRUATION

Abnormalities in the menstrual cycle may be caused by stress, endocrine dysfunction, overwork, change of climate, chronic disease, or other pathological conditions. Amenorrhea, menorrhagia, metrorrhagia, dysmenorrhea, and anovulatory menstruation are some common abnormalities.

- *Amenorrhea* is a permanent or temporary suppression of menstruation. This occurs as a normal condition before puberty, during pregnancy, between periods, sometimes during lactation, and following menopause. The absence of menstruation may be congenital, or may be due to the removal of the uterus. It may also be caused by an obstruction of the cervix or vagina, so that there is no external flow. A debilitating disease, severe anemia, thyroid imbalance, psychic upsets and excessive exercise can also cause amenorrhea.
- *Menorrhagia* is prolonged or excessive bleeding during the menstrual period.
- *Metrorrhagia* is bleeding from the uterus at a time other than the menstrual period.
- *Dysmenorrhea* is painful menstruation. The pain may be due to physical or emotional causes.
- *Anovulatory menstruation* is menstruation which takes place when the ovary has failed to expel or discharge the egg. Without ovulation, fertilization of the egg cannot occur; this is one of the causes of infertility in women.

INFERTILITY

Although infertility is generally considered to be a gynecological problem, it is a factor which has complicated childbearing for many women. Infertility is usually due to several factors rather than a single cause. Systemic, local, nutritional, glandular, and emotional factors can affect both men and women. Failure to ovulate, obstructions in the genital tract, especially in the cervix or fallopian tubes, or disturbances in the development of the uterus and its lining which interfere with the implantation and growth of a fertilized ovum are a few causes of infertility in women. Research is continuing into both physical and psychological causes of infertility. New techniques in diagnosis and treatment have enabled many "infertile" women to conceive.

SUGGESTED ACTIVITIES

- Prepare a panel discussion for class presentation on the causes and treatment of menorrhagia, metrorrhagia and dysmenorrhea. Refer to textbooks in gynecological nursing.
- Prepare a detailed written report on one of the following. Document your report with reading references.
  — Ovulation
  — The Uterine Lining Changes During the Menstrual Cycle
  — Hormones Which Regulate the Female Reproductive Organs
- Describe the feedback mechanisms of the hypothalmic-pituitary-ovarian axis.
- Define the following:
  — Menarche
  — Menstruation
  — Ovulation
  — Ovarian hormones
  — Gonadotropins
  — Follicular phase
  — Luteal phase
  — Proliferative phase
  — Secretory phase
- Diagram the rise and fall of the following hormones throughout the menstrual cycle: (a) gonadotropins and their releasing factors; and (b) the ovarian hormones.

REVIEW

A. Multiple Choice. Select the best answer.

1. The reproductive organs of the female begin to develop and grow
   a. during the first year of life
   b. during puberty
   c. during gestation
   d. during adolescence

2. Gonadotropic hormones are secreted by the
   a. graafian follicle
   b. pituitary gland
   c. corpus luteum
   d. hypothalamus

3. When ovulation does not occur, menstruation is termed
   a. anovulatory
   b. menorrhagia
   c. dysmenorrhea
   d. amenorrhea

4. The reproductive system becomes capable of functioning
   a. during puberty
   b. during adolescence
   c. in adulthood
   d. before birth

5. The beginning of the first menstrual cycle is known as
   a. metorrhagia   c. dysmenorrhea
   b. menarche   d. amenorrhea

B. Match the function in column I to the hormone in column II.

Column I	Column II
1. increases the number and length of the blood vessels in the endometrium and stimulates uterine secretions	a. estrogen
	b. FSH
	c. LH
2. stimulates the corpus luteum to secrete female sex hormones	d. progesterone
3. stimulates the glands of the endometrium to thicken	
4. stimulates development of the graafian follicle; causes rupture of the follicle	

C. Briefly answer the following questions.

1. What physical changes occur during puberty?

2. How are the processes of ovulation and menstruation interrelated?

3. What events occur during a normal 28-day menstrual cycle and when do they occur?

4. At what time during the menstrual cycle is a woman most likely to conceive?

5. Of what does the menstrual flow consist?

6. Name three causes of irregular menstrual cycles.

7. Where does the ovum mature in the ovary? What is this structure called after ovulation?

D. Outline a care plan for a woman who suspects she is going into the menopause phase of her life. She needs physiological and psychological support as well as patient education.

UNIT 4

THE MALE REPRODUCTIVE SYSTEM

OBJECTIVES

After studying this unit, the student should be able to:

- Identify the internal and external organs of the male reproductive system.
- Explain the primary function of each part of the male reproductive system.
- State reasons for male sterility.
- List the functions of testosterone.

Modern obstetrics concerns itself with more than just the growth and delivery of a baby. It incorporates a sharing by both man and woman from the time of conception and includes the heredity and environmental influence they will both have on their child. It is, therefore, important for the nurse to have an understanding of the father's function and role in the creation of his baby so that the nurse may be a source of information to the family unit.

EXTERNAL REPRODUCTIVE ORGANS

The external organs of reproduction in the male are the penis and the scrotum. The reproductive cells and their accompanying secretions are produced and carried to the outside by these organs.

The *penis* is the male organ of copulation. It consists of erectile parts known as cavernous bodies and a urethra through which semen is released. The cavernous bodies contain spaces which are usually empty, allowing the penis to be flaccid. When these spaces fill with blood, the penis becomes enlarged, turgid (swollen) and erect. The flow of blood is controlled by the automatic nervous system and varies with psychic and physical stimulation. The slightly enlarged structure at the end of the penis which contains the orifice of the urethra is called the *glans penis.* It is enclosed by a fold of skin called the *prepuce* or *foreskin.* Part of this skin may be removed for hygienic or religious reasons or because the prepuce may fit too tightly. This removal of skin is called *circumcision* and is usually performed by an obstetrician or rabbi a few days after birth.

The *scrotum* is a pouch of loose skin and superficial fascia which is divided into two lateral portions. Involuntary muscle fibers called dartos lie within this superficial fascia. The dartos and the superficial fascia divide the scrotum internally into right and left compartments; each compartment contains a testis, epididymis and associated structures. The dartos are subject to temperature conditions. Heat causes the dartos to relax, allowing the scrotum to elongate and become *flaccid* (limp). This keeps the sperm away from the heat of the body. Sperm must be kept approximately six degrees cooler than body temperature or it cannot survive. Cold causes the dartos to contract, pulling the scrotum upward and closer to the body for warmth. The contracting-and-relaxing mechanism allows sperm to remain at the most satisfactory temperature.

INTERNAL REPRODUCTIVE ORGANS

The male's internal reproductive organs are: (1) the testes, which contain the seminiferous tubules, (2) seminal ducts for transporting the sperm from the testes, (3) seminal vesicle glands, (4) the prostate gland, and (5) the bulbourethral (Cowper's) glands. *Semen* is a mixture of secretions from the testes, the prostate gland, the seminal vesicles, and the bulbourethral (Cowper's) glands.

The *testes* are the primary sex organs of the male; they produce spermatozoa (sperm) and the male sex hormone, *testosterone*. The testes are suspended in the scrotum by spermatic cords and average 4 to 5 centimeters in length and 10.5 to 14 grams in weight. Each testis is divided into lobes. Each lobe contains seminiferous tubules. The lining of these tubules consist of *spermatogenic* (sperm-producing) cells which produce sperm. Millions of sperm are produced in each testis. This spermatozoa production begins between the ages of 9 and 14 and continues throughout the life of the male. The seminiferous tubules join repeatedly and form the single, coiled tube called the epididymis.

The *epididymis* is a coiled tube, 13 to 20 feet long, located on and beside the posterior surface of each testis. It is the principal storehouse for sperm. It also adds an essential secretion to the fluid in which spermatozoa are activated and stored (semen). Starting in the epididymis, secretions are added to the semen as the sperm travels.

From the epididymis, the semen passes through the ductus deferens or vas deferens. The *vas deferens* is a slim muscular tube approximately 45.7 centimeters in length (18 inches) which carries the semen to the urethra. The urethra serves two purposes in the male — as a passage for semen and as a passage for urine.

Surrounding the urethra at the base of the bladder is the *prostate gland*, which adds a milky secretion to the semen. This milky fluid is highly alkaline and neutralizes the acidic fluid from the testes in a way that stimulates the sperm to action. Sperm are immobile in acidic media but very active in alkaline media.

Behind the prostate gland are two seminal vesicle glands; they also produce fluid. Their ducts join the vas deferens to form ejaculatory ducts. The two ejaculatory ducts then empty the semen (containing sperm) into the urethra, figure 4-1.

The two *bulbourethral glands* or *Cowper's glands* lie below the prostate on either side of the urethra. They also add secretions to the semen through ducts that open into the urethra. The urethra carries the sperm and secretions to the outside.

The secretions of the various glands help to lubricate the movement of the penis; this allows the vagina to massage the penis and create the necessary sexual stimulation to cause a release of the semen. Without this lubrication, there is an abrasive effect which causes pain, inhibits the sexual desire, and blocks the completion of the sexual act.

COPULATION

Copulation or *coitus* is the sexual act; sperm is delivered to the cervix of the female uterus by

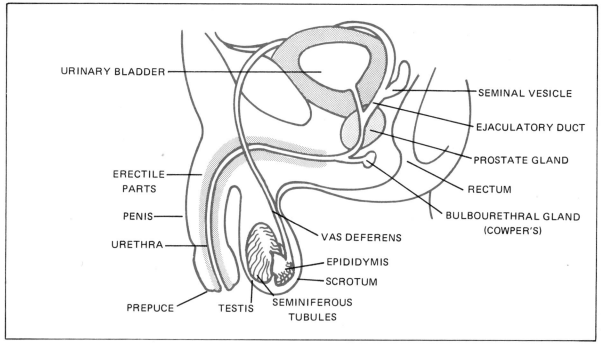

Figure 4-1

The male reproductive system in relation to the bladder and rectum (side view vertical section)

the erect penis. *Ejaculation* is the forcible release of semen from the penis. The amount of semen may vary from 1.5 to 4 milliliters per ejaculation.

The penis becomes enlarged and erect and ejaculates seminal fluid with psychic or physical stimulation. This may occur irregularly during sleep (known as wet dreams); as a result of masturbation; or during sexual intercourse. *Masturbation* is stimulation of the sex organs by means other than sexual intercourse.

Impotent is a term used when the adult male cannot have an erection or an ejaculation. The cause may be physical, such as a debilitating disease, fever or fatigue, or it may be due to psychological factors such as fear, stress, or psychosis. Treatment for impotency depends upon the cause. A medical and/or psychological evaluation is often beneficial.

SPERMATOZOA

The testes of the male produce billions of spermatozoa or sperm. *Sperm* is the mature sex cell of the male. Each sperm is a single cell made up of a head, a midsection, and a tail, figure 4-2. The head is composed chiefly of the nucleus. It carries the genes, which are responsible for transmitting traits of the male (father). The head of the sperm also carries the chromosome which determines the sex of the baby. The tail of the sperm (or flagellum) is responsible for motility. As long as the sperm remains alive, the tail moves back and forth propelling the sperm forward at a velocity of about three inches per hour. This movement allows the sperm to advance into the uterus and up through the fallopian tubes in search of the ovum. Each copulation releases about 150 million sperm along with

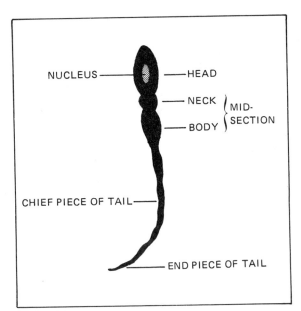

NUCLEUS —————— HEAD

——— NECK ⎫ MID-
——— BODY ⎭ SECTION

CHIEF PIECE OF TAIL ———

——— END PIECE OF TAIL

Figure 4-2

Each sperm consists of a head, a midsection, and a tail

secretions from the epididymis, seminal vesicles, prostate and bulbourethral glands. However, only one sperm fertilizes the female ovum. The ovum is about 90,000 times as large as the sperm. The ovum and the sperm each contribute exactly half of the baby's total hereditary qualities.

HORMONE REGULATION

The testes of a male remain dormant until they are stimulated by the gonadotropic hormones from the pituitary gland. This occurs between the ages of 9 and 14 years. This stage of development is called puberty. The pituitary gland begins to secrete both the follicle-stimulating hormone (FSH) and the luteinizing hormone (LH) which are responsible for testicular growth and function. This testicular growth and function stimulates the release of the primary male sex hormone, *testosterone*. Testosterone is derived from the interstitial cells of the testes and is secreted directly into the bloodstream. Testosterone contributes to:

- Development of secondary sexual characteristics such as hair distribution and growth, changes in body contour, and voice changes.
- Sex urge and behavior.
- Development, maintenance and functioning of accessory sex organs, such as the seminal ducts, seminal vesicles and prostate gland.

Adolescence is the name given to this time of change; it extends from puberty to maturity. The reproductive organs of the male continue to function throughout his life. They do, however, diminish in activity to varying degrees in old age, as do all body systems.

STERILITY

About one out of every 30 males is sterile. Sterility may be defined as the lack of *viable* (capable of growing and developing) sperm; this lack results in the inability to conceive. The most frequent cause of sterility is infection of the genital ducts. A few men have congenitally deficient testes that are incapable of producing normal sperm. Undescended testicles produce sterility because the spermatogenic cells cannot live at body temperature. The testes must descend into the scrotum, which is at a cooler temperature, in order to make viable sperm. Undescended testes can be corrected surgically, usually before the boy reaches puberty.

Male sterility can also occur when the number of viable sperm falls below 20 million in a single ejaculation. Although it takes only one sperm to fertilize an ovum, it is believed that a large number of sperm are necessary to provide enzymes or other substances that help the single fertilizing sperm reach the ovum. The enzyme, known as *hyaluronidase*, must be present in sufficient quantity to dissolve the layer of cells surrounding the ovum.

Purposeful sterilization can be accomplished by a relatively simple operation known as a *vasectomy*. Usually done as an office procedure, this operation prevents the sperm from traveling beyond the vas deferens. However, it does not interfere with the secretions from the other glands along the seminal pathway. The operation involves tying, cutting, or cauterizing the vas deferens. The man who has had a vasectomy can still experience an erection and ejaculation; however, the semen does not contain the fertilizing agent, sperm.

SUGGESTED ACTIVITIES

* Prepare a written report on the causes of male sterility.
* Discuss the psychological reasons that might cause male impotency.
* Discuss the pros and cons of vasectomy as a means of birth control.
* Describe the physiology of the male reproductive system.
* Discuss the role and responsibility of the male in family planning.

REVIEW

A. Multiple Choice. Select the best answer.

1. During puberty, the testes of the male are stimulated to produce male sex hormones by
   a. gonadotropic hormones
   b. estrogen
   c. progesterone
   d. testosterone

2. The seminiferous tubules are located within the
   a. ejaculatory ducts
   b. bulbourethral glands
   c. prostate gland
   d. testes

3. The thin muscular tube that carries the semen to the urethra is the
   a. epididymis
   b. vas deferens
   c. seminal duct
   d. seminal vesicles

4. The gland that produces an alkaline, milky fluid which neutralizes and stimulates sperm action is the
   a. seminal vesicle gland
   b. bulbourethral (Cowper's) gland
   c. prostate gland
   d. pituitary

5. Inherited traits of the father and sex of the baby are determined by the
   a. genes in the sperm nucleus
   b. female ovum
   c. body of the sperm
   d. neck of the sperm

6. The most frequent cause of sterility in the male is
   a. low sperm count
   b. congenitally deficient testes
   c. undescended testes
   d. infection of the genital ducts

7. Undescended testicles can cause sterility because
   a. they will not produce sperm
   b. spermatogenic cells cannot live at body temperature
   c. sperm produced in undescended testicles are not in sufficient quantity
   d. undescended testicles are incapable of producing sperm

8. The function of testosterone is that
   a. it contributes to the development of secondary sexual characteristics
   b. it contributes to the sex urge and sexual behavior
   c. it contributes to the development, maintenance and functioning of accessory sex organs
   d. all of these

9. The mature sex cell of the male is called
   a. seminal vesicle   c. testosterone
   b. sperm   d. bulbourethral gland

10. A vasectomy is a surgical operation which prevents sperm from traveling beyond the
    a. epididymis   c. vas deferens
    b. testis   d. scrotum

B. Label the parts of the male reproductive system on the following diagram.

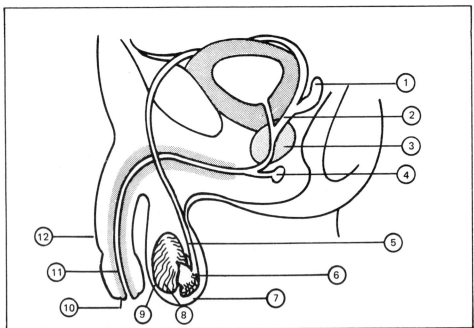

UNIT 5

CONCEPTION

OBJECTIVES

After studying this unit, the student should be able to:

- Describe the process of conception.
- Explain how traits are inherited in terms of sex-linked and sex-limited traits.
- Explain how traits are inherited in terms of dominant and recessive traits.
- Distinguish between identical and fraternal twins.

During intercourse, sperm is ejaculated from the male penis into the vagina. Microscopic in size, but numbering more than 150 million, these sperm move by means of long thin tails. They quickly move from the vagina to the uterus and then to the fallopian tube in search of the female ovum, figure 5-1. In spite of the excessive number of sperm, only one sperm fertilizes one egg. Multiple births occur when more than one egg is fertilized or when one fertilized egg divides into more than one embryo.

CONCEPTION

The human life cycle begins when the head and neck of the sperm enter the ovum, figure 5-2. This usually takes place in the outer third of the fallopian tube. The resulting fertilized egg is called a *zygote*, figure 5-3. The zygote is one cell with one nucleus, containing all the necessary elements for the future development of the offspring.

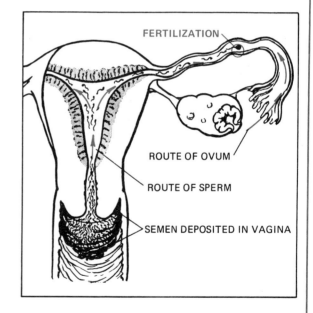

FERTILIZATION

ROUTE OF OVUM

ROUTE OF SPERM

SEMEN DEPOSITED IN VAGINA

Figure 5-1

Conception usually occurs in the fallopian tube (Courtesy of DeLee's Obstetrics for Nurses, W.B. Saunders Co.)

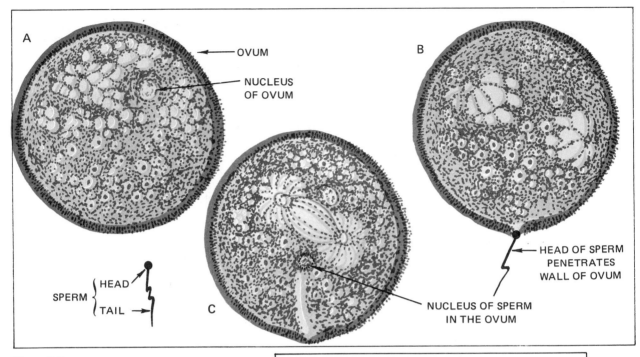

A

OVUM

NUCLEUS
OF OVUM

B

HEAD OF SPERM
PENETRATES
WALL OF OVUM

C

NUCLEUS OF SPERM
IN THE OVUM

SPERM { HEAD

TAIL

Figure 5-2
Fertilization: Sperm unites with ovum

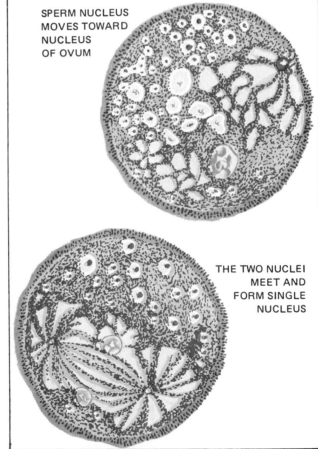

SPERM NUCLEUS
MOVES TOWARD
NUCLEUS
OF OVUM

THE TWO NUCLEI
MEET AND
FORM SINGLE
NUCLEUS

Figure 5-3
Formation of the zygote

CLEAVAGE

Soon after the nucleus of the sperm has merged with the nucleus of the ovum, a series of cell divisions begins, figure 5-4. This process of cell division is called *cleavage* and usually starts while the fertilized egg is in the fallopian tube.

The first division of the fertilized ovum results in two *blastomeres.* Prior to the division, each chromosome doubles its hereditary material. It then splits lengthwise to provide two equal half-chromosomes that regroup into two distinct nuclei, one of which goes with each half of the divided egg. Thus, right from the beginning each cell of the developing baby contains an equal number of chromosomes from each of the parents. It is these chromosomes that carry genes.

The first cleavage takes about 36 hours; each succeeding division takes slightly less time. The multiplying continues at a fairly constant rate. The egg does not increase in size (bulk) as the cell division and multiplication continue.

The fertilized ovum gradually takes on the appearance of a mulberry, and is called a *morula.* During cell division, the fertilized ovum is traveling down the fallopian tube to the uterus; this passage takes seven to nine days. When it reaches

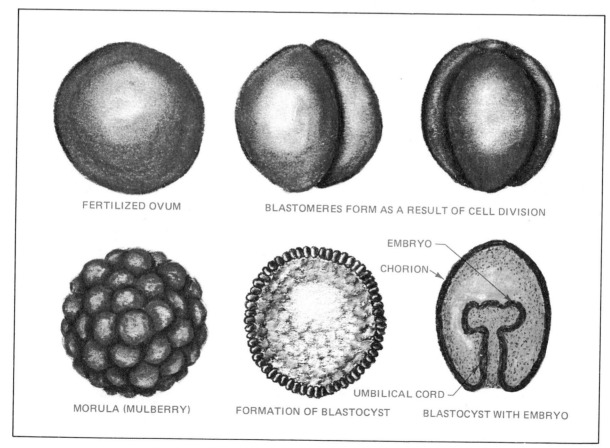

FERTILIZED OVUM

BLASTOMERES FORM AS A RESULT OF CELL DIVISION

MORULA (MULBERRY)

FORMATION OF BLASTOCYST

EMBRYO

CHORION

UMBILICAL CORD

BLASTOCYST WITH EMBRYO

Figure 5-4

Stages in embryonic development

the uterus, it is called an *embryo* until the eighth week of development. After the eighth week, it is called a *fetus*.

IMPLANTATION

After the morula enters the uterus, it becomes a hollow ball filled with fluid and is now termed a *blastocyst.* The blastocyst burrows into the uterine mucosa which has been prepared for it, figure 5-5. The disks of the cells near the outer rim develop into the embryo; the rim itself forms the fetal membrane. The rim, called the *trophoblast,* becomes the placenta and the covering (chorion) that nourishes and protects the developing fetus. The chorion, the placenta, and the amnion (bag of waters) play an important role but are not physically part of the fetus.

In other words, the blastocyst comes into direct contact with the lining of the uterus (endometrium) and adheres to it. The endometrium is now called the *decidua* due to increased thickening and enlargement of cells. Enzymes in the cells digest the uterine tissue until the embedded mass has broken into the walls of some of the maternal vessels; strands of cells are bathed in blood. Fingerlike projections (chorionic villi), which contain blood vessels, connected to the embryo, sprout from the outer cells and extend into the blood-filled spaces. The embryo receives oxygen and nourishment and disposes of waste products through these villi. While the blastocyst is becoming embedded, the inner mass of cells multiplies and the fetal membranes begin to develop. The blastocyst expands and some of the cells around the hollow ball congregate on one side. This thickened mass of cells forms the *blastoderm.* It is these cells that progressively develop into the fetus.

The blastoderm is made up of two distinct layers of cells. The original outer and thicker layer called the *ectoderm* develops into the brain,

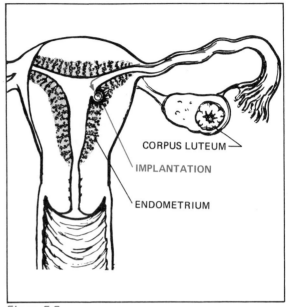

CORPUS LUTEUM

IMPLANTATION

ENDOMETRIUM

Figure 5-5

Implantation: fertilized ovum attaches to endometrium (Courtesy of DeLee's Obstetrics for Nurses, W.B. Saunders Co.)

the spinal cord, all the nerves and sensory organs, and the skin. The newer and innermost layer called the *endoderm* becomes the lining of the entire digestive tract from the pharynx down through the esophagus, stomach, liver and intestines to the anus. The intermediate layer called the *mesoderm* appears later which gives rise to the skeleton, muscles and many internal organs. These three layers of cells appear in the development of all higher animals.

DETERMINATION OF SEX

Each mature ovum has 23 chromosomes, one of which is the X, or female sex factor. Mature sperm cells develop in the testes of the male from the age of puberty. The head of the sperm has the nucleus of the cell; it contains 23 chromosomes, one of which is the Y or male sex factor.

Female
Child

— 22 chromosomes + X factor from ovum = 23 chromosomes

+

22 chromosomes + X factor from sperm = 44 + 2X factors

Male
Child

— 22 chromosomes + X factor from ovum = 23 chromosomes

+

22 chromosomes + Y factor from sperm = 44 + X + Y factors

Figure 5-6

How sex is determined

Usually equal numbers of each type of sperm are produced in the testes.

The zygote resulting from conception contains 46 chromosomes: 23 chromosomes (includes a sex factor) from each parent. If the ovum has been fertilized by a sperm carrying the X sex factor, the resulting offspring is female. If the sperm carried the Y sex factor, the offspring is male, figure 5-6.

HOW TRAITS ARE INHERITED

Geneticists (scientists who are concerned with the phenomena of heredity and its variations) have established that certain traits are transmitted through the genes. *Genes* determine hereditary traits and are found in the chromosomes. The chromosomes are made up of chains of giant molecules, a combination of protein and nucleic acid.

The nucleic acid in the chromosomes is called DNA (deoxyribonucleic acid) and contains the full genetic information needed for the formation of the human body. DNA could be called the master template for cell building. Another nucleic acid, present outside the chromosomes, is RNA (ribonucleic acid). There are three different kinds of RNA: messenger RNA, transfer RNA, and ribosomal RNA. Messenger RNA (mRNA) is copied from the DNA master template. Transfer

RNA (tRNA) seeks out the proper protein-building materials and puts them in order according to the message on the mRNA. Ribosomal RNA (rRNA) is the major component of the ribosomes, the minute particles on which the protein building takes place. *Histones* are part of the proteins present in the chromosomes. It is believed that they have a major function in all cell differentiation. *Differentiation* is the acquiring of functions which do not resemble the functions of the original cell. This means that the histones block out part of the DNA information (actually prevent the synthesis of mRNA on certain parts of the DNA) and leave open only that information needed for the cell to become a certain kind of cell (such as a liver cell, bone cell, etc.).

It is known that some physical traits are associated with the genes in the X and Y, or sex, chromosomes. These are referred to as *sex-linked* characteristics. Hemophilia and color blindness are two sex-linked characteristics, figures 5-7 and 5-8. Each of these traits is believed to be linked to the female (X) chromosome. Therefore, the characteristic can be transmitted from grandfather to grandson through the grandfather's daughter, figure 5-7. Assume that a male hemophiliac produces a daughter. She would carry one normal X chromosome from her mother and one hemophiliac X chromosome from her father.

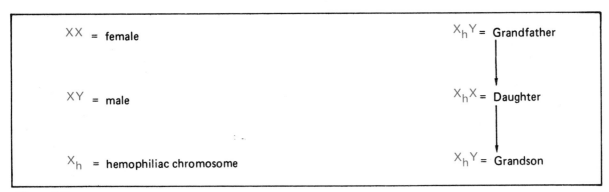

Figure 5-7

The transmission of hemophilia

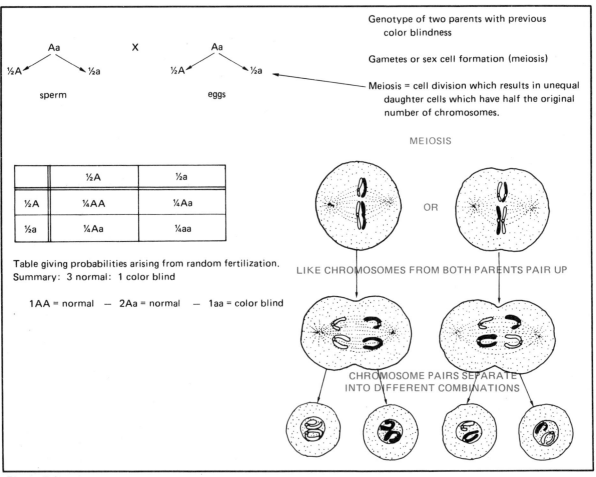

Figure 5-8

Transmission of color blindness

She would not be a hemophiliac since the healthy X chromosome would mask the hemophiliac chromosome. If, however, she had a son, he could receive either a normal or a hemophiliac X chromosome from his mother. If he received a hemophiliac chromosome, he would be a hemophiliac (since he has no healthy X chromosome to mask the hemophiliac chromosome). A female would be a hemophiliac only if she inherited a hemophiliac chromosome from both her mother and father.

Sex-limited characteristics are traits that appear in one sex only. Genes for certain traits other than sex are located on the X chromosome. When a male offspring inherits such a trait on his X chromosome, there is no matching gene on the Y chromosome. Therefore, that trait will invariably be shown. A female offspring, on the other hand, has two X chromosomes. Therefore, even if she inherits a trait , it may be masked by another more dominant gene for the same trait on the other X chromosome. For this reason, certain sex-linked characteristics appear more often in men than in women. Red-green color blindness, blood-clotting disorder, hemophilia, and baldness in men belong in this category.

In addition, traits are said to be dominant or recessive. The *dominant* trait requires only a single gene and is more likely to appear since it can mask another trait (*heterozygote*). A *recessive* trait appears only when a pair of like genes is present (*homozygote*). Some dominant traits include dark hair, brown eyes, farsightedness, astigmatism, curly hair, glaucoma, cataract, and susceptibility to rupture. Among the recessive traits are blue or gray eyes, myopia, light hair, Rh-negative blood type, diabetes mellitus, sickle cell anemia, and congenital deafness. Sometimes, characteristics may be due to two recessive traits rather than to the dominant one. Diabetes and hemophilia are transmitted by *lethal genes,* so named because their effect interferes with life.

MULTIPLE BIRTHS

Twins are described according to their origin: identical twins result from the union of one sperm and one ovum; fraternal twins result when two ova are fertilized by two sperm. In identical twins the fertilized egg divides into two embryos. There is one placenta and two amniotic sacs, figure 5-9. The twins are always the same sex. Fraternal twins may or may not be of the same sex. They have two amniotic sacs and separate or fused placentas, figure 5-10. Heredity has been recognized as a factor in the production of identical twins. The age of the mother seems to be a factor in the production of fraternal twins. In older women more than one ovum may be released during ovulation.

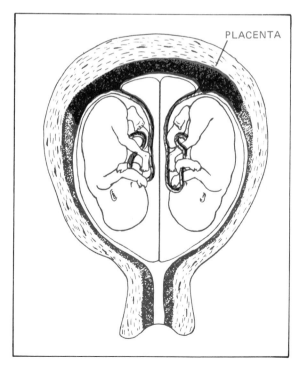

PLACENTA

Figure 5-9

Identical twins: two sacs — one placenta

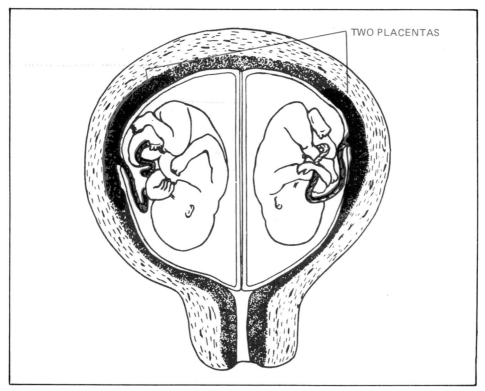

Figure 5-10

Fraternal twins: two sacs — two placentas

SUGGESTED ACTIVITIES

- Prepare a report on the history of genetics. How can genetics contribute to the health of the generations of the future?

- Investigate the problems which diabetics, or children of diabetics, have in raising a family.

- Construct pedigrees and analyse them for inheritance patterns.

- Explain the importance of preventive genetics in the areas of preconception, prenatal, and postnatal periods.

REVIEW

A. Multiple Choice. Select the best answer.

   1. Fertilization usually takes place in the

      a. uterus   c. ovary

      b. vagina   d. fallopian tubes

2. The number of chromosomes contained in the zygote is
    a. 46 and 2 sex factors   c. 44 and 2 sex factors
    b. 48 and 2 sex factors   d. 42 and 2 sex factors

3. The process of cell division that takes place soon after fertilization is called
    a. DNA   c. cleavage
    b. RNA   d. chromosomes

4. DNA is believed to be in the
    a. tail of the sperm   c. cytoplasm of the cell
    b. nucleus of the cell   d. wall of the ovum

5. An example of a recessive trait is
    a. dark hair   c. diabetes mellitus
    b. astigmatism   d. glaucoma

6. After fertilization, implantation takes place in the uterus in approximately
    a. 24 hours   c. 14 days
    b. 2 to 3 days   d. 7 to 9 days

B. Match the descriptions in column I with the sex factors in column II.

Column I	Column II
1. contains the genes	a. chromosomes
2. two sperm + two ova	b. fraternal twins
3. develop in the testes	c. identical twins
4. one sperm + one ovum	d. male sex chromosomes
5. fertilized ovum	e. sperm
6. determines sex of the child	f. zygote

C. Briefly answer the following questions.

1. What are histones?

2. Define sex-linked characteristics and give an example.

3. Define sex-limited characteristics and give an example.

4. How many amniotic sacs and placentas are there for identical twins? For fraternal twins?

5. Birth of identical twins depends largely upon what factor?

6. Birth of fraternal twins depends largely upon what factor?

UNIT 6

PRENATAL DEVELOPMENT

OBJECTIVES

After studying this unit, the student should be able to:

- Trace the development of the zygote from the first through the tenth lunar month.
- Explain the function of the amniotic sac and amniotic fluid.
- Identify factors detrimental to the development of the embryo and fetus.

During the first to second week after conception, the fertilized ovum forms a blastocyst while traveling down the fallopian tube. The embryo enters the uterus and becomes implanted in the endometrium and the rapid growth of the embryo begins. The period of the embryo is considered to be from the second to the eighth week after fertilization.

EMBRYONIC DEVELOPMENT

By the end of the first 28 days following conception (the first *lunar month*), traces of all organs become differentiated; rudiments of the eyes, ears, nose and limb buds are present. The embryo is about 7.5 to 10 millimeters in length. Development proceeds from head to tail. As previously stated, the sex is determined at conception, but is not yet able to be distinguished.

During the next 28 days, or second lunar month, the head becomes larger because of the development of the brain. The features appear relatively small. The external genitalia appear toward the end of this month, and the embryo is now about 2.5 to 3 centimeters in length. The circulatory system is established between the mother and the embryo through the umbilical cord attached to the embryo at the navel. The cord varies from 7 inches to 4 feet in length, averaging about 20 inches. It remains taut in utero due to about 300 quarts of blood rushing through the cord each day at the rate of about four miles per hour at the end of pregnancy. The cord contains two arteries, which take waste products from the fetus to the placenta to be excreted by the mother, and one vein, which carries nourishment and oxygen to the fetus.

THE AMNIOTIC SAC

A fluid-filled sac which develops around the embryo is called the amniotic sac. This sac is formed by the amnion which is a smooth, transparent, inner fetal membrane.

The amnion grows rapidly and by the end of the eighth week it fuses with the outer fetal membrane called the *chorion.* The chorion forms the outer walls of the blastocyst. The fusion of the amnion and the chorion forms the amniochorionic sac, which is more commonly known as the "bag of waters." The embryo is suspended in this sac in the amniotic fluid.

Amniotic fluid is slightly alkaline and about 98 percent water. It equalizes the pressure around the fetus and keeps the fetus moist. The fetus floats and moves about in the fluid which keeps it at an even temperature and cushions it from injury. The amount of fluid increases as the fetus develops. At the time of birth, the amount of fluid varies from 500 to 1000 milliliters. Amniotic fluid in amounts greater than 2000 milliliters at term is a condition called *hydramnios.* It is common in women with diabetes and cardiac conditions, and is also associated with conditions of the fetus such as congenital heart defects and gastrointestinal abnormalities.

Too little amniotic fluid is termed *oligohydramnios.* The cause of this condition is not completely understood. It may occur when there is an obstruction of the fetal urinary tract or renal agenesis. Oligohydramnios can have serious consequences for the fetus. In early pregnancy, adhesions between the amnion and parts of the fetus can cause serious deformities. Later in pregnancy, other complications include increased risk of cord compression and pulmonary hypoplasia (failure of proper lung development).

FETAL DEVELOPMENT

In a four-week-old embryo, the spine, arms and legs are all present but in undeveloped form. By the seventh week the skeleton is virtually complete, in miniature. At this early date the skeleton is made of cartilage, not bone. Much more growth and development of the various parts are still to come about before birth. *Ossification,* the transformation of the tough, elastic cartilage into hard bone, begins at

about this time (the seventh week) and continues into adolescence. For example, almost all of the 26 bones which eventually make up the skeleton of the adult foot are still cartilage at birth.

The muscles that are involved in standing erect and using the arms, hands, legs and feet have their beginning structures early in the prenatal period. They increase in size, complexity, and strength as gestation proceeds. No mother needs to be told that these muscles get an active workout in utero. The unborn baby can and does perform many bodily movements which are impossible for a newborn because the fetus floats within the sac of amniotic fluid and is thereby rendered weightless.

The embryo becomes a fetus at eight weeks gestation. Centers for bone formation are laid down in the long bones during the third lunar month, and the fingers and toes can be distinguished. The nails begin to form, and the external genitalia show some sex distinction. The fetus resembles a human form, weighs from 5 to 20 grams (1/2 ounce) and is now about 9 centimeters in length.

Should the fetus be expelled from the uterus at this time, it would not survive. This is called a *miscarriage* or an early *spontaneous abortion.* A large number of miscarriages which occur in the early months of pregnancy are believed to be caused by imperfect implantation or embryonic formation. This is nature's way of handling the problem of possibly defective offspring.

At the beginning of the second trimester of pregnancy, the fetus looks like a baby with its eyes closed. The arms and legs are short; the fingers and toes are well formed. Fingernails are beginning to grow, and the deciduous or temporary teeth are developing in the gums. During the second trimester (fourth through sixth month) the *lanugo* or downy hair begins to appear on the shoulders and back. The skin is wrinkled. The fetal heartbeat can be heard as early as the twelfth week with the fetone because the

1st Month — Length 7.5 - 10 mm (0.1 - 0.16 inch) (smaller than a BB shot). Rudiments of eyes, ears and nose appear. First traces of all organs become differentiated.

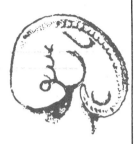

2nd Month — Length 2.5 cm (1 inch). Embryo markedly bent. Extremities rudimentary. Head disproportionately large, because of development of brain. External genitalia appear, but sex cannot be differentiated.

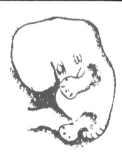

3rd Month — Length 7 - 9 cm (2.8 - 3.6 inches). Weight 5 - 20 gm (77 - 308 grains). Fingers and toes distinct, with soft nails.

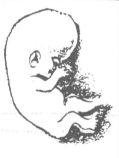

Figure 6-1

The first trimester of pregnancy (Adapted from Pelvic Anatomy for the Patient, Shering Corp.)

4th Month — Length 10 - 17 cm (3.9 - 6.7 inches). Weight 55 - 120 gm (1.9 - 4.2 ounces). Sex can be definitely differentiated. Downy hair (lanugo) appears on head.

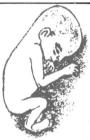

5th Month — Length 18 - 27 cm (7.1 - 10.6 inches). Weight 280 - 300 gm (9.9 - 10.6 ounces). Lanugo over entire body with small amount on head. Fetal movements usually felt by mother. Heart sounds perceptible.

6th Month — Length 28 - 34 cm (11.1 - 13.4 inches). Weight 650 gm (1.4 pounds). Skin wrinkles. Eyebrows and eyelashes appear. If born, fetus will not survive.

Figure 6-2

The fetus during the second trimester (Shering Corp.)

fetone is such a sensitive instrument. By the twentieth week, the fetal heartbeat can be heard with a fetoscope. It is about this time that the mother-to-be notices movement of the fetus. This movement is known as *quickening*.

By the end of the fifth lunar month the fetus weighs about 10 ounces and measures 10 to 13 inches in length. It is *previable* (not sufficiently developed to live outside of the fetus). Should it be born at this time, it will be extremely frail. Its expulsion from the uterus could be called a *late abortion*. Most states require a fetal death certificate if the fetus is expelled at this time. If the fetus shows any signs of life, a birth certificate is issued.

During the third trimester (seventh through tenth lunar month) the fetus becomes covered with vernix caseosa. *Vernix caseosa* is a cheese-like, greasy substance probably secreted by the sebaceous glands which acts as a protection to the skin of the fetus. Since the fetus is surrounded by the amniotic fluid, softening or *maceration* of the skin might occur if there were not this

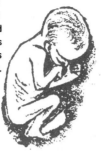

7th Month — Length 35 - 38 cm (13.8 - 15.0 inches). Weight 1200 gm (2.6 pounds). Skin red and covered with vernix. Pupillary membranes disappear from eyes. If born, fetus breathes, cries, moves but usually dies.

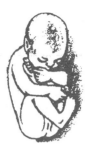

9th Month — Length 42 - 48 cm (16.6 - 18.9 inches). Weight 1700 - 2600 gm (3.7 - 5.7 pounds). Face loses wrinkled appearance due to subcutaneous fat deposit. If born, good chance to survive.

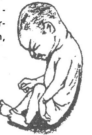

8th Month — Length 38 - 43 cm (15.0 - 17.0 inches). Weight 1600 - 1900 gm (3.5 - 4.2 pounds). Appearance of "little old man." If born, may live with proper care.

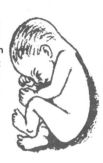

10th Month — Length 48 - 52 cm (18.9 - 20.5 inches). Weight 3000 - 3600 gm (6.6 - 7.9 pounds). Skin smooth, without lanugo (except about shoulders), ~~covered with vernix~~. Scalp hair usually dark. Fingers and toes with well-developed nails projecting beyond their tips. Eyes uniformly slate colored; impossible to predict final hue.

Figure 6-3

The fetus during the final trimester (Shering Corp.)

protective coating. Deposits of fat begin to form under the tissue-paper thin skin.

The bowel of the fetus contains a thick, dark green tenacious substance called *meconium*, which is made from bile, mucus, and *desquamated* (peeled off) epithelial cells. This will be the *neonate's* (newborn) first bowel movement.

The eighth lunar month can be called the month of storage. It is at this time that the supplies of iron, calcium, phosphorus and nitrogen needed for continuing development and immediate use in the neonatal period are being stored. The fetus is now fully developed and weighs nearly 3 pounds. It should be able to survive a premature termination of pregnancy. The amount of care required is still very great if it is to live.

In the ninth and tenth lunar months, the fetus gains weight rapidly, approximately 8 ounces per week, because of *subcutaneous* (under the skin) fat deposits. The hair and nails are fairly long. The fetus begins to shed the lanugo and may even suck the thumb. The fetus born at nine lunar months has an excellent chance of survival.

DETRIMENTS TO DEVELOPMENT

Certain factors may influence the development during the first trimester of pregnancy. Frequently, the mother-to-be is unaware of her pregnancy. She may contract infectious diseases, have x-ray studies done, or may take drugs which could affect the developing embryo. Figure 9-2 contains information regarding medications harmful to prenatal development. Thalidomide is an example of a drug which affects the embryo.

In several surveys of American and British pregnant women, it was found that nearly one-third of them took some kind of mood-changing drug: sedatives, hypnotics, and/or appetite suppressants. Babies born to drug-dependent women are found to have breathing trouble, pneumonia, brain hemorrhage, blood disease, infection and jaundice. Approximately 75 to 95 percent of babies born to heroin-addicted mothers are addicted themselves. Withdrawal symptoms begin within 24 hours after the umbilical cord is cut and the baby is deprived of its supply of heroin. Withdrawal can last several days to six months.

German measles (rubella) contracted at this time may cause cataracts, mental retardation, deafness, and abnormalities of the heart in the developing embryo. How the virus affects the developing embryo is not clear; the use of gamma globulin is not effective in preventing deformities.

In order to prevent deformities in a developing embryo, it is suggested that young girls be given the rubella vaccine before their reproductive years. In June 1969, live rubella virus vaccine was licensed for use in the United States. However, rubella vaccine should not be given to pregnant women; attenuated rubella vaccine virus can infect the embryo and result in damage to the embryo.

Syphilis is another infectious condition that may affect the development of the embryo. Mandatory premarital serological testing for venereal disease has reduced the incidence of deformities due to syphilis. However, if the fetus should be infected before the fifth month, it will probably die.

If syphilis is contracted by the mother in the later months of pregnancy and inadequately treated, it may cause congenital syphilis affecting the heart, long bones, skin, and respiratory system of the fetus. It may also cause premature delivery or a stillborn infant.

Gonorrhea is a venereal disease which may be chronic or may be acquired by the mother at the time of conception. It is generally confined to her lower genital tract, particularly the vagina and cervix. If the cervical plug has formed before the mother is infected, the gonococci may not reach the fetus. However, if a baby is born through an infected birth canal, the gonococci can cause blindness in the newborn infant unless its eyes are treated with silver nitrate or an antibiotic. Gonorrhea is generally treated with penicillin. If the mother is sensitive to penicillin, another antibiotic may be used.

Herpes virus and Chlamydia trachomatis infections are also sexually transmitted diseases which are highly contagious. Herpes infections, which are viral in origin, have been called the fastest growing sexually transmitted disease in the United States. It is a lifelong disease that has a tendency to recur again and again. Genital herpes causes blistery sores on and around the genital organs. A person can be contagious without having the blistery sores.

Women who have had genital herpes should be especially careful when they are pregnant since a baby can become infected during delivery. A pregnant woman who has had herpes should tell her doctor about it even if sores are not visible, as there may be sores inside the body. If tests show that the woman is infectious at the time of delivery, the baby can be delivered by cesarean section. This avoids the possibility of infecting the infant. If tests show that the infection is not active, the mother may be able to deliver vaginally without infecting the infant.

Scarlet fever and smallpox are two other infectious diseases that may interfere with normal embryonic development if contracted by the mother-to-be. Immediate treatment of streptococcal sore throats and proper immunization reduces the possibility of harm to the embryo.

During development of the fetus, serious problems arise if the nourishment of the mother or the oxygen level of her blood is deficient. The common cold, heavy smoking, pneumonia, extreme anemia, and heart failure are dangerous since they interfere with the circulation of adequately oxygenated blood to the placenta. If the brain of the fetus does not receive sufficient oxygen, brain damage may result. Such damage is manifested by disturbances of the central nervous system.

If the mother's diet is deficient in protein, vitamins, or minerals during pregnancy, the child's future mental and physical development may be retarded, and he or she may have a predisposition to rickets, scurvy, anemia, tetany, or dental caries.

If the mother has diabetes, there is an increased possibility of spontaneous abortion, stillbirth, and congenital defects. Babies born to diabetic mothers are usually larger than normal and hydramnios is common.

Another factor which may adversely affect the fetus is a multiple pregnancy. Because of intrauterine crowding, premature birth may result. One of the fetuses may not receive adequate supplies of minerals and vitamins. Therefore, it is likely to be less developed and smaller than the other fetus. Sometimes one survives at the cost of the other's life.

SUGGESTED ACTIVITIES

- Write a report stating the effect smoking has on the developing fetus. Document your report with a bibliography.

- Discuss how deficiencies of protein, vitamins, and minerals in the mother's diet affect the developing fetus.

- Explain the difference between a calendar month, a lunar month, and a trimester. The normal full-term pregnancy is 280 days; state this in calendar months, lunar months, and trimesters.

- Describe the following characteristics of the fetus: (a) approximate weight, and (b) length and developmental milestones at the following gestational ages.
  - 8–12 weeks   — 21–25 weeks
  - 13–16 weeks   — 26–29 weeks
  - 17–20 weeks   — 30–38 weeks

- Discuss the effects of known teratogens on the developing fetus.
  - drugs   — irradiation
  - chemicals   — infectious agents

- Describe the fetal development, which can be used for patient education, in lay terms.

REVIEW

Multiple Choice. Select the best answer.

1. The sex of the embryo is determined at
    a. two weeks   c. two days
    b. two months   d. conception

2. The embryo becomes a fetus after
   a. 8 weeks
   b. 4 weeks
   c. 16 weeks
   d. 12 weeks

3. The bag of waters is composed of the
   a. amnion and placenta
   b. placenta and uterus
   c. amnion and chorion
   d. amnion and uterus

4. The organs of the embryo become differentiated
   a. at conception
   b. during the first lunar month
   c. during the second lunar month
   d. during the third lunar month

5. Circulation is established
   a. at conception
   b. during the first lunar month
   c. during the second lunar month
   d. during the third lunar month

6. When the mother first feels fetal movement, this is called
   a. lightening
   b. quickening
   c. fluttering
   d. conception

7. A thick, dark green tenacious substance which is the newborn's first bowel movement is called
   a. bile
   b. desquamated epithelial
   c. meconium
   d. vernix caseosa

8. The month in which the fetus stores iron, calcium, phosphorus, and nitrogen for continuing development and immediate use in the neonatal period is the
   a. ninth lunar month
   b. seventh lunar month
   c. sixth lunar month
   d. eighth lunar month

9. Sexually transmitted diseases which can have an effect on the newborn are
   a. gonorrhea
   b. syphilis
   c. herpes and Chlamydia
   d. all of these

10. The umbilical cord contains two arteries which
    a. take waste products from the fetus to the placenta
    b. carry nourishment and oxygen to the fetus
    c. carry oxygen to the fetus and remove wastes
    d. none of these

11. The umbilical cord contains one vein which
    a. takes waste products from the fetus to the placenta
    b. carries nourishment and oxygen to the fetus
    c. carries oxygen to the fetus and removes wastes
    d. none of these

12. Hydramnios is a condition where
    a. the amniotic fluid is slightly alkaline
    b. amniotic fluid is in amounts greater than 2000 milliliters at term
    c. the fetus has congenital heart defects and gastrointestinal abnormalities
    d. amniotic fluid is in amounts less than 500 milliliters

13. If the mother's diet is deficient in protein, vitamins and minerals during pregnancy, the newborn may have a predisposition to
    a. rickets and scurvy   c. dental caries
    b. anemia and tetany   d. all of these

14. There is a greater chance of spontaneous abortion, stillbirth and congenital defects if the mother
    a. smokes
    b. has pneumonia during her pregnancy
    c. has diabetes
    d. has syphilis

15. The amniotic fluid
    a. equalizes the pressure around the fetus and keeps it moist
    b. cushions the fetus from injury
    c. keeps the fetus at an even temperature
    d. all of these

16. Too little amniotic fluid
    a. causes serious deformities
    b. develops small gestational age babies
    c. has no effect
    d. develops infants with pulmonary problems

UNIT 7

MATERNAL AND FETAL CIRCULATION

OBJECTIVES

After studying this unit, the student should be able to:

* Trace the flow of blood through fetal circulation.
* State how the placenta is formed.
* Name the functions of the placenta.
* Identify the means by which nutrients and gases pass through the placenta.
* Identify changes that take place in fetal circulation at birth.

Early in pregnancy, the endometrium which lies directly beneath the embedded ovum becomes thicker. This portion of the endometrium is called the *decidua basalis.* The *chorionic villi* are fingerlike projections which have developed from fetal tissue at the base of the implanted fertilized ovum. They contain blood vessels which unite to form larger blood vessels communicating with the fetus. By the end of the third month, the placenta has been formed from the decidua basalis and chorionic villi. Through these villi, oxygen and nourishment are received from the mother and passed to the fetus by way of the umbilical cord. The umbilical cord attaches the fetus to the placenta. Waste products of the fetus are discharged through the umbilical cord to the placenta.

THE PLACENTA

The placenta acts as a respiratory, nutritive, and excretory organ for the developing fetus; it connects the developing fetus to the uterine wall. The placenta develops from both embryonic and maternal tissue; that is, from the outer rim of the blastocyst and the inner lining of the uterus (endometrium).

The placenta is a fleshy organ which at term measures about 8 inches in diameter, is one inch thick and weighs about 1/6 of the baby's weight or slightly over one pound. It resembles a plant sending roots into the earth for nourishment. When the plant is pulled up, particles of earth cling to the roots. Likewise, a thin layer of the uterine wall clings to the chorionic villi when the placenta detaches after delivery.

Placental Transfer

Intensive studies of the transfer of nourishment from maternal to fetal circulation have been made. It appears that nourishing materials pass from the maternal side of the placenta (the decidua basalis) to the fetal side (the chorionic

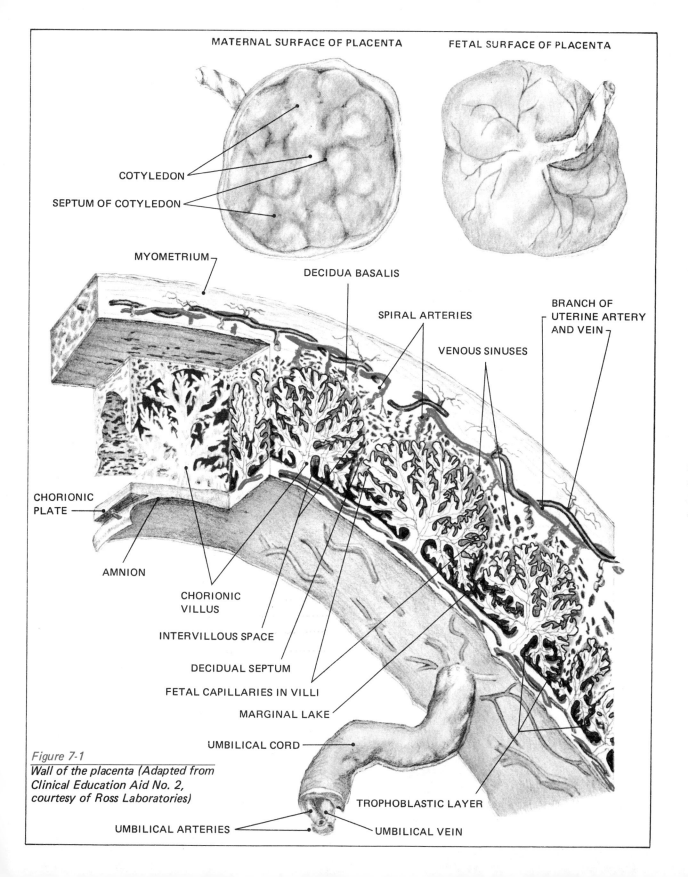

MATERNAL SURFACE OF PLACENTA

FETAL SURFACE OF PLACENTA

COTYLEDON

SEPTUM OF COTYLEDON

MYOMETRIUM

DECIDUA BASALIS

SPIRAL ARTERIES

VENOUS SINUSES

BRANCH OF UTERINE ARTERY AND VEIN

CHORIONIC PLATE

AMNION

CHORIONIC VILLUS

INTERVILLOUS SPACE

DECIDUAL SEPTUM

FETAL CAPILLARIES IN VILLI

MARGINAL LAKE

UMBILICAL CORD

TROPHOBLASTIC LAYER

UMBILICAL ARTERIES

UMBILICAL VEIN

Figure 7-1
Wall of the placenta (Adapted from Clinical Education Aid No. 2, courtesy of Ross Laboratories)

villi) by osmosis; waste products pass from the fetus to the mother's bloodstream in the same manner. There is no intermixing of maternal and fetal blood because of the layer of cells separating the fetal placenta from the maternal tissue and maternal blood vessels. It is believed that calcium, phosphorus, amino acids, glucose, fats and certain bacteria, viruses, drugs, and antibodies pass through this layer of cells into the fetal circulation.

The blood circulating in the fetus is never as rich in oxygen as the blood in the adult. The oxygen and carbon dioxide pass through the placenta by *diffusion;* that is, when the solutions of two gases at different concentrations are separated by a permeable membrane, the gas molecules pass through the membrane in both directions until the concentrations on both sides are equal. In this way the oxygen from the maternal side passes through the placenta to the fetal side; carbon dioxide and waste products pass from the fetal side to the maternal side.

The new life within the mother needs increased amounts of oxygen to grow from one cell to billions of cells in just nine months. The placenta is the connection through which the mother feeds the fetus. It also filters out harmful substances such as bacteria. However, it cannot filter out all harmful material. For example, smoking can increase the risk of spontaneous abortion and premature birth. Nicotine in the mother's bloodstream can impair the heart rate, blood pressure, oxygen supply, acid balance, and may cause the placental blood vessels to narrow and diminish the supply of nourishment to the unborn baby.

FETAL CIRCULATION

Certain fetal capillaries transfer waste products to the maternal circulation while others accept nourishment into the fetal circulation. The capillaries merge in the fetal side of the placenta, eventually meeting to form the umbilical vein and arteries which communicate with the fetus. The arteries transport waste materials from the fetus, and the vein supplies oxygen and nutrients to the fetus.

The two arteries and a vein are enclosed in the umbilical cord, which is about 20 inches long. The surface of the cord is an extension of the amnion. The blood vessels inside the cord are protected by a mucoid substance called *Wharton's jelly.*

The arterial (oxygenated) blood flows up the cord through the umbilical vein and passes into the ascending (inferior) vena cava partly through the liver, but chiefly through the special fetal structure, the *ductus venosus,* figure 7-2. The large liver of the newborn has been attributed to the supply of fresh blood from the umbilical vein.

From the ascending vena cava, the blood flows into the right auricle of the heart and passes through another fetal structure, the *foramen ovale,* directly to the left auricle. It goes from the left auricle to the left ventricle and leaves the heart through the aorta. The blood goes to the arms and head and returns to the heart, passing through the descending (superior) vena cava to the right auricle, but instead of passing through the foramen ovale, the current is now directed downward into the right ventricle and leaves the heart through the pulmonary arteries. Some of the blood goes to the lungs but most of it flows through another fetal structure, the *ductus arteriosus,* into the aorta.

Since the fetus receives oxygen from the placenta, its lungs do not function. The blood must be shunted around its lungs with only a small amount going through them to nourish the tissues, not to secure oxygen.

The blood in the aorta, except that which supplies the head and arms, passes downward to

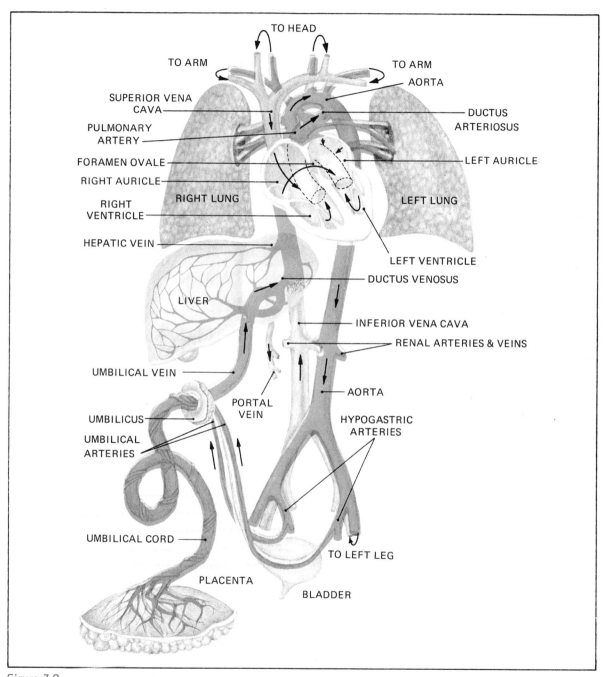

Figure 7-2
Fetal circulation (Adapted from Nursing Education Aid No. 1, courtesy of Ross Laboratories)

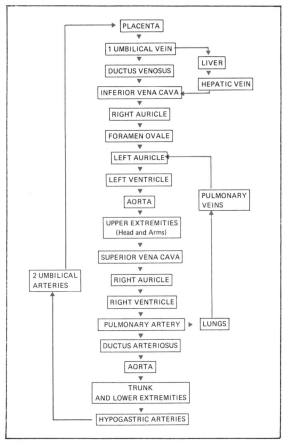

Figure 7-3

Schematic diagram of fetal circulation

supply the trunk and lower extremities. The greater part of this blood flows through the hypogastric arteries and back through the umbilical arteries of the cord to the placenta where it is again oxygenated. A small amount passes back into the ascending vena cava to mingle with fresh blood from the umbilical vein and again makes the circuit of the fetal body.

Circulation Changes at Birth

At birth, the infant's lung function is established; several of the vessels are no longer of use. The umbilical arteries become filled with clotted blood and are converted into fibrous cords. The umbilical vein in the baby's body becomes a round ligament of the liver. After the cord is tied and cut, a large amount of blood returns to the heart from the lungs. The more or less equal pressure in the auricles causes the foramen ovale to close and it eventually disappears. The ductus venosus and arteriosus shrivel up and are converted to fibrous ligaments within two to three months. The closure of the foramen ovale changes the course of the blood flow to that of normal adult human circulation.

SUGGESTED ACTIVITIES

- Describe three changes that take place in the fetal circulation system at birth. Include what may happen to the infant if ductus venosus and ductus arteriosus do not close.

- Prepare a diagram showing the difference between fetal circulation and adult circulation.

REVIEW

A. Multiple Choice. Select the best answer.

1. At birth, the course of fetal blood circulation is changed to normal adult human circulation by the closing of the
   a. foramen ovale
   b. ductus venosus
   c. ductus arteriosus

2. The transfer of nutrients from the maternal side of the placenta to the fetal side occurs by
   a. intermixing of maternal and fetal blood
   b. diffusion
   c. osmosis

3. Oxygen and carbon dioxide pass through the placenta by means of
   a. osmosis
   b. fetal lungs
   c. diffusion

4. The umbilical cord contains
   a. two veins and one artery
   b. one vein and two arteries
   c. one artery and one vein

5. The vessel in the umbilical cord that carries nourishment and oxygen from the placenta to the fetus is the
   a. one vein
   b. one artery
   c. two veins

B. Match the descriptions in column I to the correct structures in column II.

Column I	Column II
1. a short blood vessel between the pulmonary artery and aorta of the fetus	a. chorionic villi
2. special fetal structure for passing fetal blood from the umbilical vein into the inferior vena cava	b. decidua basalis
3. thickened portion of the endometrium lying directly beneath the embedded ovum	c. ductus arteriosus
4. opening between the right and left auricles of the fetal heart	d. ductus venosus
5. fingerlike projections that have developed from the outer wall of the fertilized egg	e. foramen ovale

C. Briefly answer the following questions.

    1. What is the function of the placenta?

    2. How is the placenta formed?

    3. Trace the flow of fetal blood from the placenta through the fetal circulation and back to the placenta.

_____

Self-Evaluation

A. Identify the organs indicated on the diagrams of the female and male reproductive systems.

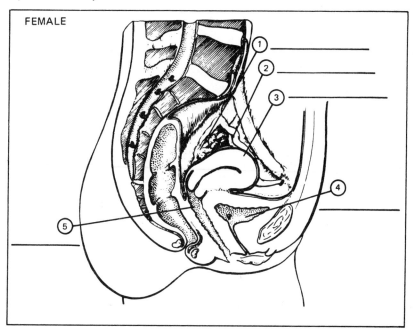

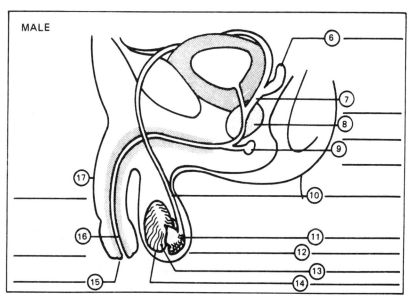

B. Multiple Choice. Select the best answer.

1. Sperm develop in the
    a. scrotum   c. testes
    b. penis   d. bladder

2. Ova develop in the
    a. fallopian tubes   c. uterus
    b. ovaries   d. clitoris

3. Each ovum and each sperm contains
    a. 22 chromosomes   c. 23 chromosomes
    b. 44 chromosomes   d. 46 chromosomes

4. Hemophilia is transmitted by
    a. DNA   c. dominant trait
    b. sex-linked gene   d. histones

5. Fraternal twins result from the union of
    a. one sperm and one ovum   c. two sperm and one ovum
    b. two sperm and two ova   d. two ova and one sperm

6. Cleavage is a term for
    a. cell division   c. implantation in the uterus
    b. fertilization   d. formation of the placenta

7. The placenta develops from
    a. the zygote
    b. the uterine mucosa
    c. cleavage
    d. embryonic and maternal tissue

8. The skin of the fetus is protected from maceration by
    a. amniotic fluid   c. lanugo
    b. vernix caseosa   d. subcutaneous fat

9. The month of storage is the
    a. tenth month   c. eighth month
    b. ninth month   d. first month

10. Meconium is composed of
    a. undigested food
    b. digested food
    c. bile, mucus, and epithelial cells
    d. bile and blood

11. The primary male sex hormone that contributes to the development
    of secondary sex characteristics is
    a. progesterone   c. testosterone
    b. estrogen   d. androgen

12. Two ovarian hormones significant in regulating the female repro-
    ductive organs are
    a. testosterone and amnion
    b. estrogen and progesterone
    c. progesterone and testosterone
    d. estrogen and testosterone

13. Prolonged or excessive bleeding during the menstrual period is called
    a. amenorrhea   c. metorrhagia
    b. menorrhagia   d. dysmenorrhea

14. The neck of the uterus is called the
    a. corpus   c. cervix
    b. fundus   d. endometrium

15. When a mature ovum is released by the ovary, the process is called
    a. ovulation   c. conception
    b. menstruation   d. implantation

C. Match the obstetrical terms in column II with correct descriptions in column I

Column I	Column II
1. after eighth week of development	a. genetics
2. downy hair	b. sex-linked
3. thin transparent sac	c. sex-limited
4. study of heredity	d. cleavage
5. protects skin of fetus	e. zygote
6. peel off in scales	f. embryo
7. softening of the skin	g. fetus
8. trait passed from grandfather to grandson	h. amnion
9. cell division	i. maceration
10. fertilized ovum	j. desquamate
11. contains testes and keeps sperm at lower than body temperature	k. deciduous
12. tube which carries seminal fluid and sperm to urethra	l. lanugo
13. storehouse for sperm	m. vernix caseosa
14. produces an alkaline, milky fluid which neutralizes and stimulates sperm action	n. testes
15. foreskin of penis	o. scrotum
16. first eight weeks of development	p. vas deferens
17. temporary teeth	q. epididymis
18. primary sex organ of male	r. prostate gland
19. characteristic pertaining to one sex only	s. prepuce
20. lining of the uterus	t. endometrium

D. Write a brief but complete paragraph on the following topics:

1. Describe the processes of ovulation, menstruation, and conception.

2. Describe fetal circulation.

3. Explain the process of diffusion. Give an example of diffusion in relation to placental transfer.

SECTION 2

Pregnancy and Prenatal Care

UNIT 8

SIGNS AND SYMPTOMS OF PREGNANCY

OBJECTIVES

After studying this unit, the student should be able to:

- Identify the physiological changes of pregnancy.
- Define primigravida, multigravida, primipara, and multipara.
- State how the increased blood volume affects heart action.
- Distinguish between the presumptive, probable, and positive signs of pregnancy.

This unit investigates those changes which affect the body systems of the pregnant woman. The signs of pregnancy which are classed as presumptive, probable, and positive are also described.

Early in the obstetrical nursing program, the student should learn the following definitions because these terms are used constantly in the obstetrical field.

primigravida   a woman pregnant with her first child

multigravida   a woman who has been pregnant several times

nullipara   a woman who has not borne children

primipara   a woman in labor with or having borne her first child

multipara   a woman in labor with or having borne her second child and subsequent children

PHYSIOLOGICAL CHANGES

A woman's body undergoes many physical changes during pregnancy. It is important for the nurse working with obstetrical patients to be aware of these changes.

Reproductive System

During the first three months of pregnancy the uterus changes in size and shape. It becomes

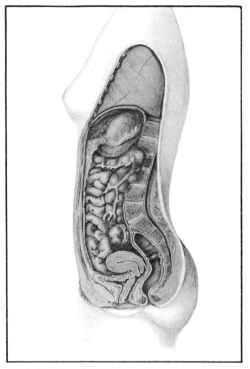

ABDOMINAL CAVITY BEFORE PREGNANCY

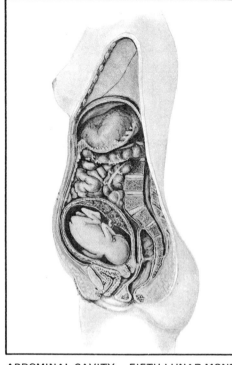

ABDOMINAL CAVITY — FIFTH LUNAR MONTH

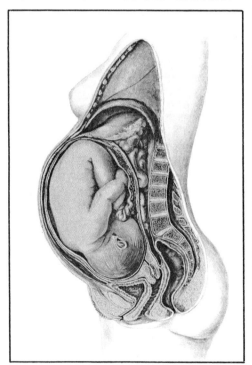

ABDOMINAL CAVITY — NINTH MONTH

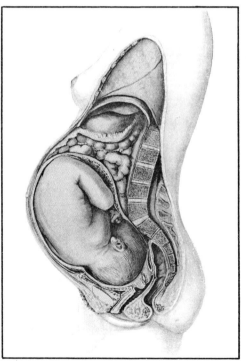

ABDOMINAL CAVITY — AT TERM

Figure 8-1

Changes in abdominal cavity (Courtesy of Maternity Center Association)

more *anteflexed* (bent forward) than usual. It eventually increases to 500 percent of the original size. Its weight increases from 2 ounces to 2 pounds. At about the sixth week of pregnancy, Hegar's sign is perceptible. *Hegar's sign* is the softening of the lower portion of the uterus. This is one of the most valuable signs of early pregnancy.

A second sign noted by vaginal examination is Goodell's sign. *Goodell's sign* is the softening of the cervix which occurs early in pregnancy.

Another early indication of pregnancy is known as *Chadwick's sign*. The tissue around the vagina and external genitals becomes thicker and softer. It takes on a bluish purple color due to the increase in blood supply to that area. During the first trimester, vaginal secretions increase and consist of a thick, white discharge.

Uterine contractions begin in the early weeks of pregnancy and continue throughout the entire period of gestation. They are painless and the patient is usually not conscious of them. These painless, intermittent contractions of the uterus are known as the *Braxton-Hicks sign*. The uterine muscles contract and relax, thereby enlarging the uterus to accommodate the growing fetus and developing power to expel the baby.

Between the fourth and fifth month of pregnancy, the fetus is small in relation to the amount of amniotic fluid. At this time ballottement can be performed. *Ballottement* is the rebounding of the floating fetus in the uterus when the fetus is lightly tapped during a vaginal examination. A gentle tap makes the fetus rise in the amniotic fluid; it then returns to its original position, tapping the examining finger. Ballottement can only be done after the fetus has grown large enough to be felt and before it becomes too large to move about freely. It is not a positive sign of pregnancy as a tumor could produce the same effect.

The Breasts

In the early months of pregnancy, the breasts become larger, firmer, and more tender. The nipple is elevated and the *areola* (pigmented area around nipple) becomes darker in color. The weight of the breasts increases approximately 1 1/2 pounds due to the increased growth and activity of the glandular tissues and a richer blood supply.

Skeletal and Muscular Systems

The skeletal system responds to pregnancy by producing a greater blood supply in the bone marrow. The ligaments holding the pelvis together at the pubic symphysis and sacroiliac articulation soften due to hormonal changes during pregnancy. This allows the pelvis to spread out, allowing more room for the passage of the baby. General muscle tone decreases.

The Skin

During pregnancy, the skin shows many changes throughout the body. In addition to increased pigmentation around the breasts, other pigmentary changes are common in pregnancy. The *linea nigra* is a dark color line running from the umbilicus to the mons veneris. *Chloasma gravidarum*, a frecklelike pigmentation of the face, often occurs during pregnancy. This pigmentation is sometimes referred to as the "mask of pregnancy"; it usually disappears after delivery. However, pigmentation of the breasts and the *striae gravidarum* (streaks on the sides of the abdomen, breasts, and thighs caused by stretching of the skin) never entirely disappear.

Circulatory System

During pregnancy, blood volume in the body increases about 30 percent; this means an increase of 500 to 1000 milliliters of blood is added to the circulatory system. The increase in the amount of blood is due largely to an increase in its water content; the blood is diluted. The hemoglobin is slightly lower in pregnant women, but it is not a true anemia due to the dilution. If the hemoglobin goes below 70 percent, however, the woman has a true anemia due to an inadequate iron supply in her diet. The increase in blood volume makes it necessary for the heart to pump about 50 percent more blood per minute than it did prior to pregnancy.

Blood volume reaches its peak during the seventh and eighth month of pregnancy and declines during the last weeks of gestation. Women with normal hearts carry this extra load without difficulty. However, for the woman with heart disease, this increase in blood volume can be of grave concern.

Palpitation of the heart is not uncommon during this period; shortness of breath may occur also. The enlarged uterus causes increased pressure on the lungs. However, a widening of the thoracic cage takes place, and this more than compensates for the uterine changes. Varicose veins are common during pregnancy, particularly in the legs, vulva, and rectum. A *varicose vein* is a vein which has become abnormally torturous and swollen as a result of prolonged increased pressure.

Urinary System

The urinary system changes during pregnancy; therefore, urine tests are important throughout pregnancy. During the course of pregnancy, the amount of urine increases and the urine has a lower specific gravity. Sugar is sometimes found in the urine due to a decreased kidney threshold for glucose. It is likely to appear in the urine after a meal. Further testing is needed to determine whether diabetes is present. Tran-

sitory *albuminuria* (presence of albumin, a simple protein, in the blood) sometimes occurs in normal pregnancy, but it can also be an indication of toxemia. Preeclampsia, which in past years was termed toxemia, refers to a disorder during gestation characterized by hypertension, albuminuria, excessive weight gain and edema. If left untreated, convulsion and coma may occur. *Cystitis* (bladder infection) often occurs in pregnancy, as does *pyelitis* (inflammation of the kidney pelvis). The ureters become dilated in pregnancy due to the pressure of the growing uterus on the ureters as they cross the pelvic brim, and to a softening of the ureteral walls as a result of endocrine influences. The ureters lose much of their muscular tone and, with the pressure of the enlarging uterus, are unable to expel the urine as satisfactorily as before.

Respiratory System

A pregnant woman must inhale much more air than the nonpregnant woman. This is due to the fact that the pregnant woman must oxygenate her own blood as well as that of the fetus. In the later months of pregnancy, the diaphragm can be displaced upward as much as one inch. The lungs are subjected to pressure from the expanding uterus and shortness of breath occurs. The lung capacity is not decreased, however, because of the slight widening of the thoracic cage.

Nervous System

The effect of pregnancy on the nervous system varies. The more emotionally unstable the woman is, the more likely the nervous system will be affected. Some women escape emotional upsets entirely while other women become sensitive and irritable. Instances of actual psychosis do occur, but these are rare.

Digestive System

Oftentimes the digestive system is taxed throughout pregnancy. During the early months, nausea is common and sometimes vomiting occurs. These symptoms generally diminish by the end of the first trimester. The appetite may be either decreased, if nausea is present, or increased in the early months. The digestive system seems to become accustomed to its new role and accepts the job it has to do to nourish the baby as well as the mother. Constipation is very common, due in part to the nervous control of the bowels, hormonal influences, and the pressure of the expanding uterus on the sigmoid and the rectum. It may also be a result of medications, such as ferrous sulfate (iron), which the mother may be taking. Constipation is often accompanied by *flatulence* (excessive gas in the gastrointestinal tract). Emptying time of the stomach is also changed due to pressure from the diaphragm and diminished tone of the stomach.

Heartburn often occurs in the second trimester. *Heartburn* is the regurgitating of acid liquid from the stomach into the esophagus; this causes a burning sensation in the esophagus. It has nothing to do with the heart. Heartburn may be caused by nervous tension, worry, fatigue, or improper diet. It can be lessened by eliminating most of the fat from the diet and eating smaller, more frequent meals.

Endocrine System

The anterior lobe of the pituitary gland secretes hormones which act on the breasts, ovaries, thyroid, and growth process. The posterior lobe of the pituitary gland secretes oxytocin, a hormone which stimulates uterine contractions. The pituitary gland is an important link in the endocrine network of pregnancy. The thyroid tends to enlarge, and as it does, its function declines, resulting in fatigue and lethargy.

Weight Gain

In the early months of pregnancy the woman may lose a little weight. This weight loss is later made up by a gain varying from 20 to 25 pounds which is usually lost after delivery. The body stores up albumin and fat to provide for the growth of the fetus; to supply energy during labor; and to furnish materials for milk in the breasts.

The average weight gain in pregnancy is about 26 pounds. It is distributed as follows: fetus 7 1/2 pounds, placenta 1 pound, amniotic fluid 2 pounds, increased uterine weight 2 pounds, increased blood volume 3 1/2 pounds, and increased breast weight 1 1/2 pounds. The remaining pounds are fat accumulation and increased amount of tissue fluid. The Committee on Maternal Nutrition of the National Research Council, and the American College of Obstetricians and Gynecologists recommend a weight gain of 24 to 28 pounds as ideal for pregnant women.

SIGNS AND SYMPTOMS

Symptoms of pregnancy are generally well defined; in most instances, diagnosis by the physician is not difficult. These symptoms are classified as:

- *presumptive* (presumed but not proven)
- *probable* (likely but not definite)
- *positive* (no doubt about it)

Presumptive Signs

1. *Cessation of Menses:* In a woman who has been menstruating regularly, the abrupt cessation of the periods is usually caused by pregnancy. This is called amenorrhea.

2. *Frequency of Urination* (micturition): During early pregnancy, frequency occurs because the enlarging uterus presses against the bladder. In midpregnancy, pressure is relieved as the uterus rises into the abdominal cavity.

3. *Morning Sickness:* Nausea and vomiting, particularly upon awakening in the morning, begins soon after the first menstrual period is missed and usually disappears by the third month of pregnancy as the woman's body adjusts. If it lasts beyond the fourth month, or when it affects the general health, it is considered a complication of pregnancy.

4. *Quickening:* The first sensation of fetal life usually is felt by the mother between the eighteenth and twentieth weeks.

5. *Changes in the Breasts:* Early in pregnancy there is enlargement of the breasts and usually some tingling in the region of the nipple which grows and becomes more erectile and dark in color.

6. *Pigmentation:* The skin turns darker and occasionally the face is almost covered with chloasma. The linea nigra makes its appearance.

7. *Chadwick's Sign:* The mucous membrane of the vagina just below the urethral orifice is a violet color after the fourth week of pregnancy.

8. *Striae gravidarum:* Shining, reddish lines on the abdomen, thighs, and breasts caused by the stretching of tissue may occur during pregnancy.

9. *General Symptoms:* During the first month of pregnancy, the woman may have a vague feeling of fatigue. She may find she requires more rest and sleep than usual; 12 hours or more is not uncommon. She may also have a dull headache, although this could be caused by reasons other than pregnancy.

Probable Signs

1. *Changes in the Abdomen:* The abdomen gradually increases in size. As it increases, the gait and carriage of the woman change. Any enlargement of the abdomen, however, whether due to tumor or fluid, may produce the same results.

2. *Hegar's Sign:* Softening of the lower uterine segment

3. *Ballottement:* Gently tapping the fetus which moves away and rebounds within the uterus.

4. *Braxton-Hicks Sign:* Painless uterine contractions occurring periodically throughout pregnancy, enlarging the uterus to accommodate the growing fetus.

5. *Hormone Tests:* Various tests, such as Friedman, Aschheim-Zondek, agglutination, and HCG (human chorionic gonadotropin). With newly developed monoclonal antibody technology, HCG can be detected in a woman's urine as early as 7 to 10 days after conception. This makes early determination of pregnancy possible in the office or clinic setting, even before a missed period. HCG can also be quantitatively measured in the mother's blood. Today there are several over-the-counter home pregnancy kits. The experience to date has been a high percentage of false negative results. This may be due to the test itself, incorrectly following the test steps, or misinterpreting the end results. This false negative reading often causes a delay in seeking prenatal care.

Positive Signs

1. *Fetal Heart Beat:* The fetal heart tones can be heard from the third month with a fetone.

Trimester	Presumptive	Probable	Positive
First 1-3 months	Amenorrhea; tender, fuller breasts; nausea and vomiting after 1st month for 6-8 weeks in 50% of women; discoloration of the vaginal mucosa; Chadwick's sign; frequency of urination; abdominal distention; increased appetite; fatigue; loss of weight; headache; constipation; increase in vaginal discharge	Enlargement of uterus; change in shape, size, and consistency of the uterus; changes in female reproductive system: Goodell's sign, Hegar's sign, positive hormone tests; Braxton-Hicks sign	Ultrasound image of fetus
Second 4-6 months	Colostrum expressed; quickening; pigmentation of skin (chloasma, linea nigra, areola of breast); heartburn, flatulence; weight gain; feeling of well-being	Ballottement	Hear fetal heart tones; feel fetal movement; see skeleton by X ray; placental souffle; funic souffle

Figure 8-2

Signs and symptoms of pregnancy

2. *Fetal Movements:* The movement of the fetus can be felt by the physician or nurse about the fourth or fifth month.
3. *Ultrasonography:* An outline of the baby, placenta, and other structures can be seen when high-frequency sound waves scan the mother's abdomen and transmit a picture to a video screen. An embryo can be identified as early as the fourth week using ultrasound.
4. *Radiography:* After the fourth month, the fetal skeleton can be seen by x-ray examination. This type of examination is used less frequently since the development of ultrasound.
5. *Funic Souffle:* A soft murmur produced by the blood flowing through the umbilical arteries.
6. *Placental Souffle:* A soft murmur produced by the blood flow in the placenta.

SUGGESTED ACTIVITIES

• Demonstrate the ability to clinically diagnose pregnancy by use of historical signs, physical exam, and laboratory data.

• List the probable, presumptive, and positive signs of pregnancy.

• Describe Goodell's, Hegar's, and Chadwick's sign according to time of occurrence. Also, describe why the change occurs.

REVIEW

Multiple Choice. Select the best answer.

1. During pregnancy, the uterus increases in size as much as
   - a. 20 percent
   - b. 50 percent
   - c. 500 percent
   - d. 100 percent

2. A positive diagnosis of pregnancy can be made with ultrasonography about the end of the
   - a. first six weeks
   - b. second month
   - c. third month
   - d. fourth month

3. A presumptive sign of pregnancy is
   - a. cessation of menses
   - b. Hegar's sign
   - c. funic souffle
   - d. Braxton-Hicks sign

4. Movement of the fetus can usually be felt by the physician about the
   - a. fourth week
   - b. eighth week
   - c. third month
   - d. fourth month

5. A probable sign of pregnancy is
   - a. quickening
   - b. Aschheim-Zondek test
   - c. amenorrhea
   - d. morning sickness

6. A primigravida is a woman
   - a. in labor with or having borne her first child
   - b. pregnant with her first child
   - c. in labor with or having borne her second or subsequent child
   - d. who has been pregnant several times

7. A multipara is a woman
   - a. in labor with or having borne her first child
   - b. pregnant with her first child
   - c. in labor with or having borne her second or subsequent child
   - d. who has been pregnant several times

8. Painless, intermittent contractions of the uterus which begin in the early weeks of pregnancy and continue throughout the entire period of gestation are called
   - a. Goodell's sign
   - b. ballottement
   - c. Braxton-Hicks sign
   - d. Hegar's sign

9. The recommended weight gain for most pregnant women is
   - a. 18 to 20 pounds
   - b. 30 to 34 pounds
   - c. 22 to 27 pounds
   - d. 25 to 30 pounds

10. Skin changes that occur during pregnancy are
    a. linea nigra and striae gravidarum
    b. chloasma gravidarum
    c. Hegar's sign
    d. a and b
    e. all of these

11. During pregnancy, blood volume in the body increases about
    a. 1 percent   c. 10 percent
    b. 3 percent   d. 20 percent

12. Oxytocin is a hormone which stimulates uterine contractions and is secreted from the
    a. anterior lobe of the pituitary gland
    b. posterior lobe of the pituitary gland
    c. thyroid gland
    d. thymus gland

13. Changes in the urinary system which might occur during pregnancy are
    1. sugar in the urine in trace amounts
    2. transitory albuminuria
    3. nitrates in the urine
    4. blood in the urine
    a. 1 and 2   c. 1, 2 and 4
    b. 3 and 4   d. 1, 2, 3 and 4

14. Preeclampsia is characterized by
    1. hypertension
    2. sugar in the urine
    3. albuminuria
    4. excessive weight gain and edema
    a. 1 only   c. 1, 3 and 4
    b. 1 and 2   d. 4 only

15. Heartburn which frequently occurs during pregnancy can be lessened by
    1. eliminating most of the fat from the diet
    2. eliminating most of the sugar from the diet
    3. eliminating large meals and eating smaller, more frequent meals
    4. lessening nervous tension, worry and fatigue
    a. 1 and 2   c. 2 only
    b. 1, 3 and 4   d. 1, 2, 3 and 4

16. Outline a care plan for a primigravida in her first trimester.

UNIT 9

NURSING CARE AND MEDICAL SUPERVISION

OBJECTIVES

After studying this unit, the student should be able to:

- Identify the components of the nursing process and their application to patient care.
- Describe how to prepare a pregnant patient for a physical and obstetrical examination.
- Calculate the expected date of confinement using Naegle's rule.
- Explain the reasons for procedures related to prenatal medical care.
- List the danger signals which the patient should immediately report to the physician.
- Identify medications that, if taken during pregnancy, can affect the fetus or neonate.

Care of the pregnant woman before delivery of the infant is called *prenatal* or *antepartal care*. It is the foundation for the normal development of the baby and for the general good health of the mother. The guidance and supervision help the woman pass through pregnancy with a minimum of mental and physical discomfort and a maximum of mental and physical fitness. It is in the area of prenatal care that the nurse can be of great assistance to the mother-to-be and the unborn child.

THE ROLE OF THE NURSING PROCESS IN OBSTETRICAL CARE

The *nursing process* is the framework upon which nursing care of the child-bearing family is based. It involves the application of a logical problem-solving method in order to meet the needs of individual patients. The nursing process is composed of four separate but interrelated steps: assessment, planning, implementation (or intervention), and evaluation. It is not a static process, but one which changes as the needs of the patient change.

HOW TO S.O.A.P. NOTES

Subjective

- Describe the patient's complaint with a short quote.
- Be aware of the patient's past medical history and current condition. It may relate to the present complaint.
- Give a description of the symptoms with regard to:

— onset
— character
— location
— radiation
— duration
— frequency
— severity
— associated phenomenon
— aggravating or alleviating factors
— prior history or treatment of the same symptom

Objective

- Vital signs
- Exam appropriate to system involved
- Lab data if available or indicated

Assessment

List the findings from the subjective and objective observations at your level of understanding.   Include the patient's complaint, pertinent physical findings, and important incidental findings, that is, history of drug allergy, high blood pressure, family history of heart disease, and health risk factors, for example, smoking.

Plan

Document and give rational reasons concerning what you plan to do for each problem. Your plan should include:
— information gathering — lab or other diagnostic tests
— treatment — medical and nonmedical therapeutic modalities
— patient education
— follow-up

Assessment

Assessment of the obstetrical patient involves a systematic and orderly identification of the patient's needs or problems. To identify these needs or problem areas, the nurse must first gather information about the patient. The data gathered is based on both subjective and objective observations. The data may be obtained from various sources, including the patient and other family members, other members of the health care team, and the patient's chart. Methods of collecting the data include direct observation, interviewing, and examination.

Observation involves both objective and subjective data collection. Objective data would include those observations that are made by the nurse, without benefit of interpretation. For example, a nurse might observe that her patient was taking short, frequent breaths and wringing her hands during a prenatal office visit. This would be considered objective data since it is a statement of what is seen, heard, smelled, tasted, or felt. If the patient were to tell the nurse, "I can't seem to catch my breath sometimes and I'm afraid something's wrong," this would be a subjective observation because it is based on information given by the patient. From both of these observations, the nurse might draw certain conclusions about the patient's physiological and emotional status.

Interviewing may be both formal and informal. Asking the patient for background information on her health in order to obtain a personal history record is an example of formal interviewing. This health history will help the nurse understand the patient and define her individual needs.

Informal interviewing occurs when the nurse talks with the patient while giving nursing care. This interaction is often the beginning of a close relationship between the nurse and the patient, and important information about the patient's feelings and problems may result from this informal exchange.

The third component of data collection is examination. During a physical examination of the patient, the nurse will obtain additional facts about the patient, such as her temperature, pulse, respiration rate, and blood pressure. These observations would then be recorded on the patient's chart as part of the objective data obtained.

Planning

The data collected during this assessment phase is then organized, usually according to basic human needs, so that a nursing care plan can be developed. Maslow has identified these needs, in order of priority, as physiological needs, safety and security needs, love and belonging needs, self-esteem, and self-actualization needs. The needs of highest priority, such as the physiological needs of air, food, drink, and rest, must be met before such needs as self-actualization can be fulfilled. The nurse usually considers the patient's developmental level, too, in organizing the data collected. The patient's mastery of certain developmental "tasks" will greatly influence the goals established for nursing care.

As data is collected, the nurse usually becomes aware of certain patient problems. In the case of the mother who was wringing her hands and experiencing shortness of breath, the nurse might identify anxiety as one of the patient's problems. This would be considered a nursing diagnosis.

A part of the planning process is the writing of a nursing care plan. Outlining a plan of care for the patient is beneficial because the nurse can then see the care process in terms of the "total patient." A written care plan also enables a nurse to take over the care of a patient from another nurse without losing continuity of care. The nurse may also derive a sense of satisfaction from the fact that specific goals of patient care have been achieved. The nursing care plan ensures that the best possible nursing care is delivered, and provides a tool by which future, related problems may be identified and resolved.

The physician's orders and recommendations, together with the nurse's assessments, will form the bases for this care plan. The following should be considered in the development of a nursing care plan:

- nursing responsibilities
- problems which may affect the method of carrying out a nursing technique or fulfilling a nursing responsibility
- problems concerning the information to be given to a patient or family members
- problems which may affect interpersonal relationships between the patient and members of the health care team
- suggestions for approaches to problems geared specifically for individual patients

The nursing care plan will include a statement of specific patient problems to which priorities have been assigned, the approach to be used to resolve the problem, the goals of the planned nursing care, and the means by which the health care team can determine whether these goals have been reached.

Implementation

Implementation (or intervention) is the nursing action that is taken to resolve a patient problem. Implementing the nursing plan can take the form of various nursing activities: performing a nursing procedure, offering physical or emotional comfort, counseling, or instructing a patient in some aspect of self-care. Nurses must always bear in mind the underlying rationale for whatever nursing action they take. In terms of the patient described previously, the partial nursing care plan shown in figure 9-1 might be appropriate.

Evaluation

The evaluation phase of the nursing process involves obtaining continuous feedback to determine whether the goals outlined in the nursing

PATIENT PROBLEM/ NURSING DIAGNOSIS (ASSESSMENT)	GOAL(S) (PLANNING)	NURSING INTERVENTION (IMPLEMENTATION)	RATIONALE FOR ACTION
Anxiety	By the end of her office visit, patient will express the knowledge that her breathlessness is a normal and expected discomfort associated with pregnancy	Explain to the patient, in terms she can understand, the usual cause for shortness of breath in pregnancy and its effects, if any, on her baby.	Knowledge of the cause of her breathlessness (usually pressure exerted on the diaphragm by the growing uterus) should alleviate the mother's anxiety about her condition and its effect on her baby.
		Instruct the patient to sleep in a semi-Fowler's position, supported by two or three pillows.	A semi-upright position reduces the pressure of the uterus on the diaphragm, thereby making the patient more comfortable and promoting rest.

Figure 9-1

Process for formulating a nursing care plan

care plan were reached. This feedback will help determine whether the nursing care plan should be modified, depending on the degree to which the goals were met. The patient has both an active and a passive role in this process. Does she feel her needs have been met? Are there observable signs that her anxiety has been allayed? Based on the observations of other members of the health care team, have the patient's needs been met? Answering these questions will help the nurse determine the effectiveness of the nursing care plan, and will guide the nurse in modifying it, if necessary. If the goals have not been met, or if they have only been partially met, the nursing process is used again to develop another care plan. This care plan too, will be evaluated for its effectiveness, and the cycle of assessment, planning, implementation, and evaluation will be an ongoing process throughout the course of the patient's care. Let's use the following example as an illustration.

Evaluation and Treatment of Mild Iron Deficiency Anemia

Definition of Problem. Anemia in pregnancy is defined as a hemoglobin level of less than 10.0g/dl or hematocrit level of less than 30–31 percent. Although anemia is defined as hemoglobin level of less than 12.0g/dl, in the nonpregnant woman, the difference in values is due to the greater expansion of plasma volume. Compared with the increase in hemoglobin and hematocrit levels, they reach their lowest point during the second trimester. Then they stabilize or increase slightly near term. Iron-deficiency anemia occurs not only when the amount of iron required by the pregnancy exceeds what can be provided by the maternal iron stores but also because of the absorption of iron from the maternal GI tract.

Data Base

- Subjective observations (chart of patient's own words)

1. History of closely spaced pregnancies
2. Poor dietary intake of iron or failure to take prescribed iron supplementation
3. Patient may be symptomatic or asymptomatic
4. Possible fatigue, dizziness, headache, and palpitations
5. Patient complains of mouth soreness

- Objective Observations (chart of nurse's comments)
  1. Patient shows possible pallor and pale conjunctiva
  2. Tachycardia
  3. Hemoglobin level below 10.0 gm or hematocrit below 31 percent

Assessment. A presumptive diagnosis is based on clinical data, in the absence of other pathology.

Plan

- Diagnostic Tests
  1. Hemogram to be done on all initial prenatal visits
  2. Hemogram routinely repeated at 30–32 weeks gestation
- Treatment
  1. If hematocrit is 37% or greater
     a) No treatment required
     b) Repeat at 30–32 weeks gestation
  2. If hematocrit is 31–36 percent
     a) Review diet
     b) Encourage the intake of daily prenatal vitamin with Fe and folic acid
     c) Repeat Hct. at 30–32 weeks gestation
  3. If hematocrit is 30% or below
     a) Review diet
     b) Treat with ferrous sulfate 300 mg. TID, and prenatal vitamins as above
     c) Repeat Hct. in 2–4 weeks. If Hct. is not responding to treatment, consult with physician.

     d) Obtain indices, CBC, serum iron reticulocyte count
     e) Check for bleeding, parasites
- Education
  1. Inform patient of foods high in iron and folic acid.
  2. Stress importance of good nutrition.
  3. Encourage patient to take prenatal vitamin supplements daily.
  4. Explain reason for iron/folic acid deficiency in latter pregnancy.

The next three units deal with prenatal care: medical supervision; normal care, diet, and exercise; and complications of pregnancy. These aspects should not be considered apart from each other, since each affects the others. The patient's initial visit to the physician is discussed first, since this is generally the time when prenatal care begins.

FIRST VISIT TO THE PHYSICIAN

The pregnant woman usually visits the doctor after she has missed one menstrual period. It is likely that some probable signs of pregnancy have been noticed. The nurse can do much to allay any fears or embarrassment of the patient. The attitude must be one of helpful care and understanding. As the patient proceeds through the examinations and tests of this first visit, the nurse should explain the procedures to help put the patient at ease.

Medical and Obstetrical History

The purpose of the medical and obstetrical history is to provide the doctor with an accurate record of the patient's past and present health. Questioning should be carried out in an orderly, systematic manner. Personal history is recorded and inquiries are made regarding family history with special reference to any condition likely to affect childbearing.

Patient Medical and Obstetrical History

1. Introduction
2. Patient Identification (name, age, sex, race, appearance)
3. Reason for visit
4. Present symptoms (common discomforts of pregnancy, bleeding problems, etc.)
5. Past Medical History:
   — illness
   — hospitalizations
   — surgeries
   — childhood illness
   — medication (OTC and street drugs)
   — tobacco use
   — alcohol use
   — allergies
   — exposures (occupational, travel)
   — contraceptive history
   — immunizations
   — transfusions
   — trauma
   — gyn and menstrual history (menarche, frequency, duration, flow, and pain)
   — past pregnancy history (term, premature, abortion, living, complications during pregnancy or delivery)
6. Family History
   — health of parents, siblings, and grandparents
   — chronic disease
   — genetic history
7. Social History:
   — cultural and religious background
   — financial/income, resource, insurance
   — living situation/marital status, family support system
   — occupation/satisfaction, stress, exposure
   — schooling
   — hobbies, interest, and exercise
   — typical day/sleep, diet
8. Closing
   — patient concerns
   — questions

If the patient is taking any medications, this fact should be brought to the doctor's attention. The doctor decides whether the medication should be continued during pregnancy.

New regulations require that all prescription drugs be labeled to indicate their effect on fetal development. They must also indicate the short-term and long-term effects they have on the mother and child. Physicians should advise the women about any potential hazards associated with taking a particular drug. Figure 9-2 lists some medications which affect fetal development.

Until the early 1960s, it was assumed that the placenta screened all harmful substances for the fetus. The Thalidomide tragedy of the sixties, however, dramatically altered that assumption. It is very difficult to trace the connection between drugs and birth defects because animals are used as experimental subjects, not humans. Although information obtained from animal studies is valuable, it cannot always be applied to humans. It is also difficult to isolate a single drug used in pregnancy. Most women consume numerous over-the-counter drugs and prescription medications during a pregnancy. The issue is further complicated by the fact that a drug may be harmful only when used at a particular time during a pregnancy, or only in conjunction with other drugs.

Despite the difficulties and complexities of tracing the specific effects of particular drugs, we do know that virtually all drugs and medications cross the placenta and reach the baby. If any medication is administered during pregnancy, the advantages gained must outweigh any risk associated with its use.

The FDA has established five categories of drugs based on their potential for causing birth defects in infants born to women who use the drug during pregnancy. By law, the label must supply all available information on the teratogenicity. The categories are as follows:

Medication	Effect on Fetus or Neonate
Cortisone	Anomalies; cleft plate
Oral Progestogens, Androgens, Estrogens	Masculinization and advanced bone age
Potassium iodide, Propylthiouracil	Goiter and mental retardation
Dicumarol, Coumadin	Fetal death; hemorrhage
Salicylates (large amounts)	Neonatal bleeding
Streptomycin	Possible eighth-nerve deafness
Sulfonamides	Kernicterus
Chlormycetin	"Gray" syndrome (anemia); death
Erythromycin	Liver damage
Furadantin	Hemolysis
Vitamin K preparations	Hyperbilirubinemia
Ammonium chloride	Acidosis
Reserpine (Serpasil)	Stuffy nose; respiratory obstruction
Heroin and morphine	Neonatal death
Phenobarbital (in excess)	Neonatal bleeding; death
Smoking	Birth of small babies
Sulfonylureas (oral antidiabetic drugs)	Anomalies
Meprobamate (Equanil, Miltown)	Retarded development
Thalidomide	Phocomelia; death; hearing loss
Vaccination; influenza	Increased titers of A and B strain antibodies in mothers
Antihistamines	Anomalies

Figure 9-2

How medications taken during pregnancy can affect the fetus or neonate

Category A. Well-controlled human studies have not disclosed any fetal risk.

Category B. Animal studies have not disclosed any fetal risk. These studies have suggested some risk; however, it is not confirmed in controlled studies concerning women. There are no adequate studies concerning pregnant women.

Category C. Animal studies have revealed adverse fetal effects; again, there are no adequate controlled studies in pregnant women.

Category D. There is some fetal risk, but the benefits may outweigh the risk (e.g. life-threatening illness, or no safer effective drug). Patients should be warned.

Category X. Due to fetal abnormalities in animal and human studies, the risk is not outweighed by the benefit. This is contraindicated during pregnancy.

NOTE: For more specific information regarding individual drug effects on the mother and fetus, refer to: Richard L. Berkowitz, M.D.; Donald R. Coustan, M.D.; and Tara K. Mochizuki, Pharm D., J.D., *Handbook for Prescribing Medications During Pregnancy*, 2d edition (Boston/Toronto: Little, Brown and Company, 1986).

An important part of the health record involves the patient's menstrual cycle. The following information should be recorded about the patient:

- At what age did menstruation begin?
- What is the normal menstrual cycle?
- Are the periods regular?
- Are they painful?
- How much bleeding is involved?
- When was the first day of her last menstrual period (LMP)?

The purpose of the last question is to enable the doctor to estimate the expected date of confinement (EDC). *Naegle's rule* is used for calculating the EDC by adding seven days to the first day of the last menstrual period, subtracting three calendar months from the new date, and adding one year (nine calendar months is the same as ten lunar months). Obviously, this is only an approximation and the error may be as much as two weeks in either direction. Figure 9-3 shows another means of arriving at the expected date of confinement. The top line refers to the date of menstruation; the figure below this date indicates the date when confinement may be expected. If the date of menstruation is June 1, confinement may be expected on March 8, or one day earlier during a leap year.

The length of pregnancy varies greatly — from 240 to 300 days — yet, it can be perfectly normal regardless of range. The average duration is 9 1/2 lunar months, 39 weeks, or 266 days from the time of conception. From the first day of the last normal menstruation period it is 10 lunar months, 40 weeks, or 280 days. It appears

Month	1	2	3	4	5	6	7	8	9	10	11	12	13	14	15	16	17	18	19	20	21	22	23	24	25	26	27	28	29	30	31	EDC
January	1	2	3	4	5	6	7	8	9	10	11	12	13	14	15	16	17	18	19	20	21	22	23	24	25	26	27	28	29	30	31	
October	8	9	10	11	12	13	14	15	16	17	18	19	20	21	22	23	24	25	26	27	28	29	30	31	1	2	3	4	5	6	7	Nov.
February	1	2	3	4	5	6	7	8	9	10	11	12	13	14	15	16	17	18	19	20	21	22	23	24	25	26	27	28				
November	8	9	10	11	12	13	14	15	16	17	18	19	20	21	22	23	24	25	26	27	28	29	30	1	2	3	4	5				Dec.
March	1	2	3	4	5	6	7	8	9	10	11	12	13	14	15	16	17	18	19	20	21	22	23	24	25	26	27	28	29	30	31	
December	6	7	8	9	10	11	12	13	14	15	16	17	18	19	20	21	22	23	24	25	26	27	28	29	30	31	1	2	3	4	5	Jan.
April	1	2	3	4	5	6	7	8	9	10	11	12	13	14	15	16	17	18	19	20	21	22	23	24	25	26	27	28	29	30		
January	6	7	8	9	10	11	12	13	14	15	16	17	18	19	20	21	22	23	24	25	26	27	28	29	30	31	1	2	3	4		Feb.
May	1	2	3	4	5	6	7	8	9	10	11	12	13	14	15	16	17	18	19	20	21	22	23	24	25	26	27	28	29	30	31	
February	5	6	7	8	9	10	11	12	13	14	15	16	17	18	19	20	21	22	23	24	25	26	27	28	1	2	3	4	5	6	7	Mar.
June	1	2	3	4	5	6	7	8	9	10	11	12	13	14	15	16	17	18	19	20	21	22	23	24	25	26	27	28	29	30		
March	8	9	10	11	12	13	14	15	16	17	18	19	20	21	22	23	24	25	26	27	28	29	30	31	1	2	3	4	5	6		April
July	1	2	3	4	5	6	7	8	9	10	11	12	13	14	15	16	17	18	19	20	21	22	23	24	25	26	27	28	29	30	31	
April	7	8	9	10	11	12	13	14	15	16	17	18	19	20	21	22	23	24	25	26	27	28	29	30	1	2	3	4	5	6	7	May
August	1	2	3	4	5	6	7	8	9	10	11	12	13	14	15	16	17	18	19	20	21	22	23	24	25	26	27	28	29	30	31	
May	8	9	10	11	12	13	14	15	16	17	18	19	20	21	22	23	24	25	26	27	28	29	30	31	1	2	3	4	5	6	7	June
September	1	2	3	4	5	6	7	8	9	10	11	12	13	14	15	16	17	18	19	20	21	22	23	24	25	26	27	28	29	30		
June	8	9	10	11	12	13	14	15	16	17	18	19	20	21	22	23	24	25	26	27	28	29	30	1	2	3	4	5	6	7		July
October	1	2	3	4	5	6	7	8	9	10	11	12	13	14	15	16	17	18	19	20	21	22	23	24	25	26	27	28	29	30	31	
July	8	9	10	11	12	13	14	15	16	17	18	19	20	21	22	23	24	25	26	27	28	29	30	31	1	2	3	4	5	6	7	Aug.
November	1	2	3	4	5	6	7	8	9	10	11	12	13	14	15	16	17	18	19	20	21	22	23	24	25	26	27	28	29	30		
August	8	9	10	11	12	13	14	15	16	17	18	19	20	21	22	23	24	25	26	27	28	29	30	31	1	2	3	4	5	6		Sept.
December	1	2	3	4	5	6	7	8	9	10	11	12	13	14	15	16	17	18	19	20	21	22	23	24	25	26	27	28	29	30	31	
September	7	8	9	10	11	12	13	14	15	16	17	18	19	20	21	22	23	24	25	26	27	28	29	30	1	2	3	4	5	6	7	Oct.

Figure 9-3

To calculate the period of uterogestation, use the top row to select the month and day when the last menstrual period began. The month and day immediately below this date is the estimated delivery date.

that some fetuses require slightly longer and some require slightly shorter times in the uterus for full development.

Physical Examination

After the patient's medical and obstetrical history have been obtained, the nurse prepares the patient for the physical examination by the doctor. The patient is weighed, blood pressure is taken, and both results are recorded. The nurse then accompanies the patient to the dressing room and explains the need for the patient to undress completely. The nurse shows the patient how to wear the examination gown.

It is expected that the nurse will remain with the patient during the examination to provide support as well as to assist the doctor. The pa-

tient is given a complete physical examination with special attention to the heart, lungs, pelvis, breasts, and nipples. Organic heart disease and tuberculosis are serious complications at any time, and especially during pregnancy.

Obstetrical Examination

The purposes of the internal examination are to examine the vagina and pelvic organs for signs of pregnancy; to take a cervical smear (Pap smear) for a cancer cytology test; to detect abnormalities such as cysts or infection; and to determine if the true pelvis is large enough to allow the baby to pass through at birth.

Before an internal examination is made, the patient should be asked to empty her bladder. The nurse then helps the patient onto the

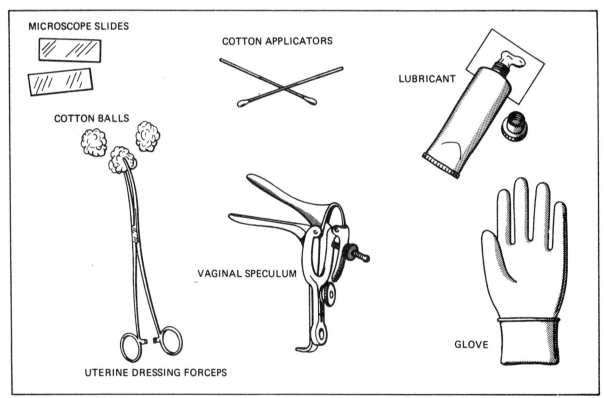

Figure 9-4

Equipment for internal examination

examination table; the patient is placed in the lithotomy position, with her feet in stirrups and draped so that there is as little immediate exposure as possible. The equipment to be used should be ready for the doctor, figure 9-4.

Laboratory Tests

During prenatal care, the urine is checked for albumin and sugar. Also, the blood is examined for hemoglobin, blood type, Rh factor, rubella antibodies and syphilis. A urine specimen is required at each visit to the doctor. Blood pressure and weight are also recorded each time.

This unit deals with early medical supervision and care of the uncomplicated pregnancy. Complications which may threaten the life of the child or the mother are covered in unit 11.

RETURN VISITS

The patient under the doctor's care returns every three or four weeks during the first seven months of pregnancy. At each visit, careful inquiries are made regarding any unusual signs or symptoms. Blood pressure is taken each time, and the urine specimen is examined for the presence of albumin or sugar.

Weight gain or loss is an important detail of prenatal care. A diet to control weight may be prescribed, but an adequate diet is important to maintain daily strength.

At each visit, many doctors examine the abdomen to determine the growth and size of the uterus; they also listen to the fetal heartbeat, which usually ranges from 120 to 160 beats per minute. Within six weeks to a month before the fetus is full term, the doctor is able to determine engagement of the presenting part.

Palpation of the Abdomen

Abdominal palpation, which doctors include in their examinations, is a useful skill for the nurse

to also acquire. As a diagnostic measure, its value is greatest after the thirteenth or fourteenth week when the uterus has risen from the pelvic cavity. The progress of a pregnancy can be determined by measuring the height of the fundus of the uterus. This can be done by calipers or by placing the hand over the fundus and estimating its height in relation to anatomical landmarks such as the symphysis pubis or umbilicus.

By twelve weeks, the fundal height is at the top of the symphysis. At sixteen weeks, the fundus can be palpated midway between the symphysis and umbilicus. By twenty weeks the fundal height has reached the umbilicus and by thirty-six weeks, it is often at the ziphoid.

Presentation and position of the developing baby can be determined by palpating its outline, figure 9-5. Sliding warmed hands down the sides of the mother's abdomen and applying gentle but deep pressure, the nurse may feel firmness

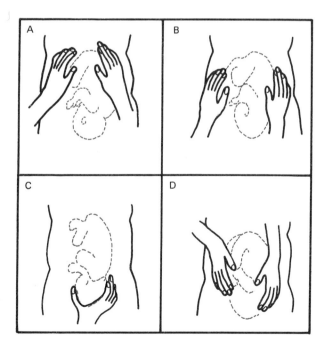

Figure 9-5
Palpating the outline of the fetus to determine its position and presentation

and resistance on one side (fetal back) and nodularity on the other (feet, elbows, etc. of the fetus). With thumb and fingers of one hand, the nurse can grasp the lower portion of the uterus just above the symphysis pubis to determine the presenting part (fetal head or breech). If it is freely movable above the brim of the pelvis, it is said to be floating; if it is firmly fixed in the pelvis, it is said to be engaged. This is called *Leopold's maneuvers.*

DANGER SIGNALS

The patient should be instructed to immediately report any of the following symptoms to the doctor. They may indicate major complications:

1. Vaginal bleeding, no matter how slight
2. Severe, continuous headache
3. Swelling of the face and hands
4. Dimness or blurring of vision
5. Flashes of light; spots before eyes
6. Pain in the abdomen and back
7. Persistent nausea or vomiting
8. Chills and fever over 100°F (37.8°C)
9. Sudden escape of fluid from the vagina
10. Painful, burning sensation on urination
11. Irritating vaginal discharge
12. Dizziness

These danger signals and the complications which they may indicate will be dealt with more fully in the unit covering complications of pregnancy.

OTC Drugs, Alcohol, Tobacco, and Caffeine

Drugs such as aspirin, acetaminophen, sedatives and tranquilizers, antihistamines, antacids, and antiemetics are frequently used in pregnancy. These drugs do not treat illness; they relieve symptoms. Other medications such as antibiotics, insulin, and steroids cure or control an illness. The benefit of these drugs will outweigh the potential hazards in most cases.

Aspirin. Even one aspirin will affect the body's ability to clot blood, and may prolong bleeding time. Two tablets will double the bleeding time. This effect can last from four to seven days after a single dose. Aspirin present in the baby's circulation at birth also prolongs bleeding time for the newborn and increases the likelihood of jaundice.

Acetaminophen. No adverse fetal effects have been reported with moderate use of acetaminophen. If, however, excessive amounts of this drug are used, there may be kidney damage in the fetus.

Alcohol. Until the mid 1970s, alcohol was thought to be harmless to the fetus. We now know that alcohol has a direct toxic effect on the developing fetus. Alcohol quickly passes through the placenta, and enters the baby's blood in the same concentration as the mother's blood. Babies born to alcoholic mothers are at risk. They suffer from Fetal Alcohol Syndrome (FAS). Lesser amounts of alcohol are also associated with some features of FAS. FAS is diagnosed when there are abnormalities in each of the following three categories:

1. Prenatal or postnatal growth retardation
2. Neurologic abnormality, developmental delay, or intellectual impairment
3. Characteristic facial dysmorphology with at least two of the following signs:
   a) microcephaly
   b) microophthalmia or short palpebral fissures
   c) poorly developed philtrum, thin upper lip or flattening of the maxillary area.

Tobacco. Tobacco smoking should also be discouraged in pregnancy. Cigarette smoke contains tars, nicotine, carbon monoxide, lead, and other substances that are harmful to both a woman and an unborn child. On an average, pregnant women who smoke give birth to lower birth weight babies. They have a greater chance of premature rupture of the membranes, premature birth, perinatal death, placenta abnormalities, and bleeding during pregnancy. These conditions are directly proportional to the amount of smoking. The effects on the woman herself are also destructive. There is a greater risk of lung cancer, cancer of the oropharyngeal cavity, esophagus and larynx, emphysema, coronary artery disease, cerebrovascular disease, and cardiac arrhythmias.

Caffeine. Caffeine present in coffee, tea, cocoa, and cola-flavored drinks are probably safe in pregnancy if consumed in moderation, provided there is the absence of peptic ulcer or hypertensive heart disease. Caffeine causes an increased production of epinephrine (adrenalin) and norepinephrine (noradrenalin). These hormones constrict peripheral blood vessels including those of the uterus. This can result in a temporary decrease of oxygen available to the fetus. According to a National Academy of Sciences report, many pregnant women take in an average of 144 milligrams of caffeine per day. This is equivalent to about one to two cups of coffee or two to three cups of tea. Caffeine readily enters the fetal blood stream, and can cause some mild tachycardia. If a pregnant woman consumes drinks or foods with caffeine, she should be advised to do so in moderation.

SUGGESTED ACTIVITIES

- Practice writing a nursing care plan for a specific patient problem.
- Practice taking the medical and obstetrical history of a student who role plays a pregnant woman.
- Practice setting up equipment and draping the patient for the obstetrical examination.
- Make a list of community resources that provide classes for the prospective parents.
- Make a chart, using the S.O.A.P. format, on a new patient. She has arrived for delivery on her due date, and has the following history:
  - Smokes one package of cigarettes a day.
  - Drinks wine, beer, or liquor once or twice a week with meals.
  - Admits to taking aspirin for headaches, which she has frequently. She has taken an aspirin within the last 12 hours.
  - Vital signs are within normal range.
- Demonstrate the ability to ascertain the fundal height by abdominal palpation and measurement. Correlate the fundal height to gestation.
- Demonstrate the ability to perform an abdominal exam. Outline the fetal structures, describe the fetal lie, presentation, position, and attitude or the Leopold's maneuver.
- Demonstrate the ability to obtain a health screening history from a patient with respect to the following:
  - patient identification
  - social history

— past medical history
— habits
— family history
— obstetrical and menstrual history
— review of systems

REVIEW

A. Multiple Choice. Select the best answer.

1. The length of pregnancy varies, but the average duration is
   a. 266 days from the time of conception
   b. 280 days from the time of conception
   c. 320 days from the last normal menstruation
   d. 240 days from the last normal menstruation

2. The woman's urine is checked for the presence of
   a. albumin and sugar   c. blood
   b. an infection   d. a venereal disease

3. Which of the following body signals does *not* need to be reported to the doctor?
   a. Vaginal bleeding   c. Frequency of urination
   b. Nausea or vomiting   d. Continuous headaches

4. Naegle's rule is used for calculating the expected date of confinement. This is done by
   a. adding 7 days to the first day of the last menstrual period, subtracting 3 calendar months from the new date and adding 1 year
   b. adding 7 days to the last day of the last menstrual period, subtracting 3 calendar months from the new date and adding 1 year
   c. subtracting 7 days from the first day of the last menstrual period, adding 3 calendar months and 1 year to that date
   d. adding 3 days to the first day of the last menstrual period, subtracting 4 calendar months from the new date and adding 1 year

5. If the first day of a woman's last menstrual period is August 21, 1982, her expected date of confinement is
   a. May 28, 1983   c. June 1, 1983
   b. May 14, 1983   d. June 7, 1983

6. A blood sample is taken during the first visit to determine
   1. blood type and Rh factor
   2. if the patient has syphilis
   3. if the patient has gonorrhea
   4. if the patient is diabetic
      a. 2 and 3   c. d only
      b. 1 and 2   d. 1, 2 and 3

7. Important information to obtain during a patient's first prenatal visit includes
   1. the age menstruation began
   2. the duration of her normal menstrual cycle
   3. the first day of her last period
   4. the medications she is taking
      a. 1 and 2   c. 4 only
      b. 1, 2, 3   d. 1, 2, 3 and 4

8. When doing an abdominal examination, the doctor is determining
   1. the growth of the uterus
   2. the position of the fetus
   3. the size of the fetus
   4. the activity of the fetus
      a. 3 only   c. 4 only
      b. 1, 2 and 3   d. 1, 2, 3 and 4

9. The initial internal examination of the vagina and pelvis is made to
   1. determine signs of pregnancy
   2. take a Pap smear
   3. determine if the true pelvis is large enough to allow the baby to pass through at birth
   4. determine the position of the fetus
      a. 1 and 2   c. 1 and 3
      b. 1, 2 and 3   d. 3 and 4

10. Medications which can have an effect on the fetus are
    1. vitamin K preparations
    2. thalidomide
    3. salicylates
    4. antihistamines
       a. 1 and 4   c. 2 and 3
       b. 1 and 2   d. 1, 2, 3 and 4

B. Matching. Match the step of the nursing process in column I with the corresponding activity in column II.

Column I

1. assessment
2. planning
3. implementation
4. evaluation

Column II

a. identifying and organizing patient needs and problems, and putting these in written form
b. giving direct nursing care
c. determining whether goals have been met
d. gathering information about the patient

C. Completion.

1. Based on knowledge of the patient and the participation of the woman or couple in childbirth preparation, _____ are developed.

2. The nurse can be assured that care has been effective when _____ _____ have been met.

UNIT 10

NORMAL PREGNANCY

OBJECTIVES

After studying this unit, the student should be able to:
- Explain what personal care is recommended during pregnancy and why.
- Identify the normal discomforts of pregnancy and explain their preventive measures and treatment.
- Using the basic four food groups, state dietary requirements of the pregnant woman.
- State the psychological concerns of the unwed mother.
- Identify the cultural groups in your area of practice, and discuss three or more health beliefs of each of the groups. And how these beliefs impact on the the quality of medical care.
- Identify reliable resource groups, where accurate information about life style, beliefs, and health practice may be obtained concerning cultural groups in your area of practice.
- Identify and discuss cultural biases, and how they relate to the ability to provide optimum health care.

The value of medical supervision and the specific examinations and tests were covered in the preceding unit. This unit deals with the physical needs of the pregnant woman, the importance of diet, the benefits of proper exercise, and the discomforts which attend normal pregnancy. The nurse needs to understand these aspects of prenatal care in order to be able to advise and assist the pregnant patient toward a normal, healthy pregnancy.

PHYSIOLOGICAL CARE

The physical care required during pregnancy is not unusual. It generally calls for moderation in normal habits and minor adjustments as pregnancy develops.

Clothing

Clothing should be practical, attractive, and nonconstricting. Stockings with elastic tops should be avoided because of their interference with venous return and the aggravating effect upon varicosities. Low-heeled shoes are more practical than high heels. However, if a patient does not develop a backache from the abnormal curving of the spine, and is able to maintain good balance, there is no medical reason for not wearing high heels. A well-fitting brassiere is recommended, and a properly fitted maternity girdle may be of some help in combatting excessive backache and pressure due to the change in posture.

Bathing

Daily bathing is encouraged. However, if the skin is sensitive, the use of soap should be restricted. Tub baths may be taken until the time labor begins unless the membranes have ruptured. Body balance is not at its best; the patient must be careful not to slip and fall in the tub. The old notion that bath water which enters the vagina can carry infection to the uterus is now believed to have little validity.

Care of the Teeth

Good oral hygiene should be practiced during pregnancy. There is no proven basis for the idea that dental problems are aggravated by pregnancy. The doctor should be consulted, however, if extensive or difficult repairs or extractions are required.

Care of the Breasts

Special care of the breasts is advised in order to increase the ability to nurse and to lessen discomfort. The breasts should be adequately supported and not bound too tightly by a brassiere which is too small. This precaution becomes most important during the last trimester and after delivery.

If the nipples are inverted or depressed, they should be massaged gently to draw them out. It is extremely important that the breasts are kept clean in order to prevent infection at nursing time. Late in pregnancy a secretion called *colostrum* exudes from the breasts. It is sometimes recommended that a woman who plans to breast-feed her baby express a few drops of colostrum from each breast every day during the last six weeks of her pregnancy. This procedure helps

to open milk ducts, thereby reducing the engorgement which often occurs when the milk first comes in.

A regular bathing routine is all the washing that nipples will require, now or later. Soap should be used sparingly because it is drying to the skin; dryness encourages cracked nipples.

Elimination

Constipation may become a problem during pregnancy. A woman who normally has a tendency toward constipation will experience increased discomfort in pregnancy due to decreased physical exertion, relaxation of the smooth muscle system all over the body, and the obstruction to the lower bowel by the presenting part of the fetus. When constipation remains a problem, the doctor may order a mild laxative. A woman should also be advised to increase the amount of fiber in her diet. Often an increase in fiber and water can greatly reduce constipation problems.

Fluid requirements are increased. A pregnant woman should drink the equivalent of at least 8 to 10 glasses of water daily for kidney regulation. The condition of the kidneys is extremely important during pregnancy; the kidneys help to filter the waste products of the fetus as well as those of the mother. The urine may have a strong smell during the first period of gestation but this is not a sign of urinary infection. It is an indication of the excessive production of hormones in the body.

Marital Relations

Sexual intercourse in moderation usually does no harm. If there is a tendency to abortion or premature labor, the question of intercourse should be discussed with the doctor.

Feminine Hygiene

Over 50 percent of pregnant women complain of an increase of vaginal secretions. If the flow of secretions is not heavy enough to necessitate wearing a pad, the patient should be informed that this is a normal state. If there is an excess, however, the doctor may order a douche. In most cases, douching in pregnancy is unnecessary.

Vaginal Infections and Sexually Transmitted Diseases

Vaginal infections are more common among pregnant women. Some of the common vaginal infections are leukorrhea and candidiasis.

The nurse should be aware of other vaginal infections which might be sexually transmitted, figure 10-1. Many sexually transmitted infections can have an adverse effect on the baby if present at the time of birth.

Sexually transmitted diseases are not commonly seen in pregnancy; however, we will cover them briefly below.

Leukorrhea. Leukorrhea is a white mucous discharge originating in the cervical canal. Normally there is an increased amount of discharge during pregnancy. Leukorrhea becomes abnormal when it becomes yellow in color and the odor and consistency change. Hormones change the vaginal pH and sometimes destroy the normal, helpful vaginal bacteria.

Candidiasis. Candidiasis is caused by a yeast organism and results in an irritating, cheesy discharge. Edema of the external genitalia is sometimes present. If the condition is left untreated during pregnancy, the baby may be contaminated while passing through the birth canal. This is how a newborn develops *thrush*, a fungus infection of the mouth.

These vaginal infections are usually mild. Their presence is noted during the internal examination, and the patient is treated accordingly.

Trichomonas Vaginalis. This is caused by a microorganism known as a trichomonad that lives in the vagina and urethra. It produces a profuse irritating discharge and causes itching of the vulva and vaginal opening.

Bacterial Vaginosis (also called *hemophilis, Gardnerella vaginalis,* and nonspecific *vaginitis*). Bacterial vaginosis is an organism that lives in the vagina. This organism causes a chalky white or gray-green vaginal discharge, which can be thick or watery. It usually produces a fishy odor, and can be accompanied by itching, dyspareunia (painful intercourse), and dysuria (painful urination).

Herpes Genitalis. Herpes genitalis is an acute primary or recurrent herpes virus infection of the cervix, vagina, or genitalis. This virus is transmitted by vaginal, anal, or oral sexual intercourse. The patient may have itching and a burning sensation at the infection site. Painful blister-like lesions can be observed. There is often vulvovaginal edema, leukorrhea, and dyspareunia. If a lesion is present at the time of labor, a Cesarean section should be performed. The herpes virus is potentially fatal for a newborn.

Condylomata Acuminata. Condylomata acuminata (genital warts) are pedunculated, elongated, and fleshy raised lesions. Large lesions may appear in cauliflower-like masses or clusters. Usually women do not have any other symptoms other than gradual appearance of the warts over the affected area. Occasionally, they can be accompanied with itching and a vaginal discharge. Condylomata acuminata are estrogen dependent lesions. Therefore, they can enlarge or become more abundant during a pregnancy.

Gonorrhea. Gonorrhea is a sexually transmitted disease caused by *Neisseria gonorrheae*, a gram-negative intracellular Diplococcus. Some infected women remain asymptomatic. However, many will complain of a purulent vaginal discharge, urinary frequency, urgency and dysuria, and pelvic pain. If a baby were to pass through a birth canal infected with gonorrhea, eye infection and possible blindness could result.

	NO. CASES IN U.S.	INFECTING AGENT	FEMALE SYMPTOMS	MALE SYMPTOMS	CONSEQUENCES TO WOMEN	TREATMENT AGENT	CURE
VIRUSES: AIDS	As of July 1987, 38,808 cases reported; 22,328 deaths	HIV (human immunodeficiency virus)	Headache, fever, night sweats, swollen lymph glands, diarrhea, weight loss, fatigue, infections	Same as female	Opportunistic infections, some cancers, death	Azidothymidine, Ribavirin	None
GENITAL HERPES	200,000 to 500,000 new cases per year; 30 to 40 million cases total	Herpes simplex virus II	Often none; blisters in or around vagina; sometimes fever or headache	Often none; sores or clusters of blisters on penis; sometimes fever or headaches	Miscarriage, birth defects, serious infection of newborn; sometimes death of baby	Acyclovir	None
GENITAL WARTS	1 million new cases per year	Human papilloma virus	Single warts or clusters of soft growths in and around vagina or anus; may be microscopic as well as visible	Warts or clusters on or around penis	Increased risk of cervical cancer	Podophyllin, 5-Fluorouracil, surgical removal	Several treatments may be needed
BACTERIA: CHLAMYDIA	4 million new cases per year	Chlamydia trachomatis bacteria	Usually none; sometimes burning at urination, vaginal discharge	Usually none; itching or burning at urination; white discharge	Pelvic inflammatory disease (PID), sterility, ectopic pregnancies	Tetracycline, erythromycin	Yes
GONORRHEA	1.8 million new cases per year	Neisseria gonorrhoeae bacteria	Often none; sometimes burning at urination, vaginal discharge, fever, abdominal pain	White discharge from penis, itching or painful urination	PID, sterility, arthritis	Penicillin, ampicillin, amoxicillin	Yes
SYPHILIS	85,000 new cases per year	Treponema pallidum bacteria	Sore (chancre) shortly after infection; fever, sore throat, or rashes	Same as female	Heart disease, brain damage, arthritis, death, damage to babies	Penicillin, erythromycin	Yes
PROTOZOA: TRICHOMONAS	Exact number of cases unknown—millions	Trichomonas vaginalis protozoa	None or yellow discharge, irritation, unpleasant odor, painful urination	None or prostitis	Urinary tract infections	Metronidazole	Yes

Figure 10-1
Sexually transmitted diseases

Chlamydia. Chlamydia trachomatis is the causative agent for the sexually transmitted disease, Chlamydia. Sixty to eighty percent of the infected women will not have symptoms. Some will have a vaginal discharge and pain when urinating. Others may exhibit symptoms of a PID (pelvic inflammatory disease), which include an elevated temperature and pelvic pain. Chlamydia can cause both eye damage and respiratory problems in an infant born through an infected birth canal. This disease has also been linked to an increased rate of prematurity and still-births.

AIDS. Acquired Immune Deficiency Syndrome is a serious disease caused by a virus that damages the body's immune system. People with AIDS are open to infections and cancers that would not be a threat to someone with a healthy immune system. More than half of all people who are diagnosed with AIDS die within two years.

A virus called *human T-cell lymphotropic virus, Type III* (HTLV-III) causes AIDS. Symptoms include fever, fatigue, loss of appetite and weight, night sweats, unexplained diarrhea, swollen glands in the neck, axilla, and groin, a dry cough, unexplained skin lesions, and persistent yeast infections. Most people infected with the AIDS virus have no symptoms and feel well. In fact, more than 90 percent of the people infected with this virus have not developed AIDS. However, people with a positive test are infectious, and can pass the virus to others through sexual contact or direct contact with infected blood.

AIDS is only spread by direct intimate contact with infected blood or semen. People contract AIDS by:

1. Engaging in sexual contact with an infected person. This person can look and feel well.
2. Sharing hypodermic needles used for illegal drug use.
3. Given blood transfusions with infected blood.
4. An infected mother can transmit AIDS to her baby during or immediately after pregnancy.

There is a concern about transmission of AIDS to medical personnel caring for AIDS patients. Risks encountered during routine nursing care appear to be minimal. The evidence seems clear that transmission by inadvertent needle sticks is much less likely to occur than with patients with hepatitis B virus. Clearly, precautions in handling needles and blood should be followed in patients with AIDS or HIV antibodies. It would be helpful to know the antibody status of all patients, but there is no mandatory or routine screening to date.

The newborn with AIDS poses a potential problem in the delivery suite, for medical staff will inevitably encounter blood and secretions that might be contaminated with HIV. Therefore, when there is a possibility of coming into direct contact with any blood from either the mother or the newborn, gloves are recommended to be used during any direct care.

The risk to health care workers from occupational exposure to persons infected with AIDS has been evaluated in several medical centers in the United States and is known to be extremely low. However, the Centers for Disease Control, with advice from health care professionals, has made recommendations to protect workers from AIDS and HIV infections. These precautions are prudent practices that help prevent the transmission of blood-borne-type infections. They should be followed routinely.

1. Use gloves where blood, blood products, or body fluids will be handled.
2. Use gowns, masks, and eye protectors for procedures that involve more extensive splashing of blood or body fluids.
3. Use pocket masks, resuscitation bags, or other ventilation devices to resuscitate a patient in order to minimize exposure.

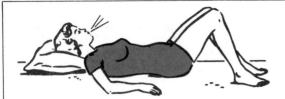

Getting ready — slowly blowing out breath until abdominal wall muscles are well contracted.

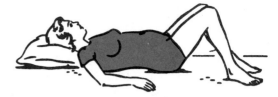

Breathing in slowly, smoothly, with abdominal wall relaxed so it is raised by inner pressure as diaphragm descends before ribs are spread sideways and breastbone lifted upward.

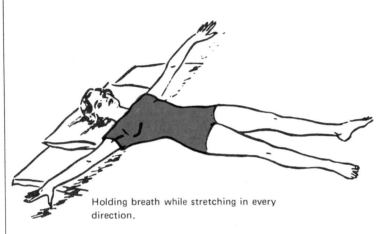

Holding breath while stretching in every direction.

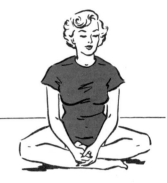

Sitting tailor fashion, at work or play whenever practical, back straight, knees as close to floor as possible.

Lying on side — all muscles loose and limp, baby's weight resting on bed, no pressure on breasts; mind on quiet, regular breathing.

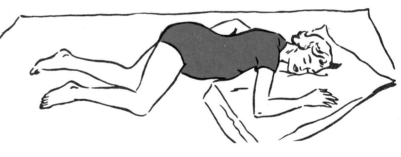

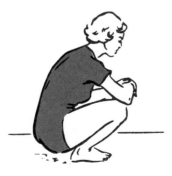

Leaning forward to rest, read or work while squatting without support.

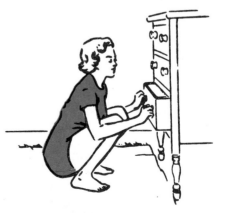

To reach low drawer or shelf.

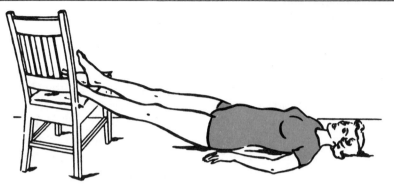

Resting with feet slightly elevated.

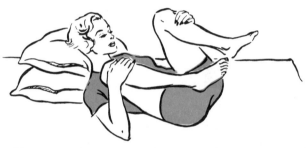

Legs pulled up beside baby; pelvis rocked up in front; pelvic floor muscles relaxed; quick, deep costal-sternal breaths — held as if for pushing, alternating with quick, shallow panting breaths — as if to avoid pushing.

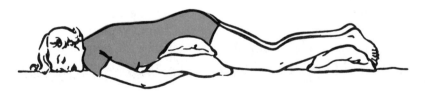

Relaxing face down, palms up, breathing naturally, to help uterus to return to good position.

◀ Figure 10-2 ▲

Exercises during pregnancy (Courtesy of Maternity Center Association)

4. Wash hands thoroughly after removing gloves, and immediately after contact with blood or body fluids.
5. Use disposable needles and syringes. Do not recap, bend, or cut needles. Place sharp instruments in a specially designated puncture-resistant container located as close as practical to the area where they are used. Handle and dispose of them with extraordinary care to prevent accidental injury.
6. Follow general guidelines for sterilization, disinfection, housekeeping, and waste disposal. Place potentially infective waste in impervious bags and dispose of them as local waste regulations require.
7. Clean up blood spills immediately with detergent and water. Use a solution of 5.25 percent sodium hypochlorite (household bleach) diluted between 1–10 and 1–100 parts water for disinfection.
8. Know the modes of transmission and prevention of these infections.

Posture and Exercise

In order to maintain her balance, the pregnant woman tends to lean backward to offset the heavy weight in front. This posture puts increased strain on the muscles and ligaments of the back and thigh causing muscular cramps and aches. Certain specific muscle exercises are helpful in maintaining the tone of the abdominal, back, and perineal muscles. The exercises shown in figure 10-2 may help to maintain good muscle tone and ease some of the discomforts of pregnancy.

CAUTION: These exercises should be performed under the direction of the doctor.

Pelvic Floor Contraction (Perineal Squeeze). During pregnancy and labor, pelvic floor muscle tone is very important. To become aware of how the muscle works, the mother should learn to tighten and relax the muscles surrounding the urethra, vagina, and anus. This may be practiced in any position. One simple method for exercising the perineal muscle can be accomplished each time urination takes place. The mother should try to halt the flow of urine midstream, then empty the bladder.

The exercise called the *perineal squeeze* can be used to tone the pelvic floor muscle: tighten up the pelvic floor muscle and hold to a slow count of five — relax — bulge muscle downward gently by holding breath and bearing down — relax — tighten again — relax. This exercise should be practiced often on a daily basis.

The perineal squeeze helps avoid involuntary loss of urine during the last few weeks of pregnancy. It helps to support the uterus and bladder in their proper position and will aid in pushing out the baby. It is also used to tighten the pelvic floor muscle back to its former state after delivery.

Activity, Rest, and Recreation

Pregnant women tire easily. Fatigue must be avoided. Normal activities in recreation and housework may be continued but should not be excessive. A woman who does her own housework needs little or no additional exercise. However, she does need fresh air, sunshine, and diversion. Walking is valuable, both for the maintenance of correct carriage and posture and for its value in getting the expectant mother into the fresh air. Any activity which incurs sudden jolts, changes of momentum, or physical trauma should be avoided. Sports may be enjoyed at a mild pace. It has been recommended by the American College of Obstetrics and Gynecologists that a pregnant woman's heart rate should not exceed 140 beats per minute during exercise. Aerobic and low impact exercise can increase a woman's sense of well-being and can help to build a certain level of endurance that may be helpful during labor.

Adequate rest periods should be planned. If a woman is employed, she should stop working six to eight weeks prior to the expected date of confinement. However, there are cases where, under the doctor's advisement, a woman may work longer.

Travel

To travel or take a trip is fine during pregnancy. However, the woman should be cautioned to avoid sitting still for long periods in a car, bus, plane, or train. She should be encouraged to walk about for a few minutes each hour or hour and a half. This helps to prevent slowdown of her circulation. If the woman is in the last four to six weeks of her pregnancy, she should consult with her doctor and be aware of alternative available care if labor should begin prematurely.

THE IMPORTANCE OF DIET

The pregnant woman who follows a well-balanced diet feels better and is more apt to retain her health than one who chooses her food thoughtlessly. Preeclampsia does not occur as often among pregnant women on excellent diets as among those on poor diets. Studies have shown a relationship between the mother's diet and the health of the baby at birth. A relationship has also been established between maternal nutrition and the subsequent mental development of the child. It appears that an insufficient quantity of protein in the diet during pregnancy may affect the quantity of brain cells in the developing fetus.

Although it is often said, "A pregnant woman must eat for two" this is not entirely true. Quality rather than quantity is the main consideration in planning a diet. During pregnancy a woman's recommended dietary allowances increase considerably. Protein demands increase from 55 grams per day to 76 grams per day; calcium from 0.8 gram per day to 1 or 2 grams per day. Eigh-teen milligrams of iron is required daily but is difficult to get in foods. An iron supplement and prenatal vitamin preparation may be prescribed by the obstetrician. During pregnancy a woman will need approximately 300 additional calories a day. This amounts to about 2100 to 2400 calories per day. The nurse should be familiar with the four basic food groups in order to give adequate dietary counseling.

Vegetables and Fruits

Four or more servings should be included from this group, especially the leafy green and yellow varieties of vegetables. Citrus fruits or tomatoes should also be included daily because vitamin C cannot be stored in the body. Vegetables are rich in iron, calcium and several vitamins. Vegetables also act as laxative agents. Their fibrous framework increases the bulk of the intestinal content and stimulates action of the intestines. Caution should be taken in the preparation and cooking of vegetables in order to maintain maximum vitamin and mineral content.

Oranges, lemons and other citrus fruits are the best sources of vitamin C. Most of these fruits also supply vitamins A and B.

Dairy Foods

The expectant mother should have at least a quart of milk daily. The high content of calcium and phosphorus make milk indispensable for good growth of bone and teeth. It is also an excellent source of protein and a tissue-building material rich in energy-providing values. Milk contains some of the most important vitamins, particularly vitamin A. Vitamin A increases resistance to infection and safeguards the development of the fetus. Other foods containing milk such as ice cream, cheese and pudding can be substituted for part of the milk requirements. However, these contain extra calories which the expectant mother may not need.

BASIC FOUR FOOD GROUPS	PRENATAL NUTRITION	NUTRITION FOR THE NURSING MOTHER
Group I	Four servings daily	Four servings daily
Leafy green and yellow vegetables		
Citrus fruits, tomatoes, raw cabbage, melon, berries in season		
Potatoes, other vegetables and fruits		
Group II		
Milk, ice cream, cheese	Nutritional equivalent of one quart milk daily	Nutritional equivalent of one quart milk daily
Group III		
Whole grain and/or enriched breads and cereals	Four servings daily unless weight gain is excessive	Four servings daily
Group IV		
Meat, poultry, fish	Two servings daily Liver at least once a week	Two servings daily Liver at least once a week
Eggs	One egg daily	One or two eggs daily
Dried beans and peas, nuts, peanut butter (meat alternates)		
Supplementary foods to complete caloric requirements:		
Butter, fortified margarine with vitamin A	If weight gain is normal, one tablespoon may be used daily	Daily
Decaffinated tea and coffee	As desired and as ordered	As desired and as ordered
Desserts, chocolate, jam, gravies, soft drinks, cream, refined cereals, white bread, salad oil	Usually avoided unless otherwise ordered	Usually avoided

Figure 10-3

Normal nutritional requirements in prenatal and postnatal care

Bread and Cereals

At least four servings of bread or cereal should be included in the diet daily. Whole wheat bread, enriched flour products, brown rice, oatmeal, and noodles are included in this group. The bread and cereal group provides carbohydrates, thiamine, riboflavin, niacin, phosphorus, and magnesium.

Meat Group

Meat is a rich source of the essential nutrient, protein. The main value of the meat group is the amino acids it provides. Amino acids are needed by the mother as well as by the fetus for the development of all the delicate and intricate systems of the body. Three or more servings of beef, pork, lamb, veal, organ meats, fish, poultry, eggs or cheese are recommended daily. Dried beans and peas or nuts may be used as alternates. Two eggs can also substitute as a serving of meat. Figure 10-3 summarizes the normal daily nutritional requirements for the pregnant woman as well as for the nursing mother. The pregnant adolescent requires more of the essential nutrients because her own body needs must also be met. She has not yet attained full maturity.

The unusual craving for certain foods during pregnancy does no harm unless eating the foods interferes with the normal diet and causes excessive weight gain. *Pica,* cravings for nonfood substances such as starch or clay, can interfere with the normal diet and can irritate the salivary glands.

Weight Gain

Usually there is little, if any, weight gain during the first three months of pregnancy. A woman gains about 3/4 to 1 pound a week during the last six months of pregnancy. Excessive weight gain should be avoided because it may predispose a woman to preeclampsia or cause complications during delivery. The recom-

ORGANS, FLUIDS	WEIGHT
Baby	7–8 pounds
Placenta	1–2 pounds
Uterus	1–2 pounds
Amniotic fluid.	1–2 pounds
Breasts	1 pound
Blood volume	3–4 pounds
Fat	5+ pounds
Tissue fluid	4+ pounds
Total	24–28 pounds

Figure 10-4

Weight gain in pregnancy

mended weight gain in pregnancy is 24 to 28 pounds, figure 10-4.

NORMAL DISCOMFORTS

Pregnancy sometimes brings common discomforts which, when recognized as normal, should cause the patient no undue alarm. Two of the most common discomforts are morning sickness and frequent urination. Additional discomforts include heartburn, distress after eating, flatulence, swelling of feet, varicose veins, hemorrhoids, leg cramps, constipation, shortness of breath, backache, vaginal discharge, itching, and salivation (mouth watering). Figure 10-5 summarizes these common patient problems and outlines the appropriate nursing actions and the rationale for these actions. It should be studied carefully.

CHILDBIRTH PREPARATION

Many doctors today recommend that an expectant mother and father attend prepared childbirth classes in the last nine to twelve weeks of pregnancy. If a woman understands what is happening within her body, she will be less fearful and less tense. This enables her to relax more with her labor and help effectively with delivery. A supportive person acting as a labor

KEY NUTRIENT	RDA	IMPORTANT FUNCTIONS	IMPORTANT SOURCES	COMMENTS
PROTEIN				
	N*-46g P*-76-100g L*-66g	Builds & repairs tissues, helps build blood and amniotic fluid; helps form antibodies; supplies energy.	Meat, fish, poultry, eggs, milk, cheese, dried beans & peas, peanut butter, nuts, whole grains and cereals.	Fetal requirements increase by about 1/3 in late pregnancy as the baby grows.
MINERALS				
Calcium	N-800 mg P-1200 mg L-1200 mg	Helps build bones & teeth; important in blood clotting; helps regulate the use of other minerals in the body.	Milk, cheese, whole grains, vegetables, egg yolk, whole canned fish, ice cream.	Fetal requirements increase by about 2/3 in late pregnancy.
Phosphorus	N-800 mg P-1200 mg L-1200 mg	Helps build bones and teeth.	Milk, cheese, lean meats.	Calcium and phosphorus exist in a constant ratio in the blood. An excess of either limits utilization of calcium.
Iron	N-18 mg P-18+ mg L-18+ mg	Combines with protein to make hemoglobin. Provides iron for fetal storage.	Liver, red meats, egg yolk, whole grains, leafy vegetables, nuts, legumes, dried fruits, prunes, prune & apple juice.	Fetal requirements increase tenfold in last 6 weeks of pregnancy. Supplement of 30–60 mg of iron daily recommended by National Research Council.
Zinc	N-15 mg P-15 mg L-15 mg	A component of insulin. Important in growth of skeleton & nervous system.	Meat, liver, eggs & seafood, especially oysters.	Deficiency can cause fetal malformations of skeleton & nervous system.
Iodine	N-100 mcg P-125 mcg L-150 mcg	Helps control the rate of body's energy use; important in Thyroxine production.	Seafoods, iodized salt.	Deficiency may produce goiter in infant.
Magnesium	N-300 mg P-450 mg L-450 mg	Co-enzyme in energy and protein metabolism. Enzyme activator. Tissue growth, cell metabolism, muscle action.	Nuts, cocoa, green vegetables, whole grains, dried beans and peas.	Most is stored in bones. Deficiency may produce neuro-muscular dysfunctions.
FAT SOLUBLE VITAMINS				
Vitamin A	N-4000 IU P-5000 IU L-6000 IU	Bone & tissue growth, cell development. Essential in development of enamel-forming cells in gum tissue. Helps maintain health of skin & mucus membranes.	Butter, fortified margarine, green & yellow vegetables, liver.	Is toxic to the fetus in very large amounts. Can be lost with exposure to light.
Vitamin D	N-0 P-400 IU L-400 IU	Absorption of calcium & phosphorus; mineralization of bones & teeth.	Fortified milk, fortified margarine, fish liver oils, sun on skin.	Toxic to fetus in excessive amounts. Is a stable vitamin.
Vitamin E	N-12 IU P-15 IU L-15 IU	Tissue growth, cell wall integrity, red blood cell integrity.	Vegetable oils, leafy vegetables, cereals, meat, eggs, milk.	Enhances absorption of Vitamin A.

Figure 10-5

Nutrients and vitamin chart (Reprinted from Becoming Parents with permission by the Childbirth Education Association of Seattle, 1443 N.W. 54th, Seattle, WA 98107) (continued)

KEY NUTRIENT	RDA	IMPORTANT FUNCTIONS	IMPORTANT SOURCES	COMMENTS
WATER SOLUBLE VITAMINS (Interdependent on each other)				
B Vitamins Folic Acid	N-400 mcg P-800 mcg L-600 mcg	Hemoglobin synthesis. Involved in DNA & RNA synthesis. Co-enzyme in synthesis of amino acids.	Liver, green leafy vegetables, yeast.	Deficiency leads to anemia. Can be destroyed in cooking and storage. Supplement of 200–400 mcg per day is recommended by the National Research Council; oral contraception use may reduce serum level of folic acid.
Niacin	N-13 mg P-15 mg L-17–20 mg	Co-enzyme in energy & protein metabolism.	Pork, organ meats, peanuts, beans, peas, enriched grains.	Stable, only small amounts lost in food preparation.
Riboflavin	N-1.2 mg P-1.5 mg L-1.7– 1.9 mg	Co-enzyme in energy & protein metabolism.	Milk, lean meat, enriched grains.	Severe deficiencies lead to reduced growth and congenital malformations. Oral contraception use may reduce serum concentration of riboflavin.
B_1-Thiamin	N-1.0 mg P-1.3 mg L-1.3– 1.5 mg	Co-enzyme for energy metabolism.	Pork, beef, liver, whole grains, legumes.	Its availability limits the rate at which energy from glucose is produced.
B_6 (Pyridoxine)	N-2.0 mg P-2.5 mg L-2.5 mg	Important in amino acid metabolism & protein synthesis. Fetus requires more for growth.	Unprocessed cereals, grains, wheat germ, bran, nuts, seeds, legumes, corn.	Large amounts of B_6 supplements may reduce milk supply in lactating women.
B_{12}	N-3.0 mcg P-4.0 mcg L-4.0 mcg	Co-enzyme in protein metabolism. Important in formation of red blood cells.	Milk, eggs, meat, liver, cheese.	Deficiency leads to anemia and central nervous system damage. Is manufactured by microorganisms in intestinal tract. Oral contraceptives may reduce serum concentrates.
Vitamin C	N-45 mg P-60 mg L-60 mg	Tissue formation & integrity. "Cement" substance in connective and vascular substances. Increases iron absorption.	Citrus fruits, berries, melons, tomatoes, chilipeppers, green vegetables, potatoes.	Large doses in pregnancy may create a larger than normal need in infant. Benefits of large doses in preventing colds have not been confirmed.
WATER OR LIQUIDS				
	N-4 C P-6–8 C L-8+ C	Carries nutrients to cells. Carries waste products away. Provides fluid for increased blood and amniotic fluid volume, helps regulate body temperature, aids digestion.	Water, juices, milk.	Often neglected, but is an important nutrient.

*N = non-pregnant
 P = pregnant
 L = lactating

Be sure to read labels on the foods you buy. The information on labels can help you make better decisions on the right foods for your family. Labels with nutritional information tell you what you're getting for your money, and give you the information you need to plan a well-balanced diet.

Figure 10-5

Nutrients and vitamin chart (Reprinted from Becoming Parents with permission by the Childbirth Education Association of Seattle, 1443 N.W. 54th, Seattle, WA 98107) (continued)

PATIENT PROBLEM	NURSING INTERVENTION	RATIONALE
Nausea and vomiting often caused by hormonal changes during pregnancy (occurs in approximately 50% of patients) Causes: • decreased gastric emptying time (increased progesterone) • nutritional deficiency • iron supplementation or other drugs • emotional ambivalence about pregnancy • increased HCG • acute infection or other illness • fatigue	Instruct the patient in general principles of prevention: • rest • relaxation • happy frame of mind • exercise • fresh air Advise the patient of specific measures that may prevent or lessen nausea and vomiting: • limiting liquid intake upon waking or with meals • eating two or three crackers or a piece of toast immediately upon waking • lying quietly for 20–30 minutes after waking • dressing slowly • eating a regular breakfast in due time; may be advantageous to eat frequent, small meals • eating primarily carbohydrates, taking liquids and solid foods separately, and avoiding foods with strong odors and extremes of temperature • resting after meals • taking sedatives, as ordered by physician • taking medication to control nausea and vomiting, as ordered by physician	A lowered state of anxiety and a healthy environment decrease the chance of nausea and vomiting. Dry, carbohydrate food is easily digestible. Limiting the amount of food in the stomach helps to improve the usually slowed gastric motility in pregnant patients. Decreasing agitation by moving slowly and avoiding unnecessary stimuli is often helpful.
Heartburn Causes: • gastric reflux—relaxation of the cardiac sphincter (progesterone) • decreased hydrochloric acid and pepsin secretion in the stomach (estrogen) • displacement of stomach and duodenum by enlarging uterus • emotional problems	Discuss with the patient ways to prevent heartburn: • eating frequent, small amounts of food • avoiding greasy foods • taking an antacid preparation, as ordered by physician Advise patient to avoid sodium bicarbonate.	Eating small amounts and avoiding greasy foods decreases gastric acidity. Sodium bicarbonate may cause fluid retention because of its sodium content.

Figure 10-6

Common problems associated with pregnancy (continued)

PATIENT PROBLEM	NURSING INTERVENTION	RATIONALE
Distress after eating Causes: • decreased gastric emptying time (increased progesterone) • nutritional deficiency • iron supplementation or other drugs • emotional ambivalence about pregnancy • increased HCG • acute infection or other illness • fatigue	Instruct the patient to: • eat slowly • chew food thoroughly • eat small amounts • rest after meals	Improves digestive process
Flatulence Causes: • ingestion of gas-forming foods • decreased exercise • decreased motility of the gut • compression of the uterus on the gut • constipation • fecal impaction	Identify for the patient some common gas-forming foods and discuss the importance of regular bowel movements with her. Advise the patient of the importance of exercise and rest. Advise the patient that a suppository may be ordered by the physician.	Regular bowel movements, avoidance of gas-forming foods, and adequate rest and exercise all contribute to the normal functioning of the digestive system. Constipation may be the cause of flatulence; a stool-softener or laxative suppository may be prescribed for the constipation.
Constipation Causes: • decreased GI tract motility • increased absorption of water from the bowel • pressure of the uterus on the bowel • decreased physical exercise • decreased fluid intake • inadequate food roughage in diet • dry stool due to iron therapy • fecal impaction	Review the patient's diet for adequate amounts of fluids, fresh fruits, vegetables, and fiber; discuss the importance of these foods with the patient. Discuss the importance of regular bowel movements with the patient. Advise the patient that a stool softener, mild laxative, or suppository may be ordered by her physician.	Fluids, fresh fruits, vegetables, and fiber foods aid in digestion A relaxed, regular routine for bowel movements decreases the incidence of constipation. A laxative or stool-softener (suppository) will aid in bowel evacuation.
Hemorrhoids Causes: • all the causes under varicosities apply	Discuss with the patient ways to prevent constipation.	Constipation increases the need for straining, placing additional pressure on the hemorrhoid.

Figure 10-6

Common problems associated with pregnancy (continued)

PATIENT PROBLEM	NURSING INTERVENTION	RATIONALE
• straining at stool due to predisposition to hemorrhoid formation	If hemorrhoids are present, instruct the patient to: • gently push hemorrhoids back into rectum • elevate hips on a pillow • apply cold witch hazel compresses • take Sitz baths	Pushing hemorrhoids back into the rectum decreases irritation. Elevating the hips relieves pressure. Cold witch hazel compresses and Sitz baths help decrease discomfort and promote healing.
Mouth watering	Reassure the patient that this is a normal occurrence in pregnancy and that it usually disappears on its own. Advise patient to eat several small meals per day, rather than large ones.	During pregnancy, the salivary glands increase production. In a few women, this increase may be excessive. Knowledge of the condition and its usual disappearance over time will decrease patient anxiety. Eating several small feedings a day will help prevent excessive salivation which is the first step in the digestive process.
Swelling of the feet Causes: • sodium and water retention from hormonal influences • increased venous pressure • varicose veins with congestion • dietary protein deficiency • increased capillary permeability	Advise the patient that restricting sodium intake will help prevent swelling. Advise the patient to elevate her feet and legs whenever possible. Warn the patient that persistent swelling should be reported to her physician.	Sodium can cause fluid retention. Foot and leg elevation helps promote blood return from the legs. Persistent swelling is a sign of preeclampsia and should be investigated promptly.
Varicose veins (aching, pain) Causes: • increased blood volume adds additional pressure on the venous circulation • increased stasis of blood in the lower limbs due to pressure of the enlarged uterus on the venous circulation • congenital predisposition to weakness in the vascular walls • inactivity and poor muscle tone decreases optimum blood circulation	Instruct the patient to: • avoid constrictions of any type (e.g., tightly fitting clothing) • rest with feet and legs elevated • move about while standing rather than remaining stationary • use elastic stockings, if indicated, and elevate legs for aching pain	Constrictions impair blood circulation. Elevation of the legs helps promote blood return from the legs. Movement and exercise promote blood circulation. Elastic stockings provide support to weak-walled veins.

Figure 10-6

Common problems associated with pregnancy (continued)

PATIENT PROBLEM	NURSING INTERVENTION	RATIONALE
• prolonged standing causes venous pooling in lower limbs and pelvis • obesity places increased pressure on blood circulation		
Leg cramps (numbness and tingling) Causes: • a diet, containing large amounts of milk and milk products, can disturb the body's calcium and phosphorus balance. Increased phosphorus causes a predisposition to leg cramps. • fatigue or muscle strain on extremities • blood vessel occlusion in the legs • sudden stretching of the leg and foot or pointing the toes	Monitor the patient for adequate intake of vitamin B complex and calcium; if determined to be inadequate, instruct the patient to drink milk regularly in order to increase calcium intake. Discuss with the patient measures to prevent or alleviate leg cramps: • rest to avoid fatigue • place a hot water bottle on affected area • extend affected leg and flex ankle, pointing toes to knees • adequate exercise • elevate the legs	A lack of calcium and vitamin B complex is thought to be a cause of leg cramps. Muscle fatigue may cause leg cramps. Warmth helps to relax a cramped muscle. Stretching the calf muscle by flexing the ankle and extending the leg will decrease muscle spasm. Adequate exercise promotes circulation. Elevation of the legs helps promote blood return from legs.
Backache Causes: • relaxation of body joints from the hormonal influence of estrogen and relaxin • muscle strain from increased weight of the growing uterus • excessive weight causes added strain on back muscles • exaggerated lordosis can cause aching and numbness of the upper extremities • wearing high heeled shoes causes postural change • fatigue and muscle tension will cause back pain	Discuss with the patient measures to alleviate or prevent backpain: • adequate rest to avoid fatigue • good posture and body alignment • proper shoes • exercise to strengthen muscles	As the patient's body weight, shape, and balance change, posture may be altered, causing muscle strain. Exercises designed to strengthen abdominal and back muscles will help maintain good posture and will prevent backache.

Figure 10-6

Common problems associated with pregnancy (continued)

PATIENT PROBLEM	NURSING INTERVENTION	RATIONALE
Shortness of breath Causes: • supine hypotensive syndrome • increased awareness of breathing • pressure from uterus on lungs expansion (This is questionable.)	Explain to the patient the usual cause of shortness of breath during pregnancy. Instruct the patient to sleep in a semi-Fowler's position, supported by two or three pillows.	Knowledge of the cause of the breathlessness (usually, pressure exerted on the diaphragm by the growing uterus) will alleviate patient's anxiety about the condition. Anxiety may exacerbate the problem. A semi-upright position reduces the pressure on the diaphragm.
Dizziness and fainting Causes: • sudden standing from a supine or sitting position will cause pooling of blood in the lower extremities • supine hypotension caused by compression of the uterus on the vena cava, resulting in decreased blood flow to the heart and brain • hypoglycemia • hyperventilation • anemia decreases the O_2-carrying capacity of the red blood cell	Instruct the patient to avoid: • rapid changes in position • standing for long periods of time • fatigue • extreme excitement and nervousness Advise the patient to: • rest on her left side • report any dizziness to her physician	Low blood pressure, which can occur in a pregnant woman if she stands for a long time or changes position rapidly, may cause dizziness or faintness. Excitement or anxiety may affect respiratory function, leading to hyperventilation and dizziness. Faintness or dizziness may also result from low blood sugar or too little iron in the blood. Resting on the left side rather than in a supine position reduces the risk of hypotension as it promotes blood return by shifting the baby's weight off the mother's inferior vena cava.
Fatigue and drowsiness Causes: • influence of increased hormone production • lack of exercise • malnutrition • anemia • psychogenic causes • excessive weight gain • infection	Explain to the patient the importance of adequate rest, particularly in the very early and late weeks of pregnancy. Advise the patient to: • experiment with pillow props to make the lying position more comfortable • practice relaxation techniques taught in childbirth education classes • interpret body signals and respond to them; if she feels tired, she should rest	Fatigue is a natural effect of hormones of pregnancy. Extra energy is needed to carry and care for the developing baby, and thus, additional rest is necessary.

Figure 10-6

Common problems associated with pregnancy (continued)

PATIENT PROBLEM	NURSING INTERVENTION	RATIONALE
Bleeding gums and nose bleeds Causes: • diet with lack of Vitamin C • increased blood volume applies additional strain to mucous membranes • increased hormones	Evaluate the patient's diet to ensure adequate intake of vitamin C. Advise the patient to: • have a dental check-up • apply pressure and/or ice to lower soft part of nose for nose bleeds • keep nasal passages lubricated	A lack of vitamin C in the diet may contribute to these conditions. Membranes become overloaded in pregnancy due to an increased volume of circulation. This may cause nose bleeds. An increased supply of hormones as well as the increase in volume of circulation may cause tenderness, swelling, and bleeding of gums. Applying ice and/or pressure to the soft part of the nose will decrease the blood flow. Dryness of the nasal passages increases the risk of nose bleeds.
Vaginal discharge Causes: • increased estrogen secretion during pregnancy causes increased production of cervical mucus—more vaginal discharge becomes evident	Explain the cause of vaginal discharges in pregnancy. Discuss cleanliness.	Increased blood supply and hormones cause the vagina to increase its normal secretions. The normal acidic atmosphere changes, too, creating a more fertile setting for common vaginal infections, including monilia.
Itchy skin Causes: • infection or allergy • stretching tissue due to an enlarging uterus • soap can contribute to dry skin, which will increase itching • dehydration	Evaluate patient's hygiene practices and the type of soap used. Advise the patient to: • take starch baths • increase fluid intake somewhat	A lack of good hygiene or the use of a drying soap may cause skin irritation. Itching may also be caused by stretching of the skin of the abdomen. An increased fluid intake may improve the elasticity of the skin.

Figure 10-6

Common problems associated with pregnancy (continued)

PATIENT PROBLEM	NURSING INTERVENTION	RATIONALE
Frequent urination Causes: • enlarging uterus stretches the base of the bladder, producing a sensation of fullness • bladder capacity is diminished by the enlarging uterus • excessive fluid intake • increased urine output by the kidney occurs in the supine position • urinary tract infection	Reassure the patient that this is a normal condition during pregnancy and that fluids should *not* be restricted in an attempt to alleviate the problem. Advise the patient to empty her bladder whenever necessary.	A frequent urge to urinate is usually caused by the growing uterus exerting pressure on the bladder; this symptom increases in the latter weeks of pregnancy when the baby drops lower into the pelvis. Fluid restriction may lead to dehydration.
Mood swings Causes: • hormone changes can affect mood • inadequate rest • inadequate diet • ambivalent feelings regarding the pregnancy and responsibility of parenting	Explain that mood swings are common during pregnancy. Encourage patient to communicate fears and feelings. Explain the importance of proper nutrition and rest.	Hormone changes may affect some women emotionally. Fear of changes in life style and adaptation to a new role may also contribute to mood alterations; expression of these feelings and fears will help allay them. Adequate rest and good nutrition will promote a state of general good health and will allow the woman to cope with emotional changes more easily.

Figure 10-6

Common problems associated with pregnancy (continued)

coach greatly enhances the experience. Many hospitals allow the husband to follow the course of labor and delivery along with his wife. It is felt that he may give emotional support, and help relax the mother-to-be so that she may take advantage of body muscle control reflexes. His presence helps reduce the fear element and tension in both the labor room and delivery room.

There are three basic components of childbirth education: (1) factual information about pregnancy, labor, and delivery; (2) physical conditioning, relaxation techniques, and breathing patterns; and (3) information about breastfeeding, postpartum experiences, and infant care.

Childbirth education is available from a variety of sources:
• classes offered by nonprofit groups such as the Childbirth Education Association
• classes taught by private instructors trained to teach expectant parents

- classes offered by public service groups such as the Red Cross
- classes offered by hospitals
- classes offered by doctors for their patients
- books, films, and tapes

Dick-Read Method of Natural Childbirth

Dr. Grantly Dick-Read, an English obstetrician, was a pioneer in the movement for natural childbirth. The Dick-Read method of childbirth is based on (1) thorough understanding of the anatomy and physiology of pregnancy and labor by the patient and (2) the use of exercises designed to strengthen useful muscles and mentally condition the patient to painless labor. The method is instituted early in pregnancy when the woman takes a training course that prepares her for labor.

Lamaze Method of Natural Childbirth

Another natural childbirth method, called psychoprophylaxis, has become very popular. Dr. Fernand Lamaze of Paris brought this technique to Western Europe in 1952. *Psychoprophylaxis* depends upon educating the mother-to-be about childbirth and training her through exercise and breathing techniques to control her activity during labor. It is an intellectual, physical, and emotional preparation for childbirth. This can be helped by good nursing support and acceptance of the laboring woman's desire to experience her own childbirth with a degree of control. A coach, usually the expectant father, also serves a vital role in helping the mother stay in control with breathing techniques and relaxation. The nurse must recognize this coach as an important team member and keep him informed of the laboring women's progress.

Childbirth, no matter how normal, is accompanied by some degree of discomfort. Exercise using the psychoprophylactic method is based on what is known as the theory of conditioned reflexes. It takes advantage of the fact that the brain can accept only one set of signals at a time. If the stronger set is one of conditioned response to exercise and control of the body muscles to expel the baby, instead of one of unpleasant pain, then it takes precedence over the signal from the uterine contractions. The fear element must be reduced to a minimum, and tension must be defeated during labor.

PREGNANCY AND BIRTH IN DIFFERENT CULTURES

In all cultures, since the beginning of time, birth has always been a special, magical event. Birth is linked to the basic spiritual concepts of creation, life, and death. It is at the center of many religious rituals. Each culture has evolved many rituals and techniques that are symbolic of that culture's world view. To a great extent, the mother's perception of her birth experience is set by her society's practices and attitudes toward birth. Our culture, for example, attempts to solve its problems scientifically and views childbirth as a medical event that can sometimes be perilous for the baby or the mother.

Almost all cultures have views on when the life force or "spirit" enters the baby. Canadian Eskimos believe the spirit enters the baby in early pregnancy. Africans believe the father's clan spirit enters the baby in early pregnancy. The mother's clan spirit does not enter until the naming ceremony after the baby's birth. Western culture varies its views on when the spirit enters the baby. The Roman Catholic Church, for example, believes the spirit enters with conception. English Common Law feels this happens at the time when the mother first feels the baby move. The question of when the spirit enters the baby is at the heart of the abortion issue.

Cultural patterns dealing with childbearing encompass all aspects of the experience, including behavior during pregnancy, labor, delivery, and the postpartum period. It is taken seriously in all cultures with an emphasis on responsibility about the parenting role. In almost every culture, there are dietary guidelines for the expectant mother. Depriving the mother of certain foods, rather than adding foods, is the most common pattern. For example, one Philippino community believes that eating a bird can keep the baby small, and eating octopus can make the fetus stick inside the mother.

Guidelines related to activity during pregnancy also vary and are very much culture related. The most common advice is to be active so that the baby does not grow too big. The Hopi and the Sanpoil Indians have a whole exercise regimen for expectant mothers.

Yale anthropologist Clellan Ford charted sixty cultures regarding their practices of discouraging sexual intercourse during pregnancy. It was found that 70 percent permitted intercourse in the second month. As pregnancy progressed, sexual activity dropped off to only 30 percent by the ninth month of pregnancy.

Cultures vary widely in terms of whether they view pregnancy and childbirth as an illness, or as a healthy, natural event. Brigitte Jordan, a medical anthropologist, notes a wide variation even in western countries. In the United States, birth is viewed as a medical procedure; in Holland, as a natural process; in Sweden, as a fulfilling personal achievement; and among the Indians of the Yucatan, as a stressful but normal part of family life.

Helping in labor and delivery is another interesting variable in cultures. In fifty-eight out of sixty cultures that anthropologist Ford studied, older women were the ones who assist the mother during childbirth. Often the women were related in some way to the laboring woman. Usually men were not allowed in the room with the mother. Marshall Klaus, an American pediatrician and bonding expert, found that not only were the majority of helpers women, but also, at least one helper remained with the woman continuously throughout labor and delivery.

The amount a mother moves around during labor and delivery also varies widely from culture to culture. The Taureg women of the Sahara walk up and down small hills while they labor. They return to their hut only to deliver their baby. In Africa, the custom is to be packed into a small hut with a large number of supporting women with very little activity.

Different birthing positions are also widespread among various cultures. Out of the seventy-six cultures in the Yale human relations area file, sixty-two have the mother give birth in a vertical rather than horizontal position. Of those, twenty-one had mothers upright on their knees, nineteen were sitting, fifteen were squatting, and seven were standing. Many cultures also provide pulling devices to help the laboring woman increase the force of her efforts to expel the baby.

Cutting the umbilical cord is another issue that has cultural variances. In the Philippines, the cord is traditionally cut with a piece of sharp bamboo and then dusted with powder. In another Philippino tribe, the cord is left long enough to touch the baby's forehead so the child will be wise.

Postpartum methods of caring for a new mother also vary greatly from one people to another. Many cultures isolate the mother and her newborn, sometimes for an extended period of time. Among the Goajiro Indians of Colombia, a well-to-do mother may remain in bed for a month after delivery. Other cultures have the woman return to her normal activities and work in less than a day after she has given birth.

Another major difference among various cultures are the patterns of closeness between the baby and mother after birth. Among the sixty-four cultures that Ford studied, one baby was weaned at six months, thirteen at eighteen months, sixteen at two years, fifteen at three years, and nineteen were unclear. In a few cultures, breastfeeding continued up to six years. Tribal cultures had a fairly long period in which the baby was nursed and carried about by the mother. As societies became industrialized, there was a tendency to shorten this period and wean the child earlier.

There are also many contrasting beliefs regarding breech births, where either buttocks or feet are presented first. Mexican-American culture considers a breech birth "a terrible sight to behold." Mexican-American midwives (Parteras) are reluctant to deliver a baby in breech position and may believe it is a curse to do so. If they are unable to manually rotate the child to a cephalic position, they will send the laboring mother to the hospital.

Some cultures believe that where a baby is born in breech position the mother is sure to die or that the child will die. Some cultures perceive breech births as "bad luck."

Conversely, in some cultures, breech babies are seen to be "lucky and wise," to "have magical gifts" and to be "ambitious."

There are an infinite number of traditional ways by which a baby and young child are protected from illness and harm believed to be caused by the "evil eye" or "evil spirits." The following table is an overview of some of the practices, derived from an ethno-cultural background:

ORIGIN	PRACTICES
Scotland	Red thread knotted into clothing
	Fragment of Bible worn on body
South Asia	Knotted hair or fragment of Koran worn on body

ORIGIN	PRACTICES
Eastern European Jews	Red ribbon woven into clothes or attached to crib
Sephardic Jews	Wearing a blue ribbon or blue bead
Italians	Wearing a red ribbon or the *corno*
Greek	Blue "eye" bead, crucifix, charms
	Phylact — a baptismal charm placed on the baby
	Cloves of garlic pinned to shirt
Tunisia	Amulets pinned on clothing consisting of tiny figures or writings from the Koran
	Charms of the fish symbol— widely used to ward off evil
Iran	Cover child with amulets— agate, blue beads
	Children may be left un-washed to protect them from the evil eye
India/Pakistan	Hindus — copper plates with magic drawings rolled in them
	Muslims — Slips of paper with verses from the Koran
	Black or red string around the baby's wrist
Guatemala	Small red bag containing herbs placed on baby or crib
Mexico	Amulet with red yarn
Philippines	Wearing of charms, amulets, medals
Puerto Rico	Mano Negro

Studying various cultural alternatives helps the nurse to view all systems with a more open mind. It is important to recognize different cultural practices and to respect the individual's right of choice. This includes (a) people that the mother chooses to have support her during labor, (b) her individual response to coping with the discomforts of labor, (c) her choice of position for delivery, and (d) her response to her newborn. It is important for the nurse to keep in mind there is *no one* right way to have a baby. Knowledge of pregnancy and birth practices of various cultures within a community (in which the nurse works) is vital for the nurse to be an effective health care provider.

THE SINGLE MOTHER

The emotional needs of the single pregnant woman are many, complex and often incompatible with each other. Unfortunately, all too little is being done to meet these needs. In an attempt to provide privacy and prevent exposure, these women may be cut off from all communication. They come to the hospital to deliver their babies and, with kindest of intentions, the staff avoids mentioning their problem. Every mother about to give birth should have an opportunity to talk about it if she wishes to do so. She may have a need to express her feelings about her pregnancy and to discuss her baby with someone who cares about her as a person. If a mother has greater needs because she is a single woman, then she must be afforded greater opportunities to meet these needs. The health care team must deal with the numerous medical, psychological, educational, and social concerns of the single mother.

It is highly probable that the unmarried woman about to deliver did not consciously choose to be in this position. However, she is fulfilling her unique function as a woman. To rob her of a sense of dignity and accomplishment at this time is inexcusable.

Pregnancy outside of marriage for the adolescent is an especially stressful situation. The young unmarried mother-to-be is particularly vulnerable since she has neither the emotional nor financial security needed to plan for an unwanted pregnancy. She may not only lose the emotional support of her parents, but may also lose her peer group's approval. This makes it very difficult to accept the pregnancy. For individuals or cultures where pregnancy is a norm, the psychological adjustment is not as severe.

To work with the single mother is a challenge. The nurse must be sensitive to changing emotions, have knowledge of the mother's family background, be honest, and create a trust necessary for interaction and effective communication.

The pregnant single woman must decide whether she will keep her baby or give the baby up for adoption. This is a very difficult task for any woman. The culture, financial and family situation, emotional maturity, and reliable support systems are factors that directly or indirectly affect her feelings and judgment. The nurse must not project personal values; rather, the nurse can reduce the mental anguish through effective communication in the difficult decision-making process. If the baby is given up for adoption, the nurse can then support the mother through the grieving process. If the woman decides to keep the baby, there are many decisions to be made; education is necessary to the well-being of baby and mother. The father should also be encouraged to participate in all discussions.

SUGGESTED ACTIVITIES

- Discuss the adjustments in body care required as pregnancy progresses.
- Practice the exercises shown in this unit so you will be able to show a pregnant patient how to perform them.

- Review the important nutrients and the basic four food groups. Which nutrients does the pregnant woman need at this time? Explain why. Which nutrients can she limit? Explain.

- Plan a diet for a normal pregnant woman.

- Plan a diet for a normal pregnant woman who dislikes milk.

- Discuss the common discomforts of pregnancy, their prevention and nursing care.

- List three sexually transmitted diseases with their adverse effects on a pregnant woman and her baby. S.O.A.P. one of the three.

- Discuss the fetal physiological response to maternal exercise.

- Discuss the current controversy surrounding the pros and cons of vigorous exercise during pregnancy.

- Demonstrate the ability to take a thorough and meaningful diet history from a patient.

- Identify at least four good sources for the following:
  - Low sodium content
  - High iron content
  - High protein content
  - Vitamins D, A, C, and B
  - Folic acid
  - Calcium (other than milk)

REVIEW

Multiple-multiple Choice. Select the best answer from the *lettered* items.

1. Morning sickness may be relieved by
   1. eating dry toast on awakening
   2. eating frequent small meals
   3. increasing liquid intake
   4. resting after meals
      a. 3 only
      b. 1, 2 and 4
      c. 3 and 4
      d. 1, 2, 3 and 4

2. Swelling or edema of the feet
   1. calls for restricted sodium intake
   2. is relieved by elevating the feet
   3. should be reported to the doctor
   4. may be relieved by changing shoes
      a. 1 and 2
      b. 1, 2 and 3
      c. 1 only
      d. 1, 2, 3 and 4

3. Itching or urticaria of the skin may be relieved by
   1. increasing calcium intake
   2. increasing fluid intake
   3. taking starch baths
   4. using milder soap
      a. 1 and 2   c. 2, 3 and 4
      b. 1 only   d. 1, 2, 3 and 4

4. During the early months of pregnancy, a woman should be sure that her diet includes
   1. an extra portion of carbohydrate food daily
   2. foods rich in iron
   3. at least one quart of milk daily
   4. 55 to 76 grams of protein daily
      a. 1, 2 and 4   c. 2 and 3
      b. 2, 3 and 4   d. 1, 2, 3 and 4

5. Milk is important to a pregnant woman's diet because it is an excellent source of
   1. body-building protein
   2. calcium which aids the development of the fetal skeleton
   3. vitamin A which increases resistance to infection
   4. iron which is necessary for a rich blood supply
      a. 2 only   c. 2 and 4
      b. 2 and 3   d. 1, 2 and 3

6. The following statements are true about diet management during pregnancy:
   1. Excessive weight gain should be avoided because it can complicate delivery.
   2. A weight gain of 22 to 27 pounds is normal during pregnancy.
   3. Preeclampsia does not occur as often among women on excellent diets.
   4. A pregnant woman must increase her calories for now she is "eating for two."
      a. 1, 2 and 3   c. 3 and 4
      b. 1 and 2   d. 1, 2 and 4

7. Psychological concerns of the single adolescent mother include
   1. possible loss of emotional support from her parents
   2. possible loss of financial support from her parents
   3. possible loss of peer group approval
   4. deciding to keep the baby or give it up for adoption
      a. 1 and 2   c. 4 only
      b. 3 only   d. 1, 2, 3 and 4

8. The main causes of constipation during pregnancy are
   1. decreased physical exertion
   2. changes in the diet
   3. relaxation of the smooth muscle system
   4. obstruction to the lower bowel by the presenting part of the fetus
      a. 1, 2 and 4   c. 1, 3 and 4
      b. 2 and 4   d. 1, 2, 3 and 4

9. Some common discomforts of pregnancy which are usually not medically serious are
   1. heartburn and flatulence
   2. shortness of breath
   3. headaches and dizziness with blurred vision
   4. vaginal discharge
      a. 1, 2 and 3   c. 1, 2 and 4
      b. 1 and 2   d. 1, 2, 3 and 4

10. Special care techniques of the breasts during pregnancy which help to increase the ability to nurse include
    1. having adequate support that is not too tight
    2. massaging nipples if inverted or depressed
    3. expressing a few drops of colostrum from the breasts each day during the last six weeks
    4. washing the breasts daily using soap sparingly
       a. 1, 2 and 4   c. 2 and 3
       b. 1, 3 and 4   d. 1, 2, 3 and 4

11. The basic components of childbirth classes are
    1. factual information about pregnancy, labor and delivery
    2. physical conditioning
    3. relaxation and breathing techniques
    4. information about breastfeeding, postpartum experiences and infant care
       a. 1, 3 and 4   c. 1, 2 and 3
       b. 1 and 3   d. 1, 2, 3 and 4

12. Fetal requirements of iron increase tenfold in the last six weeks of pregnancy. Foods high in iron include
    1. liver and red meats
    2. egg yolk
    3. dried fruits and prunes
    4. nuts and legumes
       a. 1, 3 and 4   c. 3 and 4
       b. 1 and 4   d. 1, 2, 3 and 4

13. A pregnant woman can decrease the possibility of varicose veins by
    1. avoiding any type of constriction
    2. resting with her feet and legs elevated
    3. eating foods high in calcium
    4. sleeping 12 or more hours a day
       a. 1, 2 and 3   c. 1 and 2
       b. 3 and 4   d. 2 and 3

UNIT 11

COMPLICATIONS OF PREGNANCY

OBJECTIVES

After studying this unit, the student should be able to:

- List the danger signals which may indicate complications in pregnancy.
- Describe the symptoms, prevention, and treatment of the more common complications.
- Name the tests that may be made on amniotic fluid.
- Describe the procedure for an intrauterine transfusion.

This unit discusses complications of pregnancy and those symptoms which must be called to the doctor's attention immediately.

DANGER SIGNALS

It is always desirable to be able to assure the patient that the findings on examination are normal and that she may anticipate an uneventful pregnancy. At the same time, however, the patient should be tactfully instructed regarding danger signals. Danger signals include:

- Any vaginal bleeding
- Severe, continuous headache
- Swelling of the face, fingers or feet
- Dimness or blurring of vision or spots before the eyes
- Pain in the abdomen or back
- Persistent nausea and/or vomiting
- Chills and fever

- Sudden escape of fluid from the vagina
- Blood pressure over 140/90
- Decrease in the amount of urine

Treatment is prescribed according to the severity of the situation; therapy should be individualized.

PREECLAMPSIA AND ECLAMPSIA

Preeclampsia is a condition that can be dangerous for a pregnant woman and her baby. Signs of this condition include (a) swelling of body tissues with rapid weight gain, (b) an elevated blood pressure, and (c) the presence of protein in the urine. The woman's urine output may be decreased. She may experience epigastric pain, vision changes and her reflexes may be hyperactive. *Preeclampsia* occurs in the last two or three months of gestation; it rarely occurs before the twenty-fourth week. The condition is characterized by the development of hypertension, proteinuria, and edema. The patient is often not aware of anything unusual until she becomes ill. Headache is sometimes encountered as well as visual disturbances of various degrees. The patient must be under strict doctor supervision with regular office visits and sometimes hospitalization. If the condition does not progress to eclampsia, the majority of patients return to normalcy within ten days or so after delivery.

Eclampsia is an acute toxemia of pregnancy. It is characterized by the same symptoms as preeclampsia plus spasmodic and sustained convulsions and loss of consciousness, followed by coma. It frequently results in death. Since eclampsia can be prevented by good prenatal care, it is becoming increasingly rare as more women receive adequate medical supervision during pregnancy. It occurs more often in primigravidas than in multiparas. It also occurs in women who are nutritionally deficient or who are diabetic. Women who are very young or who are over 35 years, have an increased chance of developing preeclampsia in pregnancy. Also, women who have a multiple gestation are at greater risk. This is one of the most dangerous conditions with which the obstetrician has to deal. Blood flow through the placenta is decreased with preeclampsia which causes the baby to suffer. Babies of preeclampsic mothers tend to be small in relation to the length of time they are carried; they also have a greater chance of being stillborn. The prognosis is always serious for both the mother and child.

ABORTION AND BLEEDING

Abortion is the termination of a pregnancy at any time before the fetus has obtained a stage of viability. Abortion may be subdivided into two main forms: spontaneous and induced. *Spontaneous abortion* (or miscarriage) is the termination of pregnancy through natural causes. *Induced abortion* is the termination of pregnancy with the aid of mechanical or medical agents.

A *therapeutic abortion* is the termination of pregnancy by mechanical or medical agents because a continuation of the pregnancy would be hazardous to the mother. Therapeutic abortion, unlike any other surgical operation, is governed by statute or common law in all states. However, the wording and interpretation of the laws differ widely. Some hospitals have set up abortion committees to decide the permissibility of therapeutic abortions.

Contrary to popular belief, today's abortion laws are of fairly recent origin. Before 1803, in the United States and Great Britain, abortion was either lawful or widely tolerated if performed before quickening occurred. In 1803, a general reform of British criminal law made it illegal to perform abortions prior to quickening. Canon law, established by Pope Pius IX in 1869, stated that under no circumstances is abortion justifiable. During the past 30 years, professional and lay people have increasingly favored liberation of the abortion laws. In 1969, eleven states amended their laws by extending the indications for therapeutic termination of pregnancy. By 1977 all states had re-evaluated their abortion laws; each state now abides by its own standards and regulations. Canon law remains unchanged.

A *complete abortion* is one in which the entire product of conception is expelled. An *incomplete abortion* is one in which part of the product of conception is passed, but part remains in the uterus. A *missed abortion* is one in which the fetus dies in utero, but the product of conception is retained. *Habitual abortion* is a condition in which a number of successive pregnancies are terminated by spontaneous abortion.

HYDATIDIFORM MOLE

Hydatidiform mole is an abnormal condition in which the fertilized ovum degenerates and dies; the chorionic villi convert into a mass of transparent cysts resembling a cluster of grapes which fill the uterus, figure 11-1. This condition occurs only about once in every 2000 pregnancies. Signs and symptoms that can suggest hydatidiform mole include (a) dark red or brown bleeding (b) severe nausea and vomiting, (c) an absence of fetal heart tones, (d) a larger uterus than expected for the dates, and (e) signs of preeclampsia before the twenty-fourth week of pregnancy.

Treatment consists of emptying the uterus. This may occur as a spontaneous abortion, or an induced abortion may be necessary. In some cases a hysterectomy may be performed. Follow-up care is very important. Although hydatidiform mole is usually benign, extremely malignant chorion carcinoma can sometimes add further complications. Close follow-up is needed for up to a year following hydatidiform mole. Serum chorionic gonadotropin hormone is measured frequently to be sure it is decreasing to a normal range. Pregnancy should be avoided for at least a year after a hydatidiform mole.

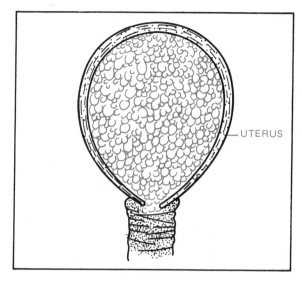

Figure 11-1
Hydatidiform mole

Evaluation of Possible Hydatidiform Mole

Definition of Problem. Hydatidiform mole is a developmental placental abnormality in which some or all the chorionic villi become edematous and degenerate into grape-like vesicles. Etiology is unknown, but it is more common in women over 40 who have had more than three births plus a history of prior hydatidiform moles. There is a higher incidence of this problem in women residing in Asia and the South Pacific than in the United States and Europe.

Data Base.

- Subjective Observations (chart of patient's own words)
  1. Vaginal bleeding, minimal, at end of first and beginning of second trimester
  2. Severe nausea and vomiting due to high HCG levels associated with hydatidiform mole
  3. Absence of fetal movement
  4. Passage of grape-like vesicles
- Objective Observations (chart of nurse's comments)
  1. Uterine size can be larger or smaller than expected by the due dates
  2. Anemia that is out of proportion to blood loss
  3. Signs of preeclampsia developing before twenty-four weeks of pregnancy. (This is very diagnostic of the mole.)
  4. Absence of FHT and inability to feel fetal parts
  5. Adnexal mass due to ovarian lutein cysts
  6. Visualization of passed grape-like vesicles

Assessment. Presumptive diagnosis of hydatidiform mole is made based on subjective symptoms and objective findings. This condition is especially confirmed with the visualization of grape-like vesicles. It is associated with elevated blood pressure and proteinuria before the twenty-fourth week of gestation.

Plan:

- Diagnostic tests
  1. Sonogram
- Treatment
  1. Refer immediately to physician
- Education
  1. Women with molar pregnancies and their families must be helped to understand and deal with
     a) Loss of pregnancy that is abnormal
     b) Possible serious complication
     c) Need to delay next pregnancy
     d) Importance of follow-up testing and close physician supervision
  2. Assist in resolution of feelings of grief, anger, and fear
  3. Help the patient and her family to understand what a molar pregnancy is, the favorable statistics for benign resolution, and what symptoms might be indicative of malignancy if they occur. Also, the importance of reporting symptoms to the physician promptly.

PLACENTA PREVIA

While spontaneous abortion is the most frequent cause of bleeding early in pregnancy, the most common cause during the later months is placenta previa. *Placenta previa* occurs when the placenta has been implanted in the lower segment of the uterus and either wholly or partially covers the cervix. There are three types of placenta previa; each type depends on the degree to which the placenta covers the internal os of the cervix, figures 11-2 and 11-3.

- Total placenta previa
- Partial placenta previa
- Low implantation of placenta

Cesarean section is the treatment of choice in the severe forms of placenta previa. Bleeding, shock, and infection are the main dangers. Blood transfusion plays an important role in the management of these cases, as does meticulous attention to antiseptic techniques.

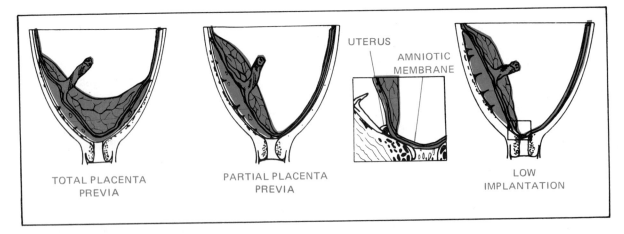

TOTAL PLACENTA PREVIA   PARTIAL PLACENTA PREVIA   UTERUS   AMNIOTIC MEMBRANE   LOW IMPLANTATION

Figure 11-2

Placenta previa — abnormal implantation (Adapted from Clinical Education Aid No. 12, Ross Laboratories)

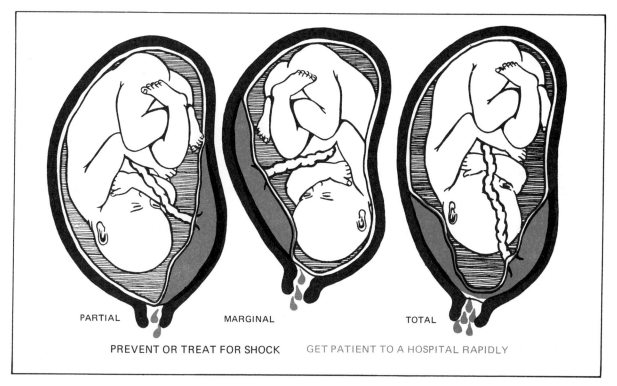

PARTIAL   MARGINAL   TOTAL

PREVENT OR TREAT FOR SHOCK   GET PATIENT TO A HOSPITAL RAPIDLY

Figure 11-3

Placenta previa and the fetus

PLACENTA ABRUPTIO

Placenta abruptio is the premature separation of the normally implanted placenta. It occurs either in the later months of pregnancy or at the beginning of labor and is characterized by both bleeding and pain, figures 11-4 and 11-5. Pressure builds up due to the bleeding behind the placenta. This causes the uterus to become rigid and painful. Placenta abruptio may be partial or complete, depending on whether all or part of the placenta becomes detached.

Treatment consists of performing a cesarean section, or rupturing the membranes so the woman delivers vaginally before the detachment increases and bleeding becomes more severe. Shock secondary to blood loss is almost always present and must be dealt with first. The prog-

nosis for the infant depends on the severity of the condition.

ECTOPIC PREGNANCY

An *ectopic pregnancy* is an extrauterine pregnancy; that is, the fertilized ovum begins to develop outside the uterus. Ninety-five percent of ectopic pregnancies occur in the fallopian tubes. Occasionally, the fertilized egg starts to develop in the ovary, or, in rare cases, within the abdominal cavity (tubal rupture). When the fertilized ovum becomes implanted within the wall of the fallopian tube, it is called a *tubal pregnancy*. Since the wall of the tube is not sufficiently elastic to allow the fertilized ovum to grow and develop, rupture of the tubal wall is the inevitable result. Symptoms prior to rupture include abdominal

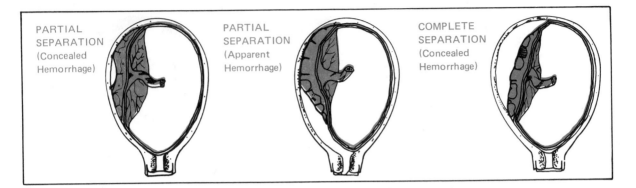

Figure 11-4

Placenta abruptio — premature separation (Clinical Education Aid No. 12, Ross Laboratories)

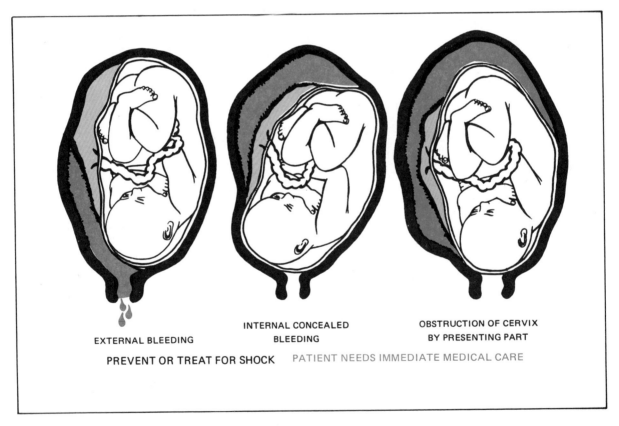

Figure 11-5

Placenta abruptio and the fetus

Complication	Cause	Symptoms	Prevention or Care

Hyperemesis gravidarum	1. Faulty nutrition
	2. Vitamin deficiency
	3. Hormones
	4. Emotional disturbances
		1. Vomiting	1. Eight hours sleep and midday rest
			2. Avoid sexual relations
			3. Avoid odors which precipitate attacks
			4. Fresh air and sunshine
			5. Proper ventilation
			6. Sedation
			7. Small amounts of food with high carbohydrate diet
			8. Vitamin B_6 and complex
			9. For more severe cases:
			  a. Complete bed rest
			  b. Extreme quiet
			  c. I.V. fluids
			  d. Sedation — phenobarbital and dramamine
			  e. Vitamin B complex
			  f. Nothing by mouth at first and later small feedings or liquids until tolerated.

Toxemias
1. Acute
  a. Preeclampsia
  b. Eclampsia
	1. True cause unknown
	2. Probable causes
	  a. Dietary deficiencies
	  b. Infection
	  c. Pressure
	  d. Endocrine imbalance of mother
	  e. Infarct of placenta
	  f. Endocrine imbalance of fetus
	  g. Rh factor of fetus
		In preeclampsia:
		1. Edema
		2. Weight gain
		3. Albuminuria
		4. Elevated blood pressure
		5. Headaches
		6. Drowsiness
		7. Dizziness
		8. Decrease in urine
		9. Casts in urine
		10. Disturbance of vision
		11. Nausea and vomiting
		12. Slight jaundice
		13. Hyperactive reflexes
		14. Epigastric pain
			1. Proper prenatal care to prevent
			2. Complete bed rest
			3. Dark room
			4. Isolation
			5. Check blood pressure
			6. Give anit-hypertensive drugs
			7. Hypertonic solutions
			8. Inhalation of oxygen
			9. Intake and output

Placenta previa	1. Placenta partially or completely over cervix
	  a. Coitus
	  b. Lifting
	  c. Falls
		1. Painless bleeding	1. Same as for bleeding
			2. Cesarean section

Figure 11-6

Complications of pregnancy (Courtesy of Maternal and Child Health, Littlefield, Adams & Co.)

Complication	Cause	Symptoms	Prevention or Care
Premature separation of placenta	1. Lifting 2. Falls 3. Without reason	1. Painful bleeding 2. Shock 3. May have no external bleeding	1. Same as for bleeding 2. Cesarean section immediately

Bleeding	1. First and second trimesters
	  a. Abortions
	  b. Chronic epithelium
	  c. Carcinoma of cervix
	  d. Varicose veins
	  e. Erosion of cervix
	2. Second and third trimesters
	  a. Placenta previa
	  b. Premature separation of placenta
	  c. Ruptured uterus
	  d. Carcinoma of cervix
	  e. Varicose veins
	  f. Erosion of cervix
		1. Bleeding
		2. Low blood pressure
		3. Shock
			1. Complete bed rest
			2. Elevate feet
			3. Check blood pressure
			4. Sedation
			
			1. Cesarean section if necessary

Abortion	1. Size and shape of uterus 2. Accidental 3. Radiation 4. Electrical shock 5. Alcohol and tobacco 6. Drugs 7. Surgical procedures 8. Coitus	1. Bleeding 2. Expulsion of fetus and placenta	1. Same as for bleeding 2. D & C if incomplete
Ectopic pregnancy	1. Growth of fetus outside of uterus 2. One in every three hundred pregnancies 3. Obstruction of uterine tubes 4. Infection	1. Missed one period 2. Nausea and vomiting 3. Stabbing, tearing pain on side 4. Bleeding with pains 5. Cervix tender and painful 6. Rupture brings dizziness, faintness, drop in blood pressure	1. Surgery 2. Antibiotics 3. Bed rest 4. Sedatives 5. Reassurance 6. Cul de sac puncture

Figure 11-6
Complications of pregnancy (Courtesy of Maternal and Child Health, Littlefield, Adams & Co.) (Continued)

pain and some vaginal bleeding. Whenever rupture of the tube occurs, the abdomen becomes tender and rigid and the pain increases. The patient may go into shock if the internal hemorrhage is massive. Upon diagnosis, surgery is indicated; usually an ectopic pregnancy becomes apparent between the second and fourth months.

HYPEREMESIS GRAVIDARUM

Hyperemesis gravidarum (excessive vomiting) is a serious complication which is rarely encountered today because of improvement in prenatal care. Symptoms include constant nausea and vomiting, loss of sleep, restlessness, and exhaustion. Weight loss is rapid and dehydration of all the body tissues is a marked sign. Hyperemesis gravidarum occurs in the first three months of pregnancy. If excessive vomiting continues, it usually indicates that a condition other than the pregnancy is the immediate cause.

The treatment of hyperemesis gravidarum generally consists of (1) stopping the dehydration and starvation that is a result of the patient's inability to ingest food, (2) improving the general psychological condition of the patient, and (3) administering medication, as ordered by the doctor.

DIABETES IN PREGNANCY

In many obstetrical practices, it is routine to screen women for gestational diabetes. This is accomplished by giving the expectant mother 50 grams of glucola at 24 to 26 weeks of her pregnancy. A blood sample is taken one hour later and evaluated. If the glucola level is above 140 mg/dl, gestational diabetes is suspected. The pregnant woman needs further testing. A three hour glucose tolerance test is then taken and evaluated. Many gestational diabetic women can be managed by diet alone; some women may need insulin. But in either case, close management throughout the pregnancy is important.

Gestational diabetes differs from insulin-dependent (type I) and non-insulin dependent; it is not usually permanent. Once the baby is delivered, the diabetes disappears. If it persists, it is reclassified usually as type II or non-insulin-dependent diabetes. Women who have diabetes before becoming pregnant are not defined as having gestational diabetes when pregnant.

Pregnancy can trigger diabetes because it produces temporary changes in the way the mother's blood sugar is regulated. Toward the end of the second trimester, the fetus begins its most dramatic growth. To give the fetus nourishment, the placenta and the mother's body pour out substances that raise the mother's blood sugar. Normally, the mother's pancreas makes extra insulin in response to the extra sugar in her blood. Insulin allows cells to use sugar for energy, and helps to keep the mother's blood sugar level within a normal range. In some pregnant women, the pancreas is unable to make enough extra insulin, causing a build up in sugar. This results in gestational diabetes. After delivery, the diabetes usually disappears; the reason for the increased insulin is gone.

Among diabetic patients there is an increased incidence of abortion, stillbirths, preeclampsia, premature labor, oversized infants, and congenital defects in the newborn. The care of the patient is usually supervised by internists as well as the obstetrician during pregnancy. The patient is examined frequently, sometimes at weekly intervals.

Diabetic women are more prone to vascular disease. This may partially explain why diabetic women are more likely to develop pregnancy induced hypertension (PIH). Urinary tract infections occur more frequently in pregnant women who are diabetic than in those who are not. This is because the presence of sugar in the urine favors the growth of bacteria.

Another complication that frequently accompanies pregnancy in a diabetic woman is *hydramnios*, an excessive accumulation of amniotic fluid surrounding the fetus in utero. It is not a serious threat to the mother but it can lead to complications as the mother approaches the time of delivery. If this complication develops, the doctor may wish to deliver the baby earlier than scheduled.

Infants delivered at term to diabetic patients have a higher mortality rate than those delivered earlier because the vascular changes in the placenta compromise the fetus. The larger size of the fetus at term may also complicate delivery. For these reasons, the obstetrician may decide to schedule an early delivery, at about the thirty-sixth week of gestation.

The baby of a mother who has high blood sugar can actually develop low blood sugar after delivery. During pregnancy, the mother's insulin does not reach the baby; the baby produces and uses its own insulin. When a mother has diabetes, the baby gets an overload of sugar, which causes the baby's pancreas to produce a greater amount of insulin. After birth, when the baby is no longer receiving sugar from the mother's system, the child takes a while to adjust the amount of insulin produced. As a result, the baby's blood sugar level can fall too low. Prolonged low blood sugar (below 30 mg/dl) can cause brain damage.

Malformations, which are often a worry for women with uncontrolled type I or type II diabetes, are not a particular problem in babies of women who have gestational diabetes. The baby's organs are formed by the tenth to the twelfth week after conception. Gestational diabetes does not usually occur until after the twentieth week.

Some women are at greater risk for developing gestational diabetes. Obesity increases the odds because excess fat causes cells to resist insulin. Therefore the cells have difficulty using blood sugar for energy. A family history of diabetes can add to the risk because the tendency to diabetes is inherited through the genes.

Severe emotional or physical stress can trigger diabetes in someone who is prone to the disease. Stress causes a rise in hormones that raise blood sugar and cause sugar that has been stored in the liver to be released into the blood.

Some women have classic symptoms of diabetes which include increased thirst, hunger, urination and weakness. Often, however, women have no obvious symptoms and feel normal. This is why the American Diabetes Association recommends testing all pregnant women between the 24th and 26th week of pregnancy as discussed earlier.

Anyone diagnosed with diabetes during pregnancy should see a diabetic specialist if her obstetrician does not specialize in diabetes. Some doctors feel a controlled meal plan alone can achieve ideal blood sugar levels. Others feel insulin is required. This depends on the woman's individual situation.

Insulin dosage and dietary management require adjustment. The woman should be alert for signs of hyperglycemia, hypoglycemia, and acidosis. She is requested to test her urine and blood four times daily. This is usually done upon rising in the morning and two hours after each meal. Tests that measure sugar levels in urine are not accurate enough for use during pregnancy and may be misleading. However, women need to test the urine for ketones. High levels of ketones in the urine is a sign that the body has switched to burning fat for energy and can be harmful to the fetus. It is also a sign that diabetes is out of control. Blood tests for sugar levels are easy to perform and relatively painless. Individual instruction must be given to each woman to learn to interpret her own results. Diet management is also on an individual basis. This is usually developed from what a woman normally likes to eat. It should include the same balance of nutrients that are considered best for pregnancy. Meals should be scheduled at regular times, keeping the same balance of protein,

ASSESSMENT	OBSERVATION	NURSING INTERVENTION
Insulin reaction (possible overdose)	Rapid development of symptoms Cold and clammy skin Trembling, twitching of lips, mental confusion Double vision Shallow breathing Loss of consciousness NPH insulin overdose has a slow reaction occurring late in day.	Check blood; it will probably be low in glucose. Give orange juice with or without sugar. Call physician for further direction.
Deficiency of Insulin Diabetic Coma (Acidosis)	Slow development of symptoms Skin hot and dry Fruity odor to breath Extreme thirst, nausea, vomiting Dull vision Deep, heavy breathing Loss of consciousness	Check blood; it will have a high sugar content. Call physician for order of regular insulin and further direction.

Figure 11-7

Insulin reaction

fat, and carbohydrates each day. A low-sodium diet may be ordered to prevent preeclampsia.

ACUTE INFECTIOUS DISEASES

Pregnant women who contract German measles (rubella) in the first trimester of pregnancy frequently give birth to infants afflicted with certain malformations such as cataracts, heart lesions, deaf-mutism, and *microcephaly* (abnormally small head). Opinions differ concerning the medical justification for therapeutic abortions in these cases.

The pregnant woman appears to be slightly more susceptible to acute upper respiratory infections than the nonpregnant woman. Therefore, the common cold, sinusitis, laryngitis, and bronchitis should never be regarded lightly.

Influenza is better controlled today with medication and is less serious than the epidemic of 1918. Although the prognosis is good, complications must be suspected when fever persists. Antibiotic drugs have decreased the danger of pneumonia in pregnancy and influenza is no longer considered a serious condition.

Measles and scarlet fever tend to cause premature labor or abortion. They do not cause congenital defects. However, women known to be pregnant should not be subjected to routine immunization against smallpox, mumps, measles, German measles, or yellow fever. Live virus vaccines when used in these immunizations can infect the fetus.

Immunizations in which killed or inactivated vaccines are used are considered safe. Such vaccines are used against influenza, epidemic typhus and typhoid, tetanus, and diphtheria.

Rabies anti-serum vaccine, killed cholera vaccine, and attenuated live oral polio vaccine or killed injectable polio vaccine may also be given to pregnant women when protection is required.

ASSESSING FETAL DISTRESS

Fetal distress can be assessed by performing various tests on amniotic fluid obtained by amniocentesis. Fetal assessment amniocentesis tests are made for chromosome studies, lecithin/sphingomyelin ratio, bilirubin, Nile blue sulfate, meconium, and the Shake test.

Amniocentesis

Amniocentesis is the method of obtaining fluid and cells from the amniotic sac (bag of waters). When fluid and fetal cells from a sample of amniotic fluid are analyzed, specific abnormalities can be identified and appropriate treatment can be initiated.

With any pregnancy there is a small chance that some birth defect will occur. The likelihood becomes greater when the woman is over age 35, or when one or both parents have a family history of genetic disorders.

Genetic testing of the amniotic fluid is a relatively new method of detecting genetic defects that might affect the fetus. Although only certain defects can be detected by amniocentesis, the benefits can be significant to couples at risk of producing a child with one of these genetic abnormalities.

Often, a family history or studies performed on a couple suggests the possibility of an abnormality in the fetus. In those cases where there is an increased risk of a specific disorder, amniocentesis may determine if the fetus is affected. When an abnormality is detected, however, the severity of the disorder cannot always be determined; it is left to the couple to decide whether they want to terminate or continue the pregnancy.

Amniocentesis is generally performed for any one of three reasons.

1. Genetic testing (chromosomal analysis for abnormalities such as Down's syndrome). This is the most common reason for an amniocentesis. It is done to determine whether there is any abnormality in the fetus itself. For this purpose, amniocentesis should be performed relatively early in the pregnancy.

   The usual reasons for genetic testing are:
   - The mother is over 35.
   - One or both parents have a family history of known specific genetic abnormalities.
   - The parents already have had a child with a genetic abnormality.

2. Testing for enzymes and proteins.
   - The fluid is tested for the presence of abnormal levels of certain enzymes which may indicate that the child is affected by some rare congenital defect (e.g., muscular dystrophy) which usually is familial.
   - The fluid is tested for alpha fetoprotein. Abnormal levels may indicate that the child is affected by a neurologic abnormality such as meningocele or anencephalus.

3. Problem pregnancy. If there is any known or suspected condition that might jeopardize the pregnancy, this procedure could help to detect the problem and might provide the doctor with information needed to plan for the last few months of pregnancy and for the delivery. For this purpose, amniocentesis is usually performed rather late in the pregnancy. Amniocentesis can also help determine the maturity of the fetus when size and menstrual dates are uncertain.

Amniocentesis can provide a wide range of information, including the sex of the unborn baby. However, it should not be used for casual screening or simply to learn the sex of the child. If there is no history of genetic abnormalities, or if no specific situation exists that requires closer investigation, there is usually no reason to perform amniocentesis. Amniocentesis carries a very slight risk of injury to the fetus and a very slight risk of causing an abortion. The physician discusses this with the mother in some detail if amniocentesis is to be considered.

Amniocentesis for genetic testing usually is done sometime between the fifteenth and eighteenth weeks of pregnancy. At this time, the procedure is simpler and safer because the uterus is large enough and there is an adequate amount of amniotic fluid. In the case of a problem pregnancy, amniocentesis usually is done later in the pregnancy, depending on the doctor's recommendation. Amniocentesis is generally performed in a hospital, but it is usually not necessary for the mother to stay overnight.

Procedure. The procedure for amniocentesis is as follows:

1. Explain the procedure to the patient and obtain an informed consent.
2. Check and record all vital signs.
3. Have the patient empty her bladder just before the doctor begins the procedure.
4. After the doctor palpates the abdomen, prep the abdomen with soap and sterile water.
5. Open amniocentesis tray on patient's bedside table and add the spinal needle and syringes.
6. Pour Betadine into the medicine glass.
7. Hold the Xylocaine bottle so the doctor can draw solution with the syringe and needle.
8. Label specimen and send it to the laboratory with a request form.
9. After completion of procedure, recheck vital signs and record in nurses notes. Attach nurses notes to prenatal record.
10. Request that the patient rest for 15 to 20 minutes after the procedure.

The amniotic fluid obtained by amniocentesis is sent to the laboratory for analysis. The following tests can be conducted on the fluid.

1. *Meconium* — Meconium obtained by amniocentesis indicates the fetus is not getting enough oxygen. This has caused the rectal sphincter muscle of the fetus to relax; it may have been acute or continuing. Meconium is, therefore, a sign of fetal distress. Its presence also interferes with other tests making them either unreliable or reliable only after difficult extraction methods.

2. *Lecithin/Sphingomyelin Ratio* — Measures fetal lung surfactant phospholipids. It approaches 100 percent reliability in determining fetal pulmonary maturity; it requires several hours for results. An L/S ratio of greater than 2:1 indicates lung maturity. This test indicates the possibility of Respiratory Distress Syndrome (RDS), also known as hyaline membrane disease.

3. *Shake Test (Rapid surfactant test)* — This test is also used to determine RDS. However, it requires only 10 minutes to obtain results. It is reliable when interpreted as "mature; low risk RDS." There are very few false positive tests; however, there are many false negative tests. If the test is negative, an L/S Ratio test must be done to obtain an accurate assessment.

4. *Amniotic Fluid Creatinine* — This test is also reliable to a high degree. It assesses fetal muscle mass and renal function. If creatinine is present in large amounts it indicates a large fetus. However, large fetuses, such as those of diabetic mothers, may have pulmonary immaturity, and growth-retarded fetuses may be mature. Therefore, false high and false low values are sometimes obtained.

5. *Amniotic Fluid Bilirubin* — Spectrophotometric measurement of bilirubin assesses fetal liver maturation. The optical density of amniotic fluid bilirubin is 450 microns (O.D. 450 μ). This test is not as reliable as L/S or creatinine for determining fetal maturity. However, it is highly important in managing Rh sensitized pregnancies as the levels of amniotic fluid bilirubin correlate with the degree of anemia in the fetus.

6. *Nile Blue Sulfate* — This substance stains the cutaneous lipid-containing cells of the fetus which increase in amount near term. The number of these cells indicates if the fetus is mature or not. As L/S ratios and creatinine are more reliable, this test is rarely used at present.

7. *Sex Determination Test* — A new procedure introduced in 1968 can tell the prospective parents the sex of the fetus. By examining the genes in the amniotic fluid which has been extracted, the sex of the fetus can be identified with 100 percent accuracy.

In addition to tests made on the amniotic fluid, other tests are used to assess the condition of the fetus.

Chorionic Villa Sampling is a procedure where samples of placenta tissue are obtained and assessed for fetal well-being. It is conducted under direct ultrasound. The patient is in a lithotomy position. A speculum is inserted into the vagina, and a tenaculum is affixed to the anterior wall of the cervix. The depth of the uterus is determined by a uterine sound. Then a catheter is directed through the cervical os into the chorionic villi site. Chorionic villa are then aspirated through the catheter into a syringe (Fig. 11-10).

The biggest advantage of chorionic villa sampling is that the procedure is performed early in the first trimester of pregnancy (9–12 weeks gestation). Since the cells do not have to be grown in the lab, laboratory results are obtained earlier. First trimester cells divide rapidly, and karyotyping is performed during the metaphase of mitosis. Therefore, if the patient chooses to terminate the pregnancy, because of the results of chorionic villa sampling, the procedure is less hazardous. It is much easier to perform at this early stage of pregnancy.

The disadvantages include a slightly higher rate of spontaneous abortion. Also, one limitation of chorionic villa sampling is that values of alpha fetoprotein levels cannot be obtained. It is felt that the information available from CVS is not as complete, or as reliable, as from amniocentesis. However, many genetic abnormalities can be determined by this procedure.

Ultrasonography

For the past ten years, and with growing frequency over the past five years, a new technology has allowed the physician to see into the uterus of the pregnant woman without exposing her and her baby to the known dangers of X rays and without pain or intrusions. The technique is called *ultrasound* (also called sonography or ultrasonography). Ultrasound uses high-frequency, inaudible sound waves which are directed into the abdomen of the pregnant woman and then reflected back to a receiver. The reflected waves give a visual "echo" of what is inside the uterus. This echo is transformed electronically into an image on a screen, figure 11-8. Bone, the densest tissue, appears as white areas in the ultrasound pictures. Muscles and less dense tissue appear in shades of gray. Fluid-filled areas give no reflection at all and appear black. From the image, the physician can learn an enormous amount about conditions in the uterus and the health of the fetus.

By far the most common use of diagnostic ultrasound is to determine true fetal age when the date of conception is unknown or mistaken

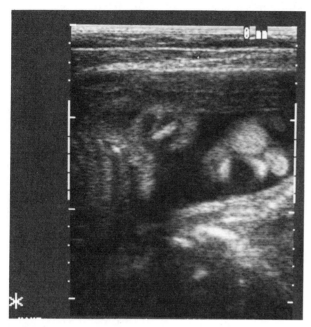

Figure 11-8

Current ultrasound technology allows highly detailed fetal imaging.

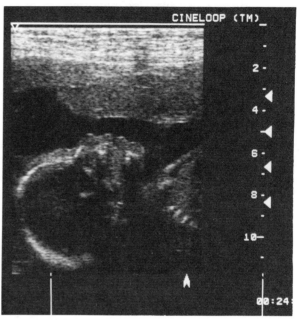

Figure 11-9

Fetal skull

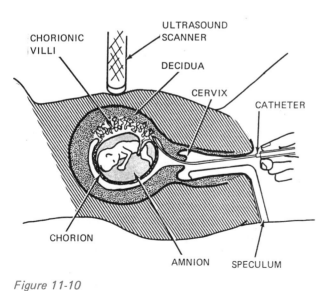

Figure 11-10

Chorionic villi sampling at 12 weeks

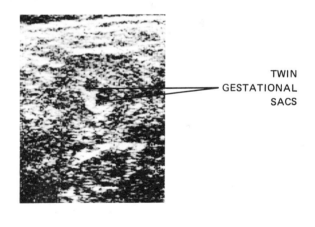

Figure 11-11

Twin gestational sacs at five weeks

by the mother. By allowing measurement of the fetal head and femur and assessment of its physical development, ultrasound can pinpoint the length of pregnancy to within a week or so. In a mother who has diabetes or high blood pressure, a series of sonograms taken every two weeks can show if the baby is growing properly. If not, the doctor can perform a cesarean to save the child. Dangerous uterine conditions such as placenta previa can be detected early. Fetal abnormalities or the presence of more than one fetus can also be diagnosed with the help of sonography, figure 11-11. There are numerous other obstetrical and gynecologic indications for ultrasound.

Ultrasound is now being used prior to amniocentesis. Sonography lets the doctor see where to insert the needle safely by locating the positions of the fetus and placenta.

Alpha Fetoprotein Test (AFP)

A measure of alpha fetoprotein may be used for prenatal detection of neural tube defects (spina bifida, anencephaly). Recent research has also shown an association between low alpha fetoprotein values and an increased risk for Down Syndrome. AFP is a screening test performed between the fifteenth and twentieth week of pregnancy by taking a sample of the mother's blood. If the test shows an abnormal value, a repeat test may be suggested. If necessary, additional diagnostic procedures such as ultrasound or amniocentesis will be used to evaluate the possibility of neural tube defects or other abnormalities.

24-Hour Urinary Estrogens

The 24-hour urinary estrogens collected in a 24-hour urine specimen are a measure of fetal-placental unit. This test is often used for fetal assessment. Estriol is an estrogen produced by the fetal-placental unit in increasing amounts as pregnancy progresses. Estriol is excreted in the mother's urine where it can be measured as necessary. Testing the level of estriol in the urine and blood can provide important information about how well the placenta is functioning. Estriol tests may be ordered for a mother with diabetes, preeclampsia, or severe hypertension, or if a baby is thought to be too small or considerably overdue. A significant drop in estriol level from one test to another may indicate the need to induce labor. The estriol level can also be tested by drawing the necessary blood sample.

Fetal Blood Sampling

The purpose of this test is to determine the status of the fetus during labor. A sample of blood is withdrawn from a small skin puncture in the presenting part of the fetus. The blood sample is then analyzed to determine fetal distress. Fetal blood sampling is discussed in unit 14.

Biophysical Profile

Biochemical assessment of the fetus has largely been replaced by biophysical and biometric evaluation. The fetal CNS is very sensitive. Hypoxia and its resultant metabolic acidosis will produce pathologic CNS depression with changes in biophysical activity. The demonstration of several biophysical activities, showing a normal pattern collectively, is reassuring of fetal well-being. A score of eight or more demonstrates probable fetal well-being.

BIOPHYSICAL PROFILE (USE OF ULTRASOUND)

	Score 2	Score 0
Fluid Assessment	One or more pockets of amnionic fluid 1cm. x 1cm. or more	No pocket greater than 1cm.
Fetal Breathing	Sustained for 30 seconds	Not sustained for 30 seconds or not present
Fetal Movement	Two gross body movements in 20 minutes	Less than two gross body movements in 20 minutes or no movement

	Score 2	Score 0
Fetal Tone	One episode of flexion/extension	No flexion/extension
Fetal Reaction	At least two FHT reactions greater than 15 beats per minute lasting 15 seconds in a 40 minute period	Less than two FHT reactions in 40 minutes

Non Stress Test

This test can be performed on the patient who is not in labor. It is based on the observation that the occurrence of fetal heart rate accelerations in response to fetal movement or uterine contractions is a reliable indicator of immediate fetal well-being. It is obtained by using an external ultrasound monitor. It is considered reactive if two or more fetal heart accelerations occur in a 10 to 20 minute period of observation. These accelerations should be greater than an increase of 15 beats per minute and should persist for 15 seconds or more. This evaluation is useful in determining fetal well-being in situations where patients are at risk for uteroplacental insufficiency (post-term pregnancy, maternal diabetes, oligohydramnios, and maternal hypertension). It is also indicated if there is a decrease or absence of normal fetal movements. In most cases, testing is instituted at thirty-two to thirty-four weeks of gestation. For more detail, see unit 14.

RH FACTOR

The *Rh factor* is an antigen found on the surface of the red blood cells. (An *antigen* is a protein substance, such as a toxin or enzyme that stimulates production of antibodies.) While searching for new erythrocyte antigens, Land-

steiner and Wiener discovered the Rh antigen in 1940. Experiments on the Rhesus monkey, after which the Rh antigen is named, showed that an important factor was present which influenced the outcome of a transfusion. About 85 percent of the white population in the United States have this antigen present; they are called Rh positive. About 15 percent lack the antigen and are called Rh negative. This percentage differs with various racial groups. The factor is of consequence only if the mother is Rh negative and the father is Rh positive.

Constant revisions in the methods of dealing with Rh are made as new antigens are constantly being discovered. It is now possible to prevent Rh-sensitization by administering an anti-Rh globulin which causes passive immunity in the patient so that she does not produce anti-Rh antibodies if she becomes pregnant with an Rh-positive fetus. RhoGAM (solution of gamma globulin, which contains a concentration of Rh antibodies), is given to the Rh-negative patient shortly after the delivery of an Rh-positive baby or after a midtrimester abortion or miscarriage. RhoGAM may be given during pregnancy at about 28 weeks gestation to prevent sensitization that may occur during fetal-maternal transfusion. Fetal-maternal transfusion occurs in less than two percent of cases.

Knowledge of the Rh factor is important in order to prevent hemolytic disease of the fetus and newborn. The physician determines whether or not an intrauterine transfusion or an exchange transfusion and phototherapy for the newborn will be required, and plans accordingly.

In the early 1950s, a British doctor named D.C.A. Bevis, ignoring the centuries-old taboo, injected a long sterile needle through the abdomen of a pregnant woman and drew out a few drops of amber-colored amniotic fluid. Analysis of the *bilirubin* (a pigment of red blood cells) in the syringe enabled Dr. Bevis to determine just how sick the fetus was. Doctors began using this technique (amniocentesis) to tell them when to induce labor prematurely so that the fetus could undergo immediate postnatal transfusion. This procedure cut the death rate from erythroblastosis fetalis in many hospitals by more than 50 percent.

Erythroblastosis Fetalis

Erythroblastosis fetalis is a hemolytic disease of the newborn. It is characterized by anemia, jaundice, enlargement of the liver and spleen, and generalized edema of the newborn. It is caused by the development of antibodies from an Rh-negative mother that react against an Rh-positive fetus. The infant's red blood cells are *hemolyzed* (broken down) and destroyed, producing severe anemia. If the anemia is severe enough, heart failure, brain damage, or death of the fetus can occur.

An Rh-negative woman may carry an Rh-positive baby as a result of mating with an Rh-positive male. In rare instances, fetal red blood cells enter the mother's circulation by passing through the placental barrier. When this happens, her body may become sensitized and develop antibodies to fend off the "foreign" invaders. These antibodies cross the placental barrier and enter the circulation of the fetus, destroying the fetal red blood cells. This destruction begins during gestation and continues after the baby is born. Usually antibodies do not develop in quantities large enough to harm the fetus until the patient has had at least one Rh-positive baby. Unit 20, Disorders of the Neonate, will discuss this condition in more detail. Treatment involves transfusing the infant with Rh-negative erythrocytes.

Intrauterine Transfusion

An *intrauterine transfusion* is the injection of Rh-negative erythrocytes into the peritoneal cavity of the fetus while it is still in the uterus. The fetus absorbs these erythrocytes in order to combat anemia.

This transfusion was developed in the fall of 1963, in Auckland, New Zealand, when Dr. A.W. Liley performed the first intrauterine transfusion for the treatment and hopeful correction of erythroblastosis fetalis. Since then, skilled workers around the world have been performing the procedure with promising results. The fetal survival rate from this procedure is approximately 50 percent.

To determine the need for an intrauterine transfusion, the physician must weigh all information carefully. Previous obstetrical history is important, as well as data from a complete physical examination, blood examinations for antibody titers, and spectrophotometric analysis of amniotic fluid. A *spectrophotometer* is an instrument for measuring the intensity of various wavelengths of light transmitted under standardized conditions by a substance under study. The tracings obtained are a summation of the topical densities of various bile pigments which appear abnormally in amniotic fluid and indicate the severity of disease in the fetus.

Preparatory Procedures. The patient is admitted to the hospital around the twenty-eighth to thirtieth week of gestation or earlier, depending upon the condition of the fetus. One of the nurse's first duties is to obtain and properly witness the legal permission form. Maternal blood samples are drawn and sent to the laboratory for a complete blood count, Rh titer, and a cross match. A blood sample is also drawn from the father so that it can be determined whether he is homozygous or heterozygous for the presence of Rh antigen in his blood cells. If he is homozygous, all of his offspring will have Rh-positive blood. If he is heterozygous, 50 percent of his offspring will be Rh negative if the mother of his children is Rh negative. All blood samples must be properly labeled and sent to the laboratory immediately.

On the day of admission, an ultrasound is taken of the patient's abdomen and the patient

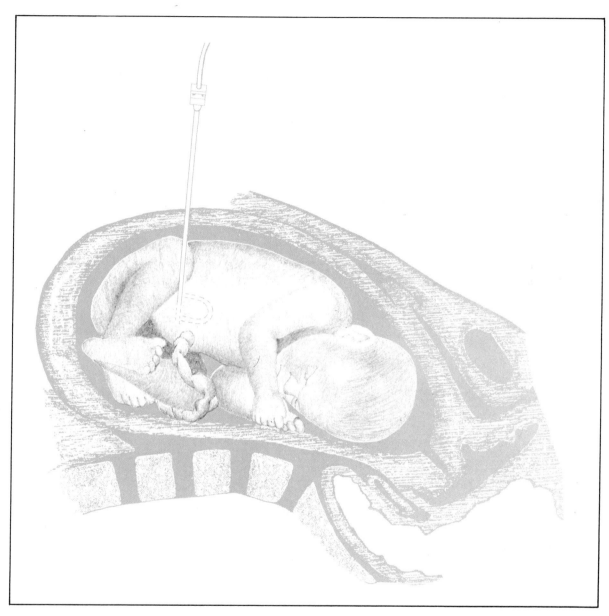

Figure 11-12

Intrauterine transfusion

undergoes amniocentesis. The amniotic fluid obtained from the amniocentesis is sent to the laboratory where a *bilirubin index* (concentration of hemoglobin pigments from disrupted fetal red cells) is determined with a spectrophotometer.

The withdrawal of fluid also allows room for the insertion of a radiopaque dye, such as diatrizoate (Hypaque) 50 percent. This contrast medium not only delineates the fetus, but, since it is swallowed by the fetus, it also outlines the fetal small intestine. At this time, another ultrasound is taken to determine the position of the fetal skeleton. The intrauterine transfusion takes place the following day.

The morning of the transfusion, the patient is allowed to have a regular breakfast. She may then be given a medication, such as meperidine hydrochloride (Demerol) and/or prochlorperazine (Compazine). The medication serves several purposes: (a) to alleviate apprehension; (b) to relieve pain, in the event pain is present; and (c) to sedate the patient since she must lie in one position for some time on an uncomfortable table.

The procedure is performed in a well-equipped room. Care and consideration must be given to the patient, and all participants should wear surgical clothing.

Aftercare. After the transfusion has been completed, the patient is returned to her room and is carefully observed for fetal activity, premature labor, peritonitis, and hemorrhage. Fetal heart tones are checked every four hours. The patient may have a liquid diet for lunch and a general diet toward evening. If necessary, Compazine may be ordered to relieve nausea and distress. Fetal complications are difficult to detect, but liver injuries, hemothorax, and sepsis have occurred as a direct result of this transfusion.

If the transfusions are successful, labor is induced with oxytocin (Pitocin) about the thirty-fifth week of gestation. The mother may receive an anesthetic to help her during delivery. After the child is born, the pediatrician carefully observes the child. Cord studies are done, and bilirubin levels are measured to determine when and how frequently exchange transfusions are necessary. It is not unusual for a transfusion to be performed within the first hour of life and repeated as necessary.

SUGGESTED ACTIVITIES

- Discuss bleeding in pregnancy and the possible causes.

- Define molar pregnancy. Compare and contrast molar pregnancy with an intrauterine pregnancy.

- Define ectopic pregnancy. List the factors that increase a woman's risk of an ectopic pregnancy.

- Define Preeclampsia and Eclampsia. Discuss the present theories regarding their etiology.

- Identify the signs and symptoms of Preeclampsia and the patients at risk.

- Describe the most common techniques of prenatal diagnosis including: (a) ultrasound, (b) amniocentesis and (c) CVS. Discuss their risks and limitations.

- Recite the danger signals of pregnancy.

- Review the chart which summarizes the complications of pregnancy. Note especially the symptoms which characterize each condition.

REVIEW

A. Multiple Choice. Select the best answer.

1. An acute infectious disease that often results in malformation of the infant is
   - a. pneumonia
   - b. polio
   - c. influenza
   - d. rubella

2. Severe anemia of the fetus that could cause its death in utero is
   - a. hyaline membrane disease
   - b. erythroblastosis fetalis
   - c. hydatidiform mole
   - d. creatinemia

3. Scarlet fever or measles contracted during pregnancy may cause
   - a. premature labor
   - b. congenital defects
   - c. acidosis
   - d. all of these

4. The termination of pregnancy through natural causes is
   - a. therapeutic abortion
   - b. complete abortion
   - c. spontaneous abortion
   - d. incomplete abortion

5. Injection of Rh-negative erythrocytes into the peritoneal cavity of the fetus is
   - a. amniocentesis
   - b. intrauterine transfusion
   - c. bilirubin sampling
   - d. none of these

B. Match the symptom in column II with the complication it may indicate in column I.

Column I	Column II
1. placenta previa	a. painful bleeding and shock
2. ectopic pregnancy	b. stabbing pain in side
3. placenta abruptio	c. painless bleeding
4. eclampsia	d. visual disturbance
5. preeclampsia	e. excessive vomiting
6. hyperemesis gravidarum	f. convulsions

C. Briefly answer the following questions.

1. Name the five tests that are made on amniotic fluid.

2. List the danger signals which may indicate a complication in pregnancy.

3. Why is labor induced for the pregnant diabetic patient?

4. List four observations to be made about the patient who has had an intrauterine transfusion.

5. What is a tubal pregnancy?

6. What is the alpha fetoprotein screen test and when is it used?

7. Describe the difference between a biochemical assessment and a biophysical profile.

SECTION 2 PREGNANCY AND PRENATAL CARE

Self-Evaluation

A. Multiple choice. Select the best answer(s). Some questions have more than one correct answer.

1. A positive sign of pregnancy is
   a. morning sickness
   b. enlargement of the uterus
   c. fetal heart tones
   d. positive Aschheim-Zondek test

2. Routine prenatal examinations made during visits to the doctor include
   a. urinalysis
   b. stool examination
   c. blood pressure
   d. weight

3. Edema with rapid weight gain, increased blood pressure and protein in the urine are signs of
   a. ectopic pregnancy
   b. preeclampsia
   c. placenta previa
   d. hyperemesis gravidarum

4. The Rh factor is of major consequence when
   a. both parents are Rh positive
   b. both parents are Rh negative
   c. the mother is Rh negative and the father is Rh positive
   d. the mother is Rh positive and the father is Rh negative

5. Morning sickness may be controlled by eating
   a. three large meals a day
   b. a high-protein diet
   c. a high-fat diet
   d. dry crackers before rising

6. Which of the following is *not* essential in the pregnant patient's diet?
   a. Citrus fruits
   b. Butter
   c. Green vegetables
   d. Eggs

7. During the prenatal period, the mother-to-be should avoid
   a. swimming
   b. constrictive, elastic-top hose
   c. travel
   d. housework

8. Weight gain during pregnancy should normally be
   a. 24–28 pounds
   b. 8–10 pounds
   c. 10–15 pounds
   d. 12–20 pounds

9. The average duration of pregnancy from the time of conception is
   a. 40 weeks
   b. 9 1/2 lunar months
   c. 10 calendar months
   d. 290 days

10. Palpation of the abdomen is of greatest diagnostic value after the
    a. fourteenth week
    b. tenth week
    c. third week
    d. twenty-eighth week

B. Identify each of the following signs and symptoms of pregnancy as *presumptive, probable* or *positive.*

1. Morning sickness
2. Positive Aschheim-Zondek test
3. Fetal heart sounds
4. Pigmentation of the abdomen
5. Frequency of urination
6. Quickening
7. Cessation of menses
8. Enlargement of the uterus

C. Associate the nursing care or preventive measures listed in column II with the normal discomforts in column I.

Column I	Column II
1. hemorrhoids	a. dry toast on awakening
2. varicose veins	b. avoid gas-forming foods
3. nausea and vomiting	c. restrict sodium intake
4. flatulence	d. elastic stockings
5. swelling of feet	e. cold witch hazel compress
6. itching	f. hot water bottle
	g. starch baths

D. Match the terms in column II with the correct descriptions in column I.

Column I	Column II
1. softening of the lower portion of the uterus body	a. amniocentesis
2. pregnant with first child	b. Braxton-Hicks sign
3. excessive vomiting	c. colostrum
4. secretion which exudes from breasts as pregnancy progresses	d. edema
5. excess accumulation of fluid in the body	e. Hegar's sign
6. puncturing the amniotic sac with a needle and syringe and withdrawing fluid	f. hyperemesis gravidarum
7. placenta which has been implanted in the lower segment of the uterus and covers the cervix	g. intrauterine transfusion
8. premature separation of the normally implanted placenta	h. multipara
9. woman in labor with or having borne her first child	i. pica
10. woman having borne her second child	j. placenta abruptio
11. antigen found on the surface of the red blood cells	k. placenta previa
12. injection of Rh-negative erythrocytes into the peritoneal cavity of the fetus while it is still in the uterus	l. primigravida
13. craving for nonfood substances	m. primipara
14. painless, intermittent uterine contractions	n. Rh factor

E. Briefly answer the following questions.

   1. Why is close medical supervision necessary for the pregnant diabetic patient?

   2. List the routine checks made at each visit to the doctor during the prenatal period. Explain why each is important.

   3. Why does frequency of urination increase in early pregnancy and decrease to practically normal in midpregnancy?

   4. List the danger signals which indicate possible complications of pregnancy.

   5. What would be the reason for having an amniocentesis done?

   6. Why would a L/S ratio or a rapid surfactant test be done on a pregnant woman in the late months of her final trimester?

   7. Name three tests, besides amniocentesis, which may be done for assessment of the fetus.

8. What is the cause of erythroblastosis fetalis and how is it treated?

9. What are the nurse's responsibilities after assisting with an amnio-centesis?

10. What are the components of the nursing process? Explain their relationship to the nursing care plan.

SECTION 3
Labor and Delivery

UNIT 12

THE STAGES AND MECHANISM OF LABOR AND DELIVERY

OBJECTIVES

After studying this unit, the student should be able to:
- Define the four stages of labor.
- List the signs and symptoms of each stage of labor.
- Explain the birth process in terms of presentation, position, and station.
- List the abbreviations for categories of presentation.
- Describe the seven movements in the mechanism of labor.

In the final two to four weeks of gestation, the fetal head sinks into the pelvis. This change of position is known as *engagement.* Its effect on the mother is called *lightening.* In lightening, the fundus of the uterus lowers, making the upper part of the abdomen flatter and lowering the waistline, figure 12-1. Breathing becomes easier, but walking and moving about are more difficult. As in early pregnancy, the pressure of the uterus causes frequency of urination.

The actual onset of labor is marked by one or more of the following signs:

- The "show"

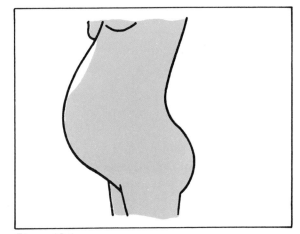

Figure 12-1
Lightening

137

- Rupture of the membranes (bag of waters)
- Regular contractions of the uterus.

The "show" is a pink vaginal discharge consisting of thick, stringy mucus streaked with blood (called the mucous plug); this is due to the rupture of capillary vessels in the cervix and lower segment of the uterus. If there is actual bleeding at any time during labor, it is abnormal and the doctor should be notified. *Rupture of the membranes (bag of waters)* is the tearing of the membranes containing the amniotic fluid which supported the baby during the term of pregnancy. The amniotic fluid may gush or trickle out the vagina, depending on the degree of tear in the amniotic sac. Rupture of the membranes may or may not occur with the onset of contractions.

The contractions of the uterus are an involuntary tightening of the uterine muscle. These contractions are often referred to as "labor pains." Each contraction ranges from 45 to 90 seconds (less than one and one-half minutes). The average contraction is about one minute long. Each contraction has three phases:

- increment — the intensity of the contractions increases
- acme — the contraction is at its height
- decrement — the intensity of the contraction diminishes

The contractions of the uterus are intermittent, with periods of relaxation between them. Contraction intervals are timed from the beginning of one to the beginning of the next contraction. The duration is measured in seconds; the intensity can be measured with a uterine monitor and is in direct relation to the progress of labor.

FALSE LABOR

It is often difficult to determine if a patient is in labor. Abdominal discomfort may occur a few days to three weeks before labor actually begins. This may be due to gas in the bowels or irregular uterine contractions. These contractions are annoying and closely resemble true labor. However, false labor contractions are irregular and the intensity does not increase with time. Also, they are usually confined to the lower abdomen. If examined, there is no marked change in the cervix. A warm bath or light activity, such as walking, will often relieve the symptoms. False labor may occur for a period of a few minutes to hours and then disappear, only to return in a similar manner, or develop into true labor contractions.

TRUE LABOR

True labor is characterized by a rhythmic, increasingly intense uterine contraction which occurs at intervals of 5 to 15 minutes; it lasts 30 seconds or more and is accompanied by typical changes in the lower portion of the body of the uterus and the cervix. The cervix, normally long and narrow, must shorten and widen. The shortening is called *effacement;* the widening, *dilatation,* figure 12-2. Effacement is measured in percentages. The higher the percentage, the thinner

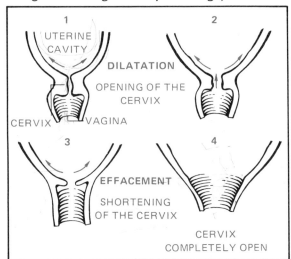

Figure 12-2

Opening of cervix during labor (1–4)

and shorter the cervix. Dilatation is measured in centimeters (2 1/2 cm = 1 inch). These changes are accomplished by the uterine contractions.

Dilatation and effacement of the cervix distinguishes true labor from false labor. The internal os of the cervix enlarges from a few millimeters in size to a diameter of about 10 centimeters, figure 12-3. At this stage, cervical dilatation is common-ly said to be "complete" or "full." The amount of dilatation and effacement of the cervix may be determined by vaginal or rectal examination.

When labor first begins, the patient usually feels an uncomfortable tenseness in her lower abdomen, back, or rectum, followed by another contraction in 20 to 30 minutes. These contractions gradually become more frequent and regular.

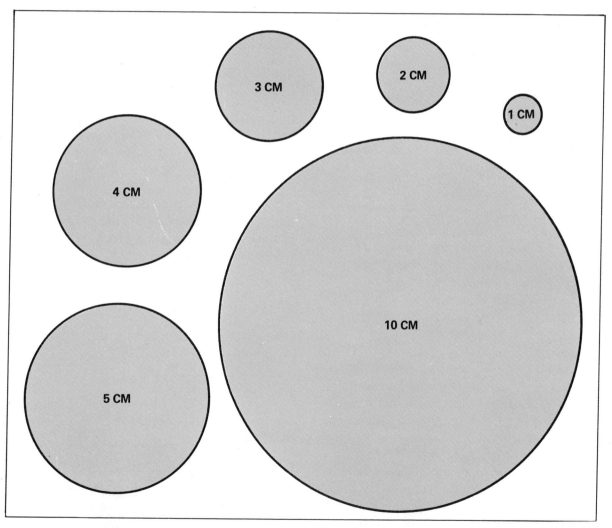

Figure 12-3

Cervical dilatation (Courtesy of Ross Laboratories)

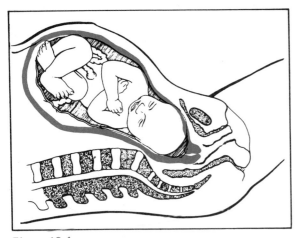

Figure 12-4

Longitudinal lie

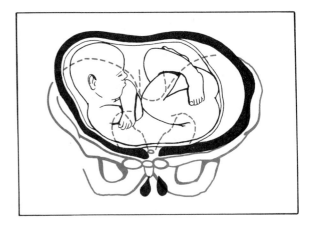

Figure 12-5

Transverse lie

FOUR STAGES OF LABOR

Labor progresses in four stages. The first stage, called the period of *dilatation and effacement,* extends from the time cervical dilatation and effacement begins until it is complete. The second stage, the period of *expulsion,* is the period between complete dilatation of the cervix to the delivery of the fetus. The third stage begins with the birth of the child and lasts until the placenta and membranes are expelled. This stage is known as the placental stage. The fourth stage of labor, recovery, begins after the birth of the placenta and lasts for the first few hours after delivery.

Before the stages of labor can be fully understood, it is important to know the relationships of the baby and birth canal. The terms *attitude, presentation, lie,* and *position* are used to describe these relationships. *Attitude* is the relationship of the fetus' body to itself. The most common attitude is flexion, and it needs the least amount of space. The head is flexed on the chest, arms are folded, legs are flexed and drawn up on the abdomen. When the head is extended, the chin will present.

Lie refers to the relation of the long axis of the baby to that of the mother. In most cases,

this axis is parallel to or in the same plane as the mother's and is called a *longitudinal lie,* figure 12-4. A much rarer occurrence is a *transverse lie,* in which the baby lies across the mother's pelvis, figure 12-5.

The *presenting* part is that part of the baby entering the internal os for delivery. In longitudinal lie, the presenting part may be either the head (cephalic presentation), or the buttocks (*breech presentation*). Cephalic presentation may be either vertex, brow or face, depending on whether the occipital area, frontal area, or

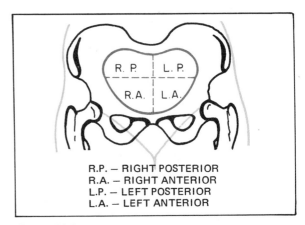

R.P. — RIGHT POSTERIOR
R.A. — RIGHT ANTERIOR
L.P. — LEFT POSTERIOR
L.A. — LEFT ANTERIOR

Figure 12-6

Pelvic quadrants

A.	Cephalic Presentations	C.	Face Presentations
	1. L.O.A. – Left occiput anterior		1. L.M.A. – Left mentum anterior
	2. L.O.T. – Left occiput transverse		2. L.M.T. – Left mentum transverse
	3. L.O.P. – Left occiput posterior		3. L.M.P. – Left mentum posterior
	4. R.O.A. – Right occiput anterior		4. R.M.A. – Right mentum anterior
	5. R.O.T. – Right occiput transverse		5. R.M.T. – Right mentum transverse
	6. R.O.P. – Right occiput posterior		6. R.M.P. – Right mentum posterior
B.	For Breech	D.	Transverse Presentations
	1. L.S.A. – Left sacrum anterior		1. L.Sc.A. – Left scapula anterior
	2. L.S.T. – Left sacrum transverse		2. L.Sc.T. – Left scapula transverse
	3. L.S.P. – Left sacrum posterior		3. L.Sc.P. – Left scapula posterior
	4. R.S.A. – Right sacrum anterior		4. R.Sc.A. – Right scapula anterior
	5. R.S.T. – Right sacrum transverse		5. R.Sc.T. – Right scapula transverse
	6. R.S.P. – Right sacrum posterior		6. R.Sc.P. – Right scapula posterior

Figure 12-7

Six positions of presentation

the chin are presenting. In transverse lie the shoulder is the presenting part. Cephalic presentations occur 96 percent of the time.

The term *position* means the relation of the presenting part of the child to the right or left side of the mother, figure 12-6. The relationship

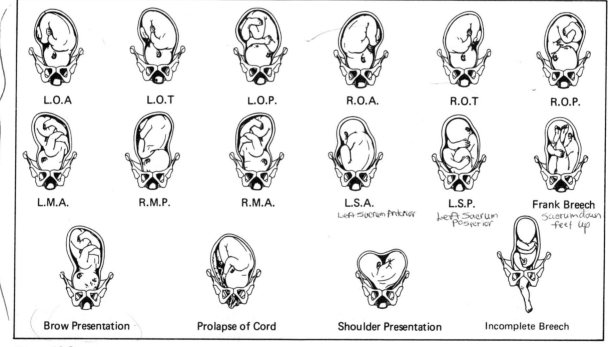

Figure 12-8

Categories of presentations (Courtesy of Ross Laboratories)

of the presenting part to the anterior, transverse, or posterior portion of the mother's pelvis is also considered in determining the position. There are six positions for each presentation, figure 12-7.

When the *occiput* (head) is the presenting part, it is identified by the letter *O*. Its position in relation to the quadrants of the mother's pelvis may be: left occiput anterior (L.O.A.), left occiput transverse (L.O.T.), or left occiput posterior (L.O.P.), figure 12-8. Similarly, if on the right, it may be right occiput anterior (R.O.A.), right occiput transverse (R.O.T.), or right occiput posterior (R.O.P.).

The sacrum (buttocks) is designated by the letter *S*, mentum (face) by the letter *M*, and scapula (shoulder) by the letter *Sc*. The presentation and position can be determined by abdominal palpation, vaginal examination, and auscultation. The left occiput anterior (L.O.A.) position is the most common position and the most favorable for the welfare of the mother and baby.

ENGAGEMENT AND STATION

When the presenting part descends and fully enters the true pelvis, it is said to be *engaged*. The degree of engagement is called *station*, figure 12-9. There are five stations:

1. Floating (presenting part high above inlet; −4, −5)
2. Fixed (presenting part in the inlet; −3, −2, −1)
3. Engaged (the largest diameter of the presenting part has reached the level of the ischial spines; 0)
4. Midplane (presenting part is between the inlet plane and maximum depth of pelvis; +1, +2, +3) *crowning*
5. On the perineum (presenting part is deep in the pelvis; +4, +5)

The degrees of engagement are determined by rectal or vaginal examination.

FIRST STAGE — DILATATION AND EFFACEMENT

Although labor varies in length, the first stage of labor in the average primipara is about 16 hours long. It may be difficult to determine exactly when true labor begins since contractions may occur before dilatation starts. Dilatation and effacement may be slow or rapid depending upon the age of the patient, her general physical condition, and the number of previous pregnancies. The membranes may rupture before the beginning of labor, or they may remain and assist in the dilatation of the cervix. If the membranes rupture at home, the patient should be

The location of the presenting part in relation to the level of the ischial spines is designated **station**, and indicates the degree of advancement of the presenting part through the pelvis.

Stations are expressed in centimeters above **(minus)** or below **(plus)** the level of the ischial spines **(zero)**. The presenting part is usually engaged when it reaches the level of the ischial spines.

Figure 12-9

Stations of presenting part (Courtesy of Ross Laboratories)

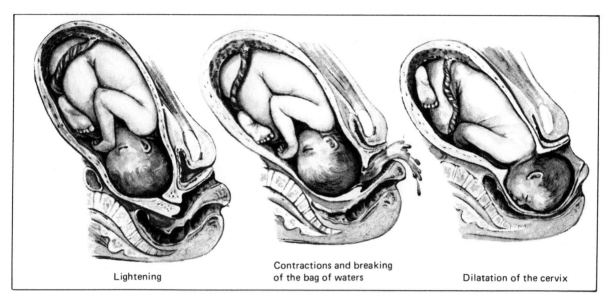

Lightening

Contractions and breaking
of the bag of waters

Dilatation of the cervix

Figure 12-10
The first stage of labor (Courtesy of Carnation Company)

brought to the hospital immediately. It is important to note the exact time the membranes rupture because there is now an entry for infection. Also *cord prolapse* (premature expulsion of the cord) could occur, causing more complications. The entire first stage is an involuntary act; the only assistance that the patient can give is to relax.

As the contractions continue through the first stage of labor, a pull is exerted on the cervix and supporting ligaments. This pulling, combined with a reduction in oxygen supply to the contracted tissue, can give rise to discomfort. The more intense the contractions, the more pull exerted on the cervix; the more often the contractions occur,

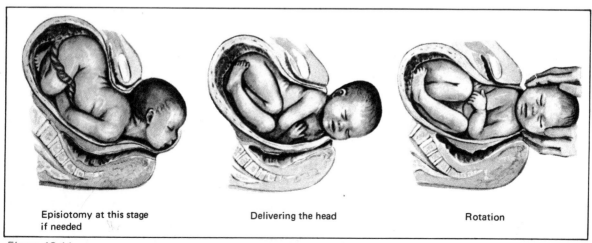

Episiotomy at this stage
if needed

Delivering the head

Rotation

Figure 12-11
The second stage of labor (Courtesy of Carnation Company)

the more frequently that pull is exerted. As the upper portion of the uterus contracts, the lower portion relaxes, allowing the baby to descend further toward the vagina. The pressure of the baby's head against the cervix stimulates the release of the hormone, oxytocin, which in turn stimulates further contractions.

In a typical pattern of labor contractions, the period from 1 to 4 centimeters is called the latent phase of labor, from 5 to 7 centimeters, the accelerated phase and from 8 to 10 centimeters, the transition phase. Each of these periods is shorter and more intense than the one before it, with the transition period being shortest and most difficult.

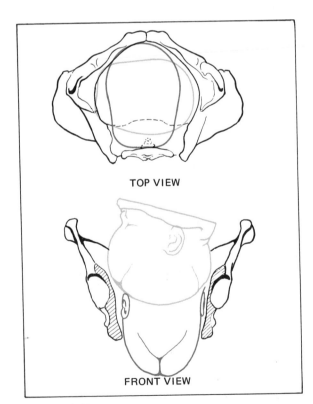

TOP VIEW

FRONT VIEW

Figure 12-12

The normal female pelvis (Courtesy of DeLee's Obstetrics for Nurses, W.B. Saunders Co.)

SECOND STAGE - EXPULSION

The position of the fetus must change as it passes through the pelvis and birth canal. Note in figure 12-12 that the long diameter of the inlet of the pelvis is side to side. The long diameter at the outlet is from front to back. Therefore, the baby's head must turn 90 degrees to emerge from the outlet. A series of movements, called the *mechanism of labor*, figure 12-13, adjusts the position of the fetus so that the smallest possible diameters of the presenting part encounter the irregular shape of the pelvic canal. Thus, the fetus encounters as little resistance as possible to its passage from the mother's body. In order of occurrence, these movements are: 1) engagement, 2) descent, 3) flexion, 4) internal rotation, 5) extension, 6) external rotation, and 7) expulsion.

Engagement

As stated earlier, *engagement* occurs when the presenting part of the fetus descends and fully enters the pelvis. In multiparas, engagement sometimes does not occur until dilatation begins.

Descent

Descent is the continuous progress of the fetus as it passes through the birth canal. It is brought about by the downward pressure of uterine contractions. Although descent is said to be continuous, it actually occurs only during contractions. Descent begins when the presenting part of the fetus fully enters the pelvis and engagement is accomplished.

Flexion

As the fetus descends and the head encounters resistance, *flexion* (condition of being bent) occurs. During flexion, the head of the fetus is bent forward causing its chin to rest on its *sternum* (breastbone). Flexion is important because the narrowest part of the head must enter the pelvic outlet. Flexion can occur either at the edge of the pelvis or when the head reaches the pelvic floor.

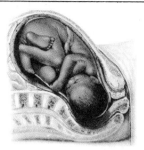
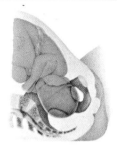

ENGAGEMENT,
DESCENT,
FLEXION

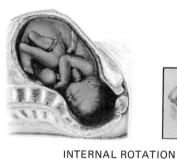

INTERNAL ROTATION

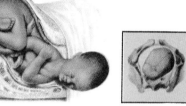

EXTERNAL ROTATION (RESTITUTION)

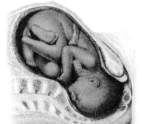

EXTENSION BEGINNING
(ROTATION COMPLETE)

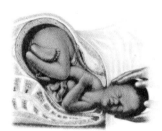

EXTERNAL ROTATION (SHOULDER ROTATION)

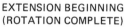
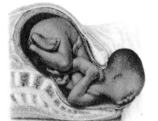
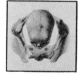

EXTENSION COMPLETE

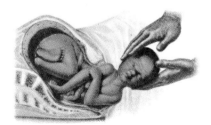

EXPULSION

Figure 12-13

Mechanism of normal labor — the process by which the baby traverses the birth canal (Courtesy of Ross
Laboratories

Internal Rotation

The third step in the mechanism of labor is internal rotation which takes place mainly during the second stage of labor. *Internal rotation* is the rotating of the head of the fetus 45 to 90 degrees to the left. The head then lies beneath the symphysis pubis. This is the most common internal rotation. If the fetus must move from a posterior position, it may have to rotate as much as 135 degrees. This means a longer labor with much more discomfort for the patient.

Extension

When the head of the fetus passes out of the pelvis and is stopped under the pubic arch, it cannot make further progress unless extension occurs. *Extension* is when the fetal head becomes unflexed and pushes upward out of the vaginal canal. The head of the fetus is actually delivered during extension.

External Rotation

After the head is delivered, it rotates back 45 to 90 degrees or until it resumes its normal relationship with the shoulders. This is called *restitution*. The baby's position in utero can be determined during restitution by observing the turn of its head. Restitution is sometimes coupled with shoulder rotation.

The rotating of the head during restitution helps to align the unborn shoulders of the fetus in anteroposterior position just beneath the pubis. This aligning of the shoulders is called *shoulder rotation*.

Expulsion

The anterior shoulder emerges first, aided by the doctor who applies a gentle but firm downward pressure on the baby's head. The doctor then raises the head gently to clear the posterior shoulder. After delivery of the shoulders the rest of the body follows. This final step, which is actually the delivery of the shoulders and body, is called *expulsion*.

The patient can actively participate in the second stage of labor. With each contraction she may be encouraged to take a deep breath, hold it, and bear down so that the abdominal muscles contract and help to expel the fetus. As the contractions lengthen in duration and become more frequent, the vaginal tissue bulges and the rectum stretches. The labia majora and labia minora separate widely; during the contraction the head of the fetus descends. A stretching and burning sensation is frequently felt when the fetal head passes over the perineum and the muscles are stretched. An *episiotomy* (an incision of the perineum) is often performed at this time to facilitate delivery. The episiotomy serves several purposes: (1) it substitutes a straight, clean surgical incision for a ragged laceration which otherwise is likely to occur; (2) it spares the baby's head from pressure against perineal obstruction; and (3) it shortens the duration of the second stage of labor. Once the head is delivered, the body is expelled with a rotational movement, and complete birth occurs. The cord attached to the newborn infant is then clamped and cut.

THIRD STAGE - PLACENTAL STAGE

The third stage of labor usually begins with a gush of blood. The placenta and its membranes are still attached to the wall of the uterus; contractions of the uterus continue for a time before the placenta separates. These contractions are less severe at first; they become stronger to expel the *afterbirth* (placenta, membranes, and umbilical cord). Bleeding from the vagina occurs at the time of separation of the placenta.

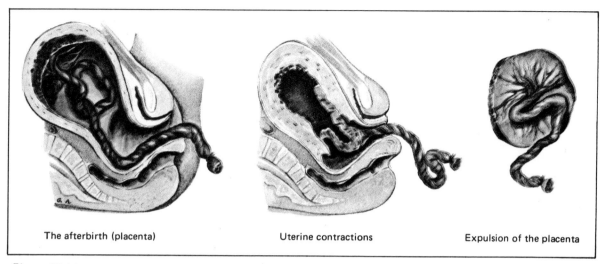

| The afterbirth (placenta) | Uterine contractions | Expulsion of the placenta |

Figure 12-14

The third stage of labor (Courtesy of Carnation Company)

With the contractions of the uterus, the placenta is expelled into the vagina, bringing the membranes after it, figure 12-14. With moderate pressure on the fundus, the placenta leaves the vagina. The fundus usually lies in the vicinity of the umbilicus (the navel). The uterus then becomes hard and firm and once more lies in the pelvis. Occasionally, the uterus may soften, rise up, and relax. This could be a symptom of hemorrhage.

CAUTION: It is most important that the uterus be carefully massaged until it remains firm. Oxytocin may be given to aid in contracting the uterus and controlling bloody discharge.

FOURTH STAGE - RECOVERY

The fourth stage consists of the first few hours after birth. The first hours following birth are a very special time for a family. The baby is usually more alert and receptive to its parents at this time than it is in the ensuing twenty-four hours.

When the mother's condition is considered stable, she is moved to a hospital bed where she continues to recover. The first hours following birth are a time when the mother must be closely watched. Her uterus is checked for firmness and location. Her normal flow of blood, excess tissue and fluids from the uterus, called *lochia*, are checked for amount and consistency. Her blood pressure, temperature and pulse are checked for stabilization and normalcy. She is asked to urinate and her bladder is checked for complete emptying.

The mother may experience some trembling of her legs which may be relieved by covering them with a warmed blanket. She may also experience a burning discomfort in her perineum which may be eased by applying an ice bag to the area. The uterus contracts for a time after delivery and may cause discomfort called "afterbirth pains." Slow, deep breathing helps to lessen these pains. Medication may also be given if necessary. The mother must continue to be carefully monitored during her entire hospital stay.

SUGGESTED ACTIVITIES

- Submit a written, documented report on one of the following:
  - Cervix in Primigravida
  - Four Stages of Labor: Nursing Care According to the Nursing Process
  - Successive Stages of Extrusion of Placenta
- Identify each category of presentation.

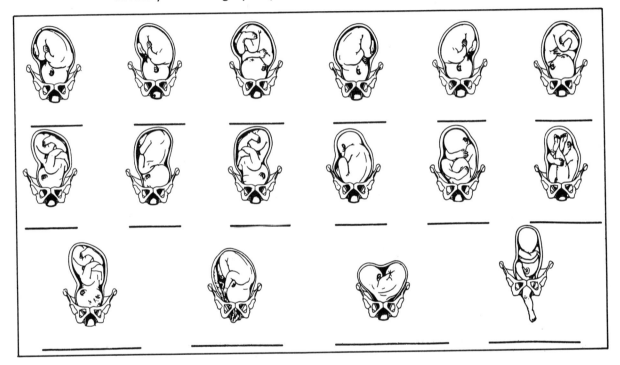

- Define labor. Describe the physiological changes in each stage.
- Identify the signs of approaching labor.
- Define station, engagement, and crowning.
- Differentiate between true labor and false labor.
- List the six cardinal movements in birth.

REVIEW

Multiple Choice. Select the best answer.

1. The widening of the cervical opening is called
   - a. effacement
   - b. engagement
   - c. dilatation
   - d. prolapse

2. The first stage of labor for a primipara usually lasts
   a. 3 to 6 hours
   b. 6 to 10 hours
   c. 10 to 16 hours
   d. 24 hours

3. Descent of the fetal head into the pelvis is called
   a. lightening
   b. effacement
   c. labor
   d. false labor

4. The patient has an active role to play during the
   a. first stage of labor
   b. second stage of labor
   c. third stage of labor
   d. all of these

5. Duration of the contractions of the uterus (called "labor pains") ranges from
   a. 10 to 45 seconds
   b. 20 to 40 seconds
   c. 45 to 90 seconds
   d. 60 to 120 seconds

6. True labor is characterized by
   a. increasingly intense uterine contractions
   b. contractions that occur at regular 5 to 15 minute intervals
   c. dilatation of the cervix
   d. all of these

7. The four stages of labor are
   a. dilatation/effacement, expulsion, placental, recovery
   b. dilatation, presentation, engagement, expulsion
   c. early, latent, transition, expulsion
   d. none of these

8. Lie refers to
   a. how deep the baby's head has dropped into the pelvis
   b. the relation of the long axis of the baby to that of the mother
   c. the baby's head being on the right or left side of the mother
   d. how long it takes for the baby to move down the birth canal.

9. When the presenting part descends fully into the true pelvis, it is said to be
   a. floating
   b. fixed
   c. engaged
   d. midplane

10. If the baby is in a head-down position, with back facing out toward the mother's abdomen and the occiput on the left side, the position is termed
    a. L.O.A.
    b. L.O.P.
    c. L.S.A.
    d. L.O.T.

11. An episiotomy is performed
    a. when the laboring woman has the urge to push
    b. when the fetal head is stretching the perineum and muscles
    c. when the vaginal tissue bulges and the rectum stretches
    d. when it appears the perineum has torn

12. The process by which the baby traverses the birth canal is called
    a. presentation   c. position
    b. station   d. mechanism of labor

13. The percentage of births that occur with a cephalic presentation is
    a. 50 percent   c. 96 percent
    b. 4 percent   d. 75 percent

14. The physician can determine the presentation and position of the baby by
    a. vaginal examination   c. auscultation
    b. abdominal palpation   d. all of these

15. The presenting part is usually engaged when it reaches the level of the
    a. ischial tuberosities c. iliac crests
    b. ischial spines   d. perineum

16. Complete the following: Provisional determination of fetal lie, position, and descent may be made by _____.

UNIT 13

MANAGEMENT OF THE PATIENT IN LABOR

OBJECTIVES

After studying this unit, the student should be able to:

- Describe the nursing care given during the first stage of labor.
- State the purpose and describe the procedure for a rectal examination, vaginal examination, perineal prep, enema, and catheterization.
- Name four factors that affect the rapidity of labor.
- List six signs of abnormal labor.

When the first hospitals were built in the Middle Ages, only the very poor were confined in them for childbearing. A 30 percent mortality rate existed due to infection and lack of knowledge in nursing techniques and isolation care. Progress in the field of science and education greatly improved conditions. In 1847, the cause and prevention of childbed fever were discovered. In the late 1800s, Pasteur's and Lister's theories on the spread of infection were accepted and obstetricians introduced aseptic techniques into maternity wards. With the advance of science and improved patient care, the obstetrical patient is given the same consideration as surgical patients.

ADMISSION PROCEDURES

Admission procedures vary among hospitals. However, the patient who is in labor undergoes examinations and care upon admission which are basically the same.

Greeting and Welcoming the Patient

Nurses should greet the expectant parents in a warm, friendly manner, and introduce themselves. If the nurse has studied the prenatal record, the background information will help personalize and individualize the greeting.

Assisting the Patient to Undress

The nurse provides the patient with a hospital gown and assists her to undress. The clothing which she intends to keep with her is tagged to make sure it is properly identified. Generally, the patient will have been notified to leave valuables at home.

Obtaining the Patient's History

When the mother-to-be is admitted to the hospital in labor, the obstetrics nurse should question the amount of sleep she has been getting, her last sleep period prior to admission — how long and how well — and her physical activity before coming to the hospital. The nurse reviews the prenatal record for the background of the patient and ascertains the following:

- Time contractions began; their frequency and duration
- Presence of show or vaginal bleeding
- State of bag of waters
- Expected date of delivery; last menstrual period (LMP)
- When patient last ate and what she ate, including fluids
- Number of pregnancies patient has had (gravida/para)
- Any complications during the pregnancy

The nurse includes miscarriages in recording the number of pregnancies and the number of children the patient has borne. *Gravida* refers to the total number of pregnancies including the present one. *Para* refers to the number of pregnancies that have continued through the period of viability (20 weeks of gestation), including any stillborn babies.

A term that may be frequently seen in hospital charting is TPAL. This refers to the number of term or completed gestational pregnancies (T), premature deliveries (P), abortions (A), and number of living children (L). It is charted simply as numbers (i.e., 3–1–0–4). These numbers indicate three term pregnancies, one premature birth, no abortions, and four living children.

EXAMINATIONS AND PROCEDURES

The first stage of labor (the dilating stage) begins with the first symptoms of true labor and ends with the complete dilatation of the cervix. Usually, the doctor examines the patient early in labor. However, for the welfare of the mother and child, the nurse must constantly be aware of all changes in the patient's condition and vital signs. This information must be accurately recorded and promptly reported to the attending physician.

Temperature, Pulse, and Respiration

Vital signs are taken and recorded every four hours while the patient is in labor. A rise in temperature may indicate an infection; an increased pulse rate may be a sign of dehydration.

✓ Report any abnormalities immediately.

Urine Specimen

A urine specimen may be analyzed immediately for blood, sugar, albumin, and amniotic fluid. If it contains blood or amniotic fluid, the doctor may order a catheterized specimen.

Blood Pressure

Blood pressure is generally taken every two hours. If preeclampsia or pregnancy-induced hypertension (PIH) is present or suspected, the blood pressure is taken more often.

✓ Report any abnormalities immediately.

Uterine Contractions

At first, as labor begins, contractions are mild; they last about 30 seconds and occur at about 20-minute intervals. As labor progresses, they increase in intensity, last longer, and occur more frequently.

Uterine contractions of labor and the dilatation of the cervix occur in an intense, wavelike pattern. The duration of muscular contractions range from 30 seconds to over one minute. Each contraction is made up of three phases: (1) a period of increasing intensity, known as *increment*, (2) a period when the contraction is at its height, called *acme*, and (3) a period of diminishing intensity, or *decrement*. The increment is longer than the other two periods combined. The nurse can actually feel the muscular action by placing one hand on the abdomen at the level of

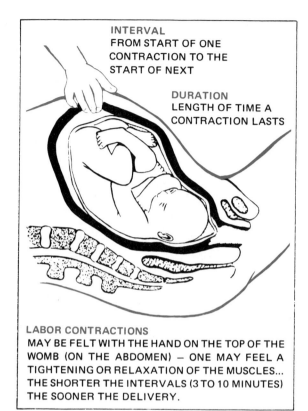

INTERVAL
FROM START OF ONE
CONTRACTION TO THE
START OF NEXT

DURATION
LENGTH OF TIME A
CONTRACTION LASTS

LABOR CONTRACTIONS
MAY BE FELT WITH THE HAND ON THE TOP OF THE
WOMB (ON THE ABDOMEN) — ONE MAY FEEL A
TIGHTENING OR RELAXATION OF THE MUSCLES...
THE SHORTER THE INTERVALS (3 TO 10 MINUTES)
THE SOONER THE DELIVERY.

Figure 13-1

Contractions of the uterus

the fundus, figure 13-1. The nurse can see the action as the abdominal wall rises and relaxes again. A contraction is timed from the beginning of one contraction to the beginning of the next contraction. The number of seconds the contraction lasts should also be noted.

Record and report the frequency, duration, and intensity of contractions. A prolonged contraction lasting more than 90 seconds could lead to fetal hypoxia and should be brought to the physician's attention.

Abdominal Palpation

The abdomen is palpated to check the position and presentation of the baby. The size of the baby can also be estimated.

Fetal Heart Tones

Fetal heart tones are heard with the use of the *fetoscope* (obstetrical stethoscope) which is worn on the examiner's head, or by using a Doppler instrument or electronic fetal monitor. The heart tones are checked between and during contractions. They normally slow down during a contraction, but return to normal as the contraction ends. The normal fetal heart rate is from 120 to 160 beats per minute. Fetal heart tones must be checked frequently during the first stage of labor. Any slowing down or speeding up of the heart tones beyond the normal limits should be reported immediately to the doctor. These changes may indicate fetal distress and the doctor may wish to augment (increase) labor.

✓ Report abnormal rate immediately.

Rectal Examination

The rectal examination may be done to determine the progress of the patient. The cervical opening can be felt to ascertain dilatation; the level of descent of the presenting part can also be determined.

• See procedure given later in this unit.

Vaginal Examination

The vaginal examination is performed to evaluate (1) the dilatation of the cervix, (2) the effacement of the cervix, (3) the station of the presenting part, and (4) the identification of the presenting part. It is also performed when physical rupture of the bag of waters (amniotomy) is required.

• See procedure given later in this unit.

Perineal Preparation

The purpose of the perineal shaving and cleansing is to remove the pubic, perineal and anal hair in preparation for delivery of the infant. Many physicians require only a mini-prep

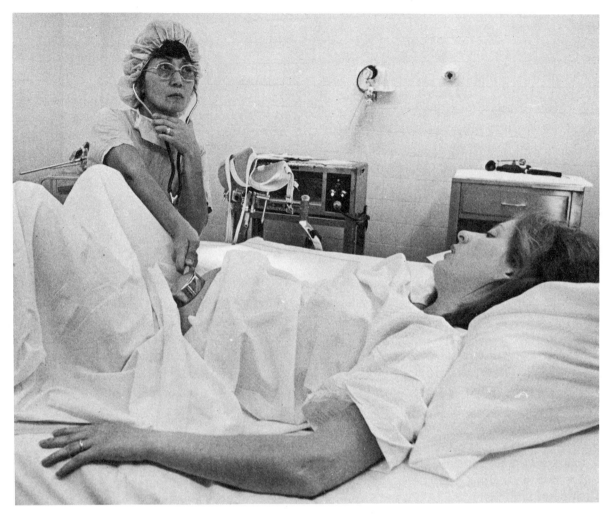

Figure 13-2

Listening for fetal heart tones

(anal and perineal area only). Perineal preparation serves to (1) make repair of the episiotomy easier, (2) insure quicker healing and cleanliness of area after delivery, (3) help prevent infection of the episiotomy, and (4) allow a better view during labor. However, recent studies have demonstrated that the infection rate is lower among women who have not been shaved. This is probably because the shaving can nick or irritate the skin, leaving openings for bacteria. For women with very long perineal hair, a scissor clip can be used as an alternative to shaving. A complete perineal shave is rarely performed in today's obstetrical practice.

Enema

If the membranes have not ruptured, an enema may be ordered by the doctor to (1) empty the rectum and prevent contamination during delivery, or (2) stimulate uterine contractions. With a multipara, the enema is usually not given if the first stage of labor is well advanced because it hastens labor.

Catheterization

It is essential that the patient void during labor. If other measures to encourage voiding fail, catheterization may be necessary. A distended bladder may hinder labor by preventing the baby's head from descending. Overdistention may also overstretch the bladder and cause a slight abrasion which favors bacterial growth and cystitis.

• See procedure given later in this unit.

A change of position during the first stage of labor can not only make a woman more comfortable, but can also enhance the progress of labor.

POSITIONS FOR THE FIRST STAGE OF LABOR

Standing and/or
Standing and Leaning Forward

Advantages

1. Takes advantage of gravity during and between contractions
2. Contractions are less painful and more productive
3. Fetus well-aligned with angle of pelvis
4. May speed labor

Disadvantages

1. Tiring for long periods
2. May not be possible with anesthesia

Walking

Advantages

1. Takes advantage of gravity
2. Contractions often less painful and more productive
3. Fetus well-aligned with angle of pelvis
4. May speed labor
5. May relieve backache
6. Encourages descent through pelvic mobility

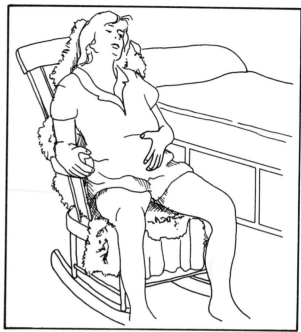

Figure 13-3

Disadvantages

1. Tiring for long periods
2. Difficult or impossible with anesthesia, analgesia, or electronic fetal monitoring

Sitting Upright, Figure 13–3

Advantages

1. Good resting position
2. Some gravity advantage
3. Can be used with electronic fetal monitoring

Disadvantage

1. Prolonged sitting associated with slower labor progress

Semi-sitting

Advantages

1. Good resting position
2. Some gravity advantage

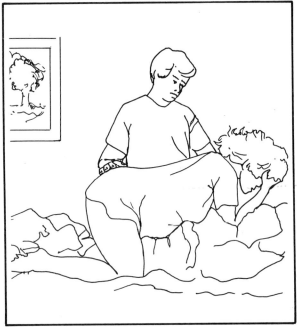

Figure 13-4

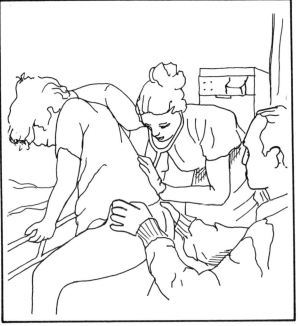

Figure 13-5

3. Can be used with fetal monitor
4. Vaginal exam possible

Disadvantages

1. Increases back pain
2. May slow labor progress if used for long periods

Hands and Knees, Figure 13-4

Advantages

1. Helps relieve backache
2. Assists rotation of baby in OP position
3. Allows pelvic rocking

Disadvantages

1. Uncomfortable and tiring for long periods
2. May interfere with external monitoring

Side-lying

Advantages

1. Good resting position
2. Convenient for interventions

3. Helps lower elevated blood pressure
4. Safe if pain medications have been used
5. Increases blood flow to placenta

Disadvantages

1. Contractions may be less effective and longer
2. Inconvenient for vaginal exams

Squatting, Figure 13-5

Advantages

1. Takes advantage of gravity
2. Relieves backache

Disadvantage

1. Tiring for long periods

Back-lying

Advantages

1. Convenient for care giver, for procedures, and vaginal exams
2. Restful

Disadvantages

1. Supine hypotension
2. Increases backache
3. Labor contractions found to be longest, most painful, and least productive

ABNORMAL SIGNS

While observing the patient in labor, the nurse must constantly be alert to indications that labor is not progressing normally. The nurse must report the following signs immediately to the doctor:

- Abnormal vaginal bleeding with pain
- Irregular, too fast, too slow, or absent fetal heart tones
- Cessation of contractions after labor has begun
- A rise in blood pressure
- Rigid uterus after contractions
- Severe headaches and dizziness
- Passage of meconium-stained fluid
- Prolapse of the umbilical cord

Prolapse of the Umbilical Cord

When the umbilical cord lies beside or below the presenting part, it is called a *prolapsed cord.* Although an infrequent complication, it is significant because of the high fetal mortality rate. Compression of the umbilical cord between the presenting part and the maternal pelvis reduces or cuts off the blood supply to the fetus; this may lead to the death of the baby.

Immediate diagnosis is most important. The only ways to diagnose a prolapsed cord are by seeing the cord outside the vulva or by feeling the cord during a vaginal examination. It may be diagnosed whenever the presenting part does not fit closely and fails to fill the inlet of the pelvis. The cord may occupy one of three positions:

- It may lie beside the presenting part at the pelvic inlet.
- It may descend into the vagina.
- It may pass out of the vagina.

The longer the cord, the more apt it is to prolapse. If the cord is seen at the vaginal entrance during labor, the nurse should place the patient in the knee-chest position and notify the physician at once. No time should be wasted. If this position is not possible, help the patient to turn onto her side and place pillows under her hips. If the cord is visible, the nurse should keep it moist with sterile wet saline dressings. Special care should be taken to not compress the cord. The nurse should never attempt to replace a prolapsed cord back into the vagina.

RAPIDITY OF LABOR

Many factors affect the rapidity with which labor and delivery are accomplished. These factors include:

- the size of the baby
- position of the baby
- mother's pelvic measurements
- rupture of the membranes
- muscle tone of mother's cervix
- quality of the contractions
- relaxation of the patient
- effect of medications on the patient
- whether the patient is primipara or multipara (the multipara generally completes labor faster)

STIMULATION OF LABOR

The doctor may *induce* (cause to begin) labor if complications of pregnancy have occurred. Such complications include preeclampsia, placenta previa, placenta abruptio, diabetes, and hydramnios. Other indications which the doctor considers are: fetal distress, the Rh factor, a multipara with a history of short labors, and a past-due (42 plus weeks gestation) baby. The simplest method of inducing labor is to rupture the membranes. This procedure is called an *amniotomy*. In some cases, it may be necessary to administer medications. If complications jeopardize the health and safety of the mother and baby, a cesarean section may be necessary.

The medication used to induce and *augment* (increase) labor is an oxytocic drug, usually Pitocin or Syntocinon. This medication increases the strength and frequency of contractions. It is usually administered through intravenous drip but can be given by an intramuscular injection or in tablet form. Induction is necessary to cause the onset of labor when the membranes have ruptured and contractions have not begun. Augmentation is necessary if contractions are not sufficiently strong enough to cause the cervix to dilate and efface once labor has actively begun.

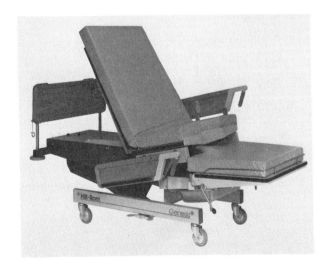

Figure 13-6

Birthing bed is often used for all stages of labor and delivery. (Courtesy of Hill-Rom Corp.)

NURSING CARE DURING THE FIRST STAGE OF LABOR

During the early part of labor the patient may be out of bed if the membranes have not ruptured. Food may or may not be given, depending upon the progress of labor and the doctor's orders. To relieve a dry mouth, ice chips or a clean, wet washcloth to suck on can be substituted for water; however, a record of fluid intake and output should be kept.

Bed linen is replaced as necessary and the mother-to-be is kept as comfortable as possible. Emotional support is necessary at this time. If the husband is not with the patient, the nurse's role becomes even more important.

The nurse should explain the examinations and procedures required during the first stage of labor. The patient will be more relaxed and more willing to accept these treatments and procedures when she knows what to expect. Specific nursing care includes the following:

- Encourage the patient with comfort, cheerfulness and sympathy. Give assurance of the progress she is making.

- Observe the character of the patient's contractions: frequency, duration, intensity.

- Observe the presence of show. In good amounts, show denotes rapid progress. The color of show usually changes from pink to red as progress is made.

- Check the pulse. If the pulse is over 100, the patient may be dehydrated.

- Check the blood pressure. Elevation may suggest preeclampsia. Report any abnormalities and recheck frequently.

- Observe the fetal heart tones. The normal rate is 120–160 beats per minute. The rate decreases after each contraction. Slowing or speeding of the fetal heart tones suggests fetal distress.
  a. Report all abnormal signs immediately.
  b. Maintain accurate records.

First Stage of Labor: From the beginning of contractions to complete dilatation of the cervix (known as the "stage of dilatation"). It usually lasts 10 to 16 hours for the primipara and 6 to 10 hours for the multipara.

PATIENT PROBLEM	NURSING INTERVENTION	RATIONALE
Slight contractions	Mother usually feels elated at this time; help prolong this feeling through encouragement.	A woman's psychological attitude and ability to remain calm and relaxed have a great effect on her ability to cooperate during labor.
	Allow her to engage in quiet activities such as reading, playing cards, watching T.V., or listening to the radio.	Pursuing familiar activities will help promote relaxation.
	Avoid bustling preparations, noises, whispering, and rattling of utensils.	
	If the membranes are intact, permit the patient to walk about and to shower if she wishes.	
Thirst	Permit fluid intake until contraindicated.	Adequate intake of fluids prevents dehydration.
Backache	Put pressure on the small of mother's back, or try rubbing her lower back briskly.	These maneuvers offer counterpressure to the force that the baby is exerting on the back as it descends into the pelvis.
	Advise the patient that pelvic rocking or arching of her back may help alleviate the backache.	
Profuse perspiration	Wash patient's hands and face with cool water.	Offers comfort through "therapeutic touch" and may help relax her.
Fear and anxiety	Reassure the parents; encourage the father to provide mother with emotional support and keep him informed of the progression of labor.	Such emotional support will help prevent the fear-tension-pain syndrome.
		Father can help to reassure the mother if he is informed.
Fear of anesthesia	Explain the effect of the agent to be used prior to administration. Use a quiet, reassuring voice.	Prior knowledge will help allay anxiety.
Full bladder	Encourage the patient to void every 3 or 4 hours.	A full bladder could interfere with the normal progress of labor.
	If catheterization is necessary, insert the catheter between contractions.	
Irritability	Accept any expression of irritability cheerfully.	The mother needs to feel supported and "accepted" during labor.
	Explain to the mother and father that an irritable reaction is normal during labor.	Increased irritability often indicates that the first stage of labor is nearly ended.

Figure 13-7

Nursing care for discomfort during the first stage of labor (Adapted from Maternal and Child Health, Littlefield, Adams & Co.)

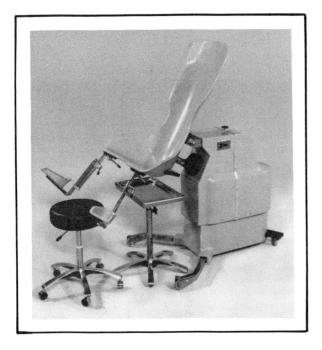

Figure 13-8
Birthing chair allows sitting/squatting positions which improves blood flow to the baby and aids in the delivery process. (Courtesy of Century Manufacturing Company)

- Urge the patient to void frequently. A distended bladder can be palpated above the symphysis pubis. Labor may be slowed by a distended bladder.
- Record the fluid and food intake.
  a. Liquids may be given up to about four to six hours before delivery, depending on the type of anesthesia to be administered.
  b. Good fluid balance forestalls dehydration and exhaustion. The doctor may order an I.V. in the case of long labor.
- Watch for signs of the second stage of labor. Maintain close observation so the doctor can be notified in sufficient time before delivery.
- When delivery seems imminent or when the perineum begins to bulge and the head of

the fetus can be seen, take the patient to the delivery room and transfer her to the delivery table for cleaning and draping. Keep charting up-to-date.

EXAMINATIONS AND PROCEDURES

RECTAL EXAMINATION

Purpose

This exam is done to determine the progress of labor: dilatation, effacement, and presentation. Usually vaginal examinations are performed but there may be times when a rectal exam is preferred.

Equipment

- 1 glove — disposable
- Lubricant

Precautions

1. Only the doctor or experienced nurse should perform this procedure.

2. Keep in mind the patient's history, and determine a possible termination of labor.

3. Keep in mind the size of the circles on the cervix dilatation chart in unit 12.

4. Check the patient during a contraction. This may indicate the rate of progress. Note the descent of the head with each contraction and if the membranes bulge with the contraction.

5. Remember the type of medication the patient has had and how often it has been given.

6. Keep in mind the difference between the external and internal os and always go by the size of the "contraction ring" or the internal os. Note other symptoms at

this time and try to determine the delivery time.

7. Prevent contamination of the vaginal area.

Procedure

1. Screen the patient and explain the procedure.

2. Turn the patient on her back or left side, knees flexed, and tell her to relax.

3. Put on the glove; lubricate index finger well and insert it into the rectum slowly and carefully, both for the comfort of the patient and to prevent reflex resistance. Press on the upper abdomen (uterus); locate the cervical opening and ascertain the dilatation, station, effacement, and presenting part.

4. After the examination, discard the glove. Clean the anus.

5. Record findings on the chart.

VAGINAL EXAMINATION

Purpose

A vaginal examination is done to ascertain the amount of cervical dilatation, presenting part, station, and effacement of the cervix, or to rupture the membranes.

Equipment

- Sterile glove
- Bacteriostatic agent
- Allis clamp or membrane hook for rupturing membranes

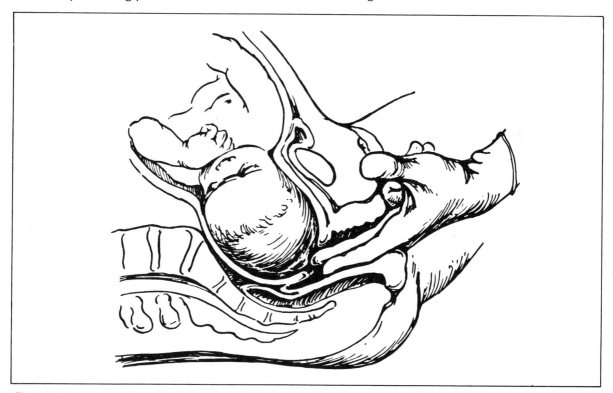

Figure 13-9

Vaginal examination of patient in labor

● Adequate lighting

Precautions
- This procedure is usually done by the patient's physician or an experienced labor nurse.
- Stay with the doctor during the procedure.

Procedure
1. Explain the procedure if the patient seems tense.
2. Pull the curtain around the patient to insure privacy.
3. Open glove packet for the doctor.
4. Pull covers to bottom of bed and drape the patient.
5. Have the patient lie on her back, knees up, soles of feet together and legs flexed apart. Have her relax.
6. Cleanse the vulva with a bacteriostatic agent.
7. The doctor, nurse, or midwife puts on a glove and inserts the examining fingers into the vagina and ascertains the dilatation, station, effacement, and presenting part.
8. If the doctor wishes to rupture the membranes, open up a long sterile Allis clamp or membrane hook (amnihook).
9. Check the fetal heart tone after the examination.
10. Cleanse the external genitals of the patient with a bacteriostatic agent after the examination.
11. If the doctor has ruptured the membranes, tell the patient that she must now remain in bed.
12. Inform the patient that she will have leakage from time to time. Slip a protective pad under her hips and have others available for her use.

CATHETERIZATION PROCEDURE

Purpose
This procedure is done to empty the bladder if the patient is unable to void. A distended bladder may hinder labor by preventing the head from descending and contributes to the patient's discomfort. Overdistention may cause stretching of the bladder so that a slight abrasion occurs which favors bacterial growth and cystitis.

Equipment
- Disposable catheterization set
- Disposable sterile gloves
- Adequate lighting
- Sterile sheet
- Sterile towels
- Zephiran or Betadine solution
- Cotton balls
- Lubricant

Procedure
1. Explain the procedure.
2. Have the patient lie on her back with her legs up, apart and flexed.
3. Screen the patient and cover her with a bath blanket, exposing only the perineal area.
4. Arrange for a bedside light (a relaxed patient and good light are important to a successful catheterization).
5. Wash hands and open the tray.
6. Pour Zephiran or Betadine solution over the cotton balls.
7. Put on the sterile gloves.
8. Place a sterile sheet under the patient's buttocks.
9. Drape the patient with sterile towels.
10. Squeeze lubricant on clean area of tray.
11. Gently expose the meatus by holding the labia open with left hand.

12. Cleanse the perineal area, using a cotton ball for one downward stroke, and discard into box. Use last cotton ball for cleaning the urinary meatus. (Squeeze excess solution out of cotton ball.)

13. Pick up catheter with right hand about 3 to 4 inches from tip; lubricate tip of catheter.

14. Gently insert the catheter into the urinary meatus until urine flows through the tubing, figure 13-10. Ask the patient to take deep breaths through her mouth. If there is any difficulty in locating the meatus, ask for assistance.

15. Hold catheter in place with left hand and place specimen bottle at end of catheter to obtain a sterile specimen. Allow excess urinary flow to collect in the large portion of the catheterization tray.

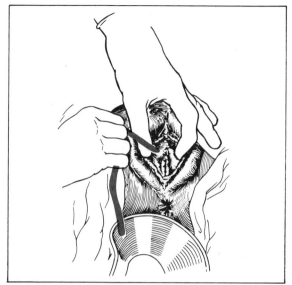

Figure 13-10

Meatus made visible by separating the labia in order to insert catheter.

SUGGESTED ACTIVITIES

- State how you would determine if the membranes are ruptured.
- List the major signs of fetal distress. Briefly describe diagnosis and management.
- List factors predisposing to and/or suggesting cephalopelvic disproportion.
- Describe ways in which the father may be encouraged to participate in the labor and birth experience.
- Describe techniques that nurses and other support people can use to enhance the comfort of the laboring woman.
- With the assistance of the instructor and permission of the patient, listen for fetal heart tones.

REVIEW

A. Multiple Choice. Select the best answer.

   1. Surgical rupture of the membranes is called

      a. amniotomy   c. Emerson Birtheez method

      b. amniocentesis   d. fetation

2. The normal rate of the fetal heart tone is
   a. 90–100 beats per minute
   b. 180 beats per minute
   c. 90–140 beats per minute
   d. 120–160 beats per minute

3. The blood pressure of a patient in uncomplicated labor is taken every
   a. 15 minutes
   b. half hour
   c. hour
   d. two hours

4. Temperature, pulse, and respirations of a patient in labor are taken every
   a. hour
   b. two hours
   c. four hours
   d. six hours

5. The term used to refer to the number of pregnancies that have continued through 20 weeks of gestation is
   a. gravida
   b. para
   c. primi
   d. parturient

6. The three phases of uterine contractions are termed
   a. increment, acme, decrement
   b. increment, intensity, duration
   c. frequency, duration, intensity
   d. onset, intensity, decrement

7. An increased pulse rate for the mother during labor may indicate
   a. fetal distress
   b. fatigue
   c. infection
   d. dehydration

8. Catheterization is sometimes done during labor if the patient is unable to void because
   1. a distended bladder may hinder labor by preventing the fetal head from descending
   2. the laboring mother has no control over her bladder
   3. an overdistended bladder may cause abrasion which can lead to cystitis
   4. overdistention of the bladder may cause severe backache
   a. 2 and 4
   b. 1, 3 and 4
   c. 1 and 3
   d. 1, 2, 3 and 4

9. A vaginal examination is done to determine
   1. dilatation of the cervix
   2. effacement
   3. station of the presenting part
   4. identification of the presenting part
   a. 1, 2 and 3
   b. 1 and 2
   c. 3 and 4
   d. 1, 2, 3 and 4

10. Nursing care during labor includes
    1. recording fluid and food intake
    2. observing character of patient's contractions
    3. checking vital signs
    4. observing fetal heart tones
       a. 1 only
       b. 3 only
       c. 1, 2 and 3
       d. 1, 2, 3 and 4

B. Briefly answer the following questions.

  1. List six signs that labor is not progressing normally.

  2. Name four factors that may affect the rapidity of labor.

UNIT 14

FETAL MONITORING

OBJECTIVES

After studying this unit, the student should be able to:

- Explain the process of direct fetal monitoring.
- Explain the process of indirect fetal monitoring.
- Define transducer.
- Name three types of external transducers used for fetal monitoring.
- Describe the procedure for obtaining a fetal blood sample.
- Name the conditions that would indicate the need for fetal monitoring.
- Name the conditions that would indicate the need for a fetal blood sample.
- Read a fetal monitor chart.

t is of interest to note that references to fetal observation for distress can be found in print as far back as the 1600s. In 1821, obstetric auscultation was described as a potentially important diagnostic tool to detect fetal life and distress during labor. Attempts to record fetal heart tones were made by Pestolozza in 1891, Seitz in 1903, and Hofbauer and Weiss in 1908. Cremer used a vaginal electrode to obtain a fetal ECG tracing in 1906. During the late 1930s and 1940s, research into fetal heart rate monitoring increased. By 1964, the Doppler device was available. The first successful recording of a fetal ECG through the abdomen was reported by Hon in 1957. The idea was then conceived to pass an electrode through the cervix and clip it to the fetal scalp in order to record the fetal ECG. Major improvements were made in 1972. Today, monitoring is done either externally or internally.

A major goal in obstetrics is to be able to assess the condition of the fetus during labor and delivery. Fetal monitoring is one method used for diagnosing fetal condition. In some hospitals, the only practical method for evaluating fetal status in the normal, uncomplicated pregnancy is regular listening with a fetal stethoscope. This method involves counting the heartbeats of the fetus. However, accuracy of the count depends upon the person counting. A fetal heart rate (FHR) greater than 160 or less than 120 beats per minute may indicate fetal distress.

If the fetal heart is listened to with a fetal stethoscope every 15 minutes for a duration of 30 seconds, only 3 percent of the available information is obtained. Modern technology permits monitoring of the FHR with a precision and endurance far exceeding the capabilities of the human ear. Newer methods of continuous *auscultation* (listening for sound within body cavities) are provided by ultrasonic devices that amplify the fetal heart sound. By using these newer approaches to evaluate the relationship of the FHR to uterine contractions, reliable and predictive information about the fetus may be obtained from the heart rate of the fetus. Even during contractions when the possibility of FHR changes and fetal stress are greatest, the fetal monitor allows doctors to follow the FHR and thereby maintain fetal surveillance. Fetal monitoring has proven to be valuable in the management of high-risk pregnancies where fetal tolerance of the stress of labor is low and the risk of fetal damage is high. Monitoring makes possible early detection of fetal distress due to umbilical cord compression, which is the most common cause of fetal distress during labor. It also helps in the early detection of abnormal uterine activity.

The following is a list of patient categories for which fetal monitoring is desirable when feasible. It is meant to be a guide in selecting patients for monitoring and represents a suggested order of preference by category. It should not be construed as a list of those who are the only patients to be monitored.

Category I

1. Abruptio placenta
2. Prolonged rupture of membranes
   a. with fever
   b. without fever
3. Amnionitis
4. Preeclampsia
5. Uterine inertia or dystocia problems

6. Fetal jeopardy or fetal distress (meconium staining alone included, unless associated with breech presentation)
7. 42 weeks or more gestation
8. Prolonged labor

Category II

1. Rh incompatibility
2. Breech position
3. Cardiovascular and renal disease (especially hypertension)
4. Diabetes
5. Other medical problems including suspected postmaturity
6. Prematurity without other complications
7. Multiparity

Category III

1. History of unexplainable death in utero
2. Hydramnios
3. Induction of labor for patient or physician convenience

Fetal monitoring is accomplished by either indirect methods using external transducers or direct methods using fetal scalp electrodes and/or an internal catheter. A *transducer* is a piece of equipment used to convert one form of energy into another form of energy. In medical terminology, a transducer receives energy produced by pressure or sound and relays it to another transducer as an electrical impulse. The second transducer can either convert the energy back to its original form or make a record of it on a recording instrument.

The sequence of the electrical impulse which reproduces the fetal heartbeat makes it possible to detect the motion of fetal heart valves and the actual sound made by fetal blood. This can be monitored either directly or indirectly using fetal electrodes, abdominal electrocardiograms, ultrasonic units or phonocardiograms.

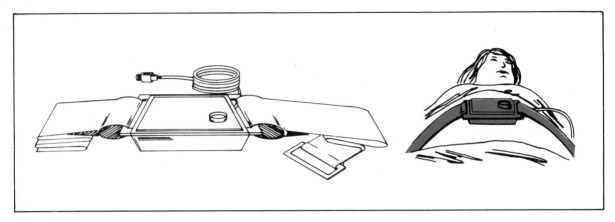

Figure 14-1

The uterine activity transducer responds to the muscle tonus in the abdominal wall.

INDIRECT METHOD

During *parturition* (childbirth) the uterus contracts periodically. These contractions may be detected by changes in the body or by the forces exerted by the uterine muscle tissue. External geometrical changes may be detected by a transducer strapped to the patient's abdomen. Such a transducer is often called a tocotransducer, or uterine activity transducer. External transducers used in indirect fetal monitoring include the uterine activity transducer, the phonotransducer, and the Doppler transducer. Indirect monitoring usually takes place early in labor but can be used throughout labor.

The Uterine Activity Transducer

The uterine activity transducer monitors uterine activity during labor and delivery by responding to the muscle tonus in the abdominal wall. The transducer is placed on the abdomen in an area where the uterine contour changes the most during a contraction — usually a little to either side of the midline. The transducer is strapped securely to the skin surface of the patient's abdomen; the strap must not be too tight for comfort. A record of the intrauterine pressure is transmitted by the transducer onto a chart.

Phonotransducer

Phonotransducer (microphone amplification) technique offers the doctor a means of screening for possible complications much earlier in labor than ever before. The phonotransducer is a combination of mechanical and electrical filtering of fetal heart activity. It is an effective means of obtaining reliable information in over 80 percent of early labor cases.

The phonotransducer is the easiest transducer to apply. The area of maximum fetal heart sound is located by using a fetal stethoscope. (The best FHR signal is usually through the back and shoulder of the fetus.) The phonotransducer is placed over the area and secured with tape or the rubber belt that comes with the unit.

The Doppler Transducer

The Doppler transducer is an ultrasonic device that monitors the fetal heart rate by detecting

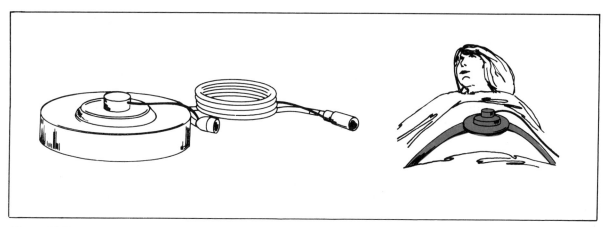

Figure 14-2

The phonotransducer is placed on the abdomen over the spot of maximum fetal heart sound.

the fetal heart movement. Its primary advantage over the phonotransducer is its relative insensitivity to talking, abdominal noises and maternal heart sound. It provides excellent information on fetal heart activity. It can be used to localize the placenta.

The Doppler transducer is placed on the abdomen. After a waiting period of 10 to 20 seconds, which is needed for the amplifier to stabilize, it is manually moved along the contour of the abdomen until the spot is found where the fetal heartbeat is the strongest. The transducer is then secured to this spot by tape or by using the rubber strap supplied with the unit. The transducer must be repositioned if the patient or fetus changes positions.

Movement of the fetal body or of an extremity produces an abrupt, short, large-amplitude signal. Other detectable movements include fetal hiccups and breathing and maternal bowel peristalsis.

Clinical situations in which the Doppler instrument has been found to be useful include

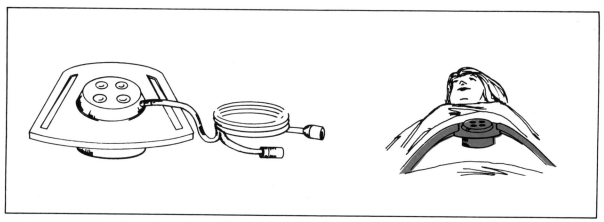

Figure 14-3

The Doppler transducer uses ultrasound to detect fetal heart movements.

early detection of pregnancy, diagnosis of fetal death in utero, detection of a remote fetal heart, intermittent observation of the rate and rhythm of the fetal pulse, placental localization, diagnosis of multiple pregnancy, the differential diagnosis of vaginal bleeding during pregnancy, and fetal monitoring in the third trimester and during labor.

An incidental discovery attributable to use of the Doppler instrument is that the average fetal pulse rate is 170 to 179 in the eighth to eleventh week of pregnancy and slows to an average of 149 by the sixteenth week.

DIRECT METHOD

The direct method of fetal monitoring involves the use of various types of EKG electrodes with or without an intrauterine catheter. The direct method is more reliable and exact than the indirect method. It permits monitoring of the fetal EKG both during and between contractions. However, it is limited because it requires skilled personnel to attach the electrode and place the catheter. Also, the patient must have ruptured membranes and the presenting part must be low enough to allow for the correct placement of the electrode. Direct fetal monitoring cannot be used with such complications as placenta previa and premature labor; neither can it be used for monitoring the second twin.

Intrauterine Catheter

Within the uterus, uterine contractions cause pressure changes in the trapped fluid. A thin, flexible polyethylene catheter filled with distilled water may be used as a fluid trap to bring these pressure changes out to a transducer which in turn translates the fluid pressure into an electrical signal. This signal gives simple, reliable information on the beginning of the uterine contraction, its duration and absolute strength.

Sterile technique is used when inserting the catheter. If a fetal scalp electrode is to be used with the catheter, the catheter is inserted before the electrode is attached. This is necessary in order to minimize the possibility of dislodging the electrode during insertion of the catheter.

- See procedure given later in this unit.

EKG Electrode

The EKG electrode is attached to the presenting part of the fetus in order to directly monitor the fetal heart rate. Sterile technique is used when attaching the electrode to the fetus. The presenting part of the fetus must be clearly identified and must be far enough into the birth canal to allow for correct placement of the electrode. *CAUTION:* Do not apply the electrode over the face or fontanels of the fetus. If membranes have not ruptured, an amniotomy must be performed.

- See procedure given later in this unit.

INTERPRETATIONS

There are many companies that manufacture monitoring systems. Each system is accompanied by specific instructions for its use. Most companies send a representative to give operating instructions to the obstetrical staff.

Every obstetrical nurse should pursue the study of fetal monitoring and the interpretations of fetal heart rate patterns. The fetal heart signal has a two-phase, galloping rhythm with a rate of 120 to 160 beats per minute. The first phase represents atrial contraction; the second reflects AV valve closure and semilunar valve opening. Pulsatile blood flow in the umbilical and other fetal vessels produces single-phase sounds which are higher pitched than the fetal heart signal. The umbilical sound is characterized also by frequent changes in location. The placental sound is complex, combining a windlike sound

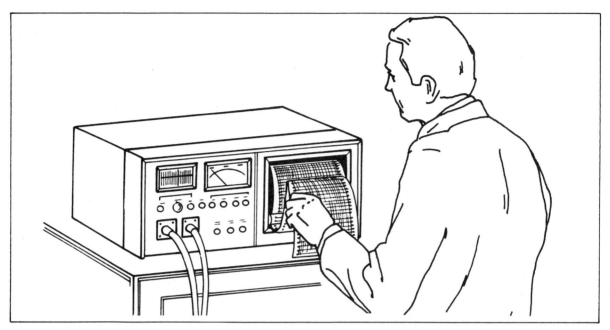

Figure 14-4

*A fetal monitor such as this records information received from some types of trans-
ducers. The transducer picks up a signal and transmits it as an electric impulse which
is recorded by the monitor.*

at the maternal pulse rate (70 to 90) and the
umbilical signal at the fetal rate (120 to 160).
The placental sound is generated only in the area
of umbilical cord insertion and cannot be detected over the remainder of the placenta.

Fetal heart rate patterns can indicate such
conditions as head compression, uteroplacental
insufficiency, cord compression, uterine contractions, and prolonged bradycardia. However,
study and practice are recommended in order to
learn how to use the monitoring equipment and
to be able to interpret the readings.

Fetal monitoring provides information concerning the fetal heart rate and the uterine
contractions. The top half of the fetal monitor
screen represents the fetal heart rate frequency.
It indicates the fetal heart rate instantaneously
with beat-to-beat recording, the baseline heart,

variability, and periodic fetal heart rate changes,
figure 14-5.

The fetal heart rate baseline is usually 120 to
160 beats per minute. A variability of the baseline reflects autonomic control. Good variability
is 3 to 10 percent of the baseline. Excessive
variability (15 percent) may be an early sign of
distress or stress. Minimal variability is 3 percent
of the baseline, figure 14-6. Loss of beat-to-beat
variability must be checked as it is a sign of nervous system hypoxia. Minimal variability could
also be an indication of prematurity, or the
presence of drugs in the fetal circulation. This is
especially true of tranquilizers, narcotics, and
phenothiazines given during labor.

A heart rate of less than 120 beats per minute
is *fetal bradycardia*. Moderate bradycardia in the
fetus is 100 to 119 beats per minute; marked

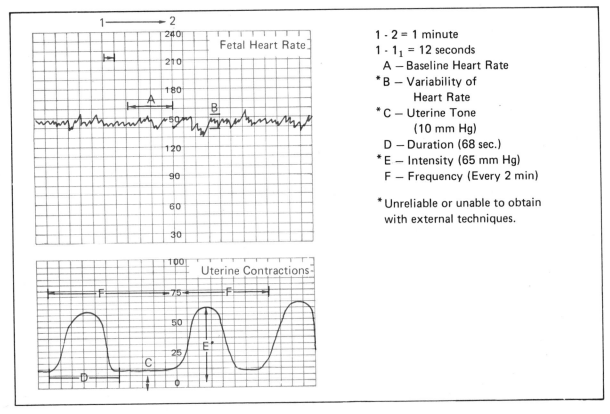

1 - 2 = 1 minute
1 - 1₁ = 12 seconds
 A — Baseline Heart Rate
*B — Variability of
        Heart Rate
*C — Uterine Tone
        (10 mm Hg)
 D — Duration (68 sec.)
*E — Intensity (65 mm Hg)
 F — Frequency (Every 2 min)

*Unreliable or unable to obtain
 with external techniques.

Figure 14-5
The top half of the monitor tracing indicates beat-to-beat recording of the FHR, baseline heart rate, variability, and periodical FHR changes. The bottom half indicates the increment, acme, and decrement of uterine contractions as well as the baseline tone, frequency, duration, and intensity of the contractions.

bradycardia is 99 beats or less per minute. Brady-cardia usually clears up at the time of delivery; however, it could be an indication of a congenital heart lesion.

Fetal tachycardia is a rapid heart rate, usually 160 or more beats per minute. It may be associated with maternal fever, dehydration and acidosis, fetal immaturity or prematurity, or mild fetal hypoxia. It is a very serious sign when associated with any uteroplacental insufficiency pattern, severe cord compression, thick meconium stain, or loss of beat-to-beat variability of the baseline. Transient rises in fetal heart rate

and referred to as *accelerations;* transient falls as *decelerations.*

The bottom half of the fetal monitor screen represents the uterine contractions. The increment, acme, and decrement of the contraction is shown as well as the baseline tone, frequency, duration, and intensity of the contraction.

Acute Fetal Distress

Fetal heart rate patterns indicating acute fetal distress are: (1) late decelerations of any severity, and (2) variable decelerations which last more

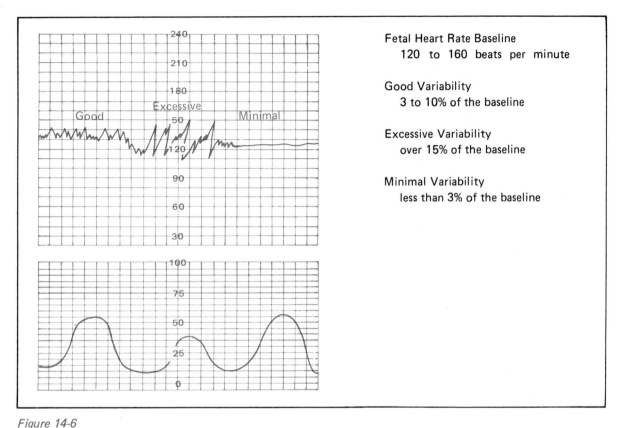

Fetal Heart Rate Baseline
 120 to 160 beats per minute

Good Variability
 3 to 10% of the baseline

Excessive Variability
 over 15% of the baseline

Minimal Variability
 less than 3% of the baseline

Figure 14-6

Baseline fetal heart rate variability. Excessive variability or loss of beat-to-beat (minimal) variability may be a sign of fetal distress. The bottom portion of the chart indicates uterine contractions.

than one minute where the fetal heart rate has dropped to 60 beats per minute or less. *Acute fetal distress* during labor may be defined as fetal compromise related to the recurring stress of the uterine contractions or umbilical cord compression. Diagnosis of fetal distress and appropriate nursing actions are shown in figure 14-7.

FETAL HEART RATE PATTERNS

Fetal heart rate patterns are a visible means of determining the condition of the fetus throughout labor. Although the majority of uterine contractions occur without fetal heart rate changes, the contractions do cause an effect on

the fetus, umbilical cord and *intervillous* (between villi) blood flow.

An irregularity of the baseline fetal heart rate appears to be an important indication of the maturity of the autonomic nervous system. If there is an increased baseline change between uterine contractions, it may indicate fetal tachycardia. Fetal tachycardia is frequently associated with immaturity, maternal fever, or minimal fetal hypoxia. Tachycardia shown late in the contracting phase of the uterus may be an early sign of fetal distress. When it is associated with late or prolonged variable deceleration and especially if minimal irregularity is present, fetal distress is occurring. Persistent pure bradycardia

DIAGNOSIS OF FETAL DISTRESS

Warning signs:

   a)   mild cord compression (variable deceleration)
   b)   tachycardia of 160 beats per minute or greater
   c)   smooth baseline FHR (i.e., absence of the normal baseline FHR variability)

Ominous signs:

   a)   cord compression (variable deceleration) which lasts longer than one minute, and drops to less than
        60 beats per minute or less, progressively worsening
   b)   uteroplacental insufficiency (late deceleration) of any magnitude, with or without tachycardia. If it
        is associated with a very smooth baseline FHR, the situation is serious. It is less serious if it is
        associated with normal baseline FHR variability.

NURSING INTERVENTION FOR FETAL DISTRESS

   1.   Change mother's position in order to relieve pressure on the umbilical cord and to correct maternal
        supine hypotension by taking the weight of the uterus off the vena cava.
   2.   Monitor FHR frequently to detect changes in pattern.
   3.   Decrease uterine activity by discontinuing administration of pitocin. Abnormally strong contrac-
        tions, or those that last for a long time, may impair placental circulation.
   4.   Administer oxygen to the mother at a rate of 6 to 7 liters per minute by a tightly fitted face mask.
   5.   Monitor mother's blood pressure.
   6.   Prepare for operative delivery. (If ominous FHR patterns persist for thirty minutes after the institu-
        tion of the above measures, immediate termination of labor may be considered.)

Figure 14-7

Diagnosis of and nursing care for fetal distress (Adapted from materials supplied by Corometrics Medical Systems Inc.)

of the baseline — not associated with other periodic fetal heart rate changes — has not been associated with depressed newborns, but pure bradycardia may be associated with congenital heart lesions. Sympathetic drugs such as adrenalin increase heart rate while parasympathetic drugs decrease the heart rate.

Acceleration occurs in about 30 percent of all labors. If the drug *atropine* is given, the occurrence is 80 percent. The accelerations are due to intermittent bursts of sympathetic activity and do not reflect any fetal jeopardy.

Decelerations are uniform in their shape; in that they tend to mirror the uterine contraction curve. As shown in figure 14-9, there are three types of decelerations:

1. Early deceleration from head compression

2. Late deceleration, which denotes utero-placental insufficiency, is always sinister

3. Variable deceleration, which is the most common type pattern, denotes umbilical cord compression

There is no treatment for early deceleration and no necessity for any treatment. However, any late deceleration is always harmful. Late decelerations are characterized by:

• Late onset in the contracting phase of the uterus

	Early Decelerations	Late Decelerations	Variable Decelerations
1. Shape	Uniform	Uniform	Variable
2. Association with baseline	None	Tachycardia-high normal (120-160)	No change unless severe then bradycardia
3. Timing	Early	Late	Variable
4. Physiology	Head Compression	Uteroplacental insufficiency	Cord Compression
5. Clinical input	Innocuous	Ominous	Variable
6. Duration	Usually < 60 seconds almost never > 90 seconds	Usually under 90 seconds	Usually <60 seconds—if longer, of clinical importance
7. Lower level of FHR	Not usually below 110—almost never below 100	Usually not under 110 —if under 110 of grave importance and particularly if associated with loss of variability	Not unusual to go below
8. Effect of O₂	None	Positive (?)	None
9. Effect of position change	Little or none	Possible	Possible
10. Effect of Atropine	Positive	None	Positive

Figure 14-8

Decelerations of fetal heart rate (Courtesy of Jack M. Schneider, M.D.)

- Consistent specific fetal heart rate pattern, uniform in shape
- Fetal heart rate that usually does not fall below 120 beats per minute, but may fall to 60 beats per minute
- Duration that is usually less than 90 seconds
- Baseline rate within normal or upper-normal range.

Late decelerations are a probable indication of uteroplacental insufficiency. Administration of high concentrations of oxygen may modify the decelerations; or they may be partially modified by administration of atropine. Other causes are hypertension and too frequent contractions.

A variable deceleration changes both in its shape and in the timing of its onset. Its shape does not reflect the smooth rise and fall of intrauterine pressure and its onset shows no consistent relationship to the contraction. It is probably due to a compressed umbilical cord and usually it is alleviated by the mother changing position. Fetal pH falls slightly in response to transitory variable decelerations but recovers within one to two minutes if there is no added injury.

OXYTOCIN CHALLENGE TEST (OCT)

The oxytocin challenge test is a means of evaluating how well the placenta is nourishing and supplying oxygen to the fetus. The test consists of giving the patient intravenous oxytocin by controlled infusion sufficient to produce 3 contractions in a 10-minute period and simultaneously recording the fetal heart rate and

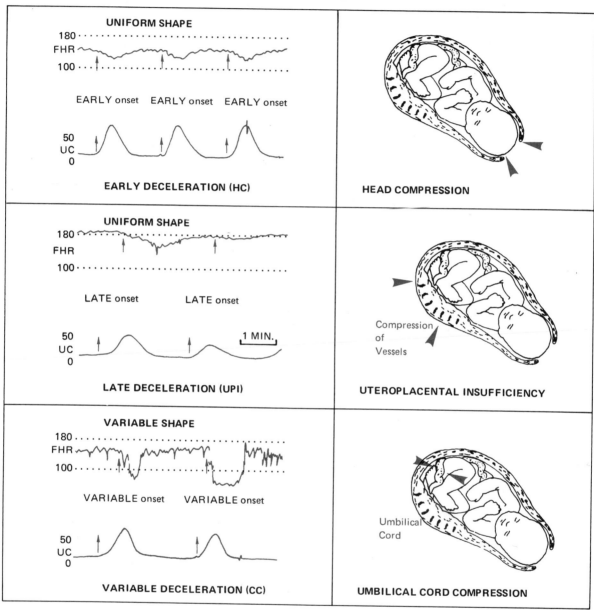

Figure 14-9

Fetal heart rate patterns

uterine contractions with an external transducer. The reaction of the fetal heart to the contractions supplies the needed information. The test may be performed as early as 28 weeks if clinically indicated. Indications are: diabetes mellitus, chronic hypertension, preeclampsia, intrauterine growth retardation, Rh sensitized pregnancy with meconium-stained amniotic fluid, maternal cyanotic heart disease, and history of previous stillborn. Contraindications are: prematurely ruptured membranes, placenta previa, previous cesarean section, or history of premature labors.

The oxytocin challenge test is not dangerous for either the mother or the baby; however, labor could begin as a result. A uterine activity transducer and a Doppler transducer are placed on the patient's abdomen and secured by the straps provided with the unit. The transducers pick up the fetal heart rate and information on the contractions. It then transmits the information to a monitor which records the information on a paper strip. A slow drip I.V. of dextrose is started, and 10–20 minutes of heart rate are recorded. After 10–20 minutes, a second I.V. containing oxytocin is started in order to make the uterus contract. The rate of infusion is controlled by a pump, increasing the rate until 3 contractions occur in a 10-minute period. There is no way to predict how long this will take. However, when 3 contractions within a 10-minute period have been recorded, the intravenous is stopped and the test results read.
CAUTION: Avoid hyperstimulation; signs are uterine contractions which are closer than every 2 minutes, increased tone of contractions, or prolonged uterine contractions. Occasionally, 10 milliunits of oxytocin per minute may be necessary. Generally, the dosage does not exceed 2.5 milliunits per minute.

If late decelerations develop, the test is called positive and suggests diminished uteroplacental reserve. If no late decelerations develop, the test is negative. If negative, the test may be repeated weekly. Tests other than negative (positive, suspicious, hyperstimulation, or unsatisfactory) can be repeated as clinically indicated.

Purpose

The oxytocin challenge test is done to determine how well the placenta is performing its function of feeding and supplying oxygen to the fetus.

Equipment

- Fetal monitor
- Uterine activity transducer and a Doppler transducer or abdominal EKG or phono-transducer
- Blood pressure equipment
- Slow drip I.V. of dextrose
- I.V. solution containing oxytocin
- I.V. pump

Procedure

1. Place patient in semi-Fowler's position to prevent supine hypotension.

2. Check blood pressure every 10 minutes to avoid supine hypotension.

3. Strap transducer to the patient's abdomen.

4. Obtain a baseline FHR (noting rate, variability, etc.) and uterine contraction pattern, if any, for 10 minutes prior to oxytocin infusion. (If 3 contractions are obtained within this 10-minute period with interpretable FHR, it is not necessary to give oxytocin.)

5. Start oxytocin, via I.V. pump, at rate ordered by the doctor.

6. Increase oxytocin every 20 minutes until contractions are 3 in 10 minutes. If late decelerations are repetitive, regardless of uterine contraction frequency, it is not necessary to increase the oxytocin.

7. Discontinue oxytocin and record until uterine contractions diminish and become farther apart or until they stop completely.

Interpretation of Test

1. *Negative* —
   (1) No late periodic FHR changes.
   (2) Usually shows FHR acceleration with fetal movement.
   (3) Implies no placental insufficiency and fetus in good environment for at least one week.

2. *Positive* — consistent and persistent late decelerations of FHR occurring repeatedly with most contractions even if frequency is less than 3 in 10 minutes.
   (1) Usually shows absence of FHR acceleration with fetal movement.
   (2) Implies placental insufficiency may be present and suggests need for intervention depending on fetal maturity.

3. *Suspicious* —
   (1) Lack of FHR acceleration with movement is suspicious.
   (2) Inconsistent but definite late deceleration that does not persist with continued contractions.
   Consider repeating the test in 24 hours or intervention if fetus is mature.

4. *Hyperstimulation* — late deceleration with hyperstimulation suggests a need to repeat the test in 24 hours with lower doses of oxytocin. However, if no decelerations occur with hyperstimulation, the test is interpreted as negative.

A good recording of the FHR and uterine contractions is needed to ensure an interpretable test. If fetal distress is indicated by a positive test or prolonged bradycardia, take the following steps.

1. Stop oxytocin.
2. Increase plain I.V. fluids.
3. Turn patient to left side.
4. Give oxygen at 6 to 7 liters per minute.
5. Place in Trendelenburg position.
6. Check blood pressure frequently.

NONSTRESS TEST (NST)

The nonstress test evaluates the fetal heart rate in response to natural uterine activity or to increased fetal activity. The significant correlation between the presence of fetal heart rate accelerations and the negative oxytocin challenge test led to the development of the nonstress test. In this test, a 10-minute period of fetal heart rate is evaluated. If the fetal heart rate reacts to fetal movements with 2 or more accelerations of at least 15 beats per minute above the baseline and lasts at least 15 seconds, an oxytocin challenge test need not be performed. The length of the test may vary in different hospitals. If the nonstress test is nonreactive and remains so for an additional 20 minutes, an oxytocin challenge test is done. The additional time for nonreaction is necessary to prevent recording only during a fetal sleep cycle, which can last up to 20 minutes. If the nonstress test is suspicious, it is repeated in 24 hours.

The value of the nonstress test is two-fold. First, it is a simpler test than the oxytocin challenge test and requires less time. Thus, it represents an economic saving to the hospital. Second, when administration of oxytocin is inadvisable, the nonstress test provides a noninvasive means of evaluating the fetus. If the woman is experiencing sufficient spontaneous uterine activity (as often happens after an amniocentesis), the nonstress test might also be used as a contraction stress test without the use of oxytocin.

Purpose

The nonstress test is used to evaluate fetal heart rate in response to fetal or uterine activity when the oxytocin challenge test is contraindicated.

Equipment

- External monitor
- Blood pressure equipment

Procedure

1. Place the woman in semi-Fowler's position with a pillow under her right hip.
2. Take the woman's blood pressure and pulse every 10 minutes.

3. Strap the monitor to the woman's abdomen at a site where the FHR can best be heard.
4. Instruct the woman to press a button on the monitor each time she feels movement. The movement is then recorded on a tape as a dot or line.
5. If there is no movement within 20 minutes, stimulate the fetus by abdominal or vaginal examination.
6. Record fetal heart rate for an additional 20 minutes.
7. Note the date, time, gestational age of fetus and reason for the test on the tape; sign the tape.

Interpretation of Test

1. Reactive in 10 minutes, figure 14-10. At least 2 accelerations of at least 15 beats per minute and lasting 15 seconds or more with fetal movement.

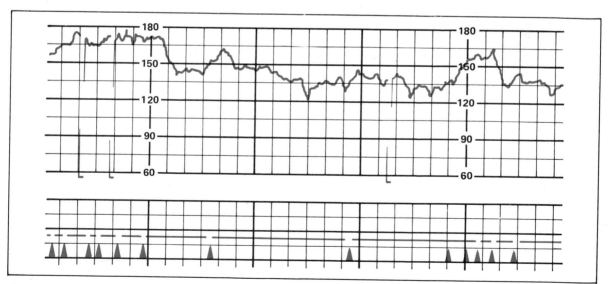

Figure 14-10

Reactive nonstress test reading with fetal movement and acceleration

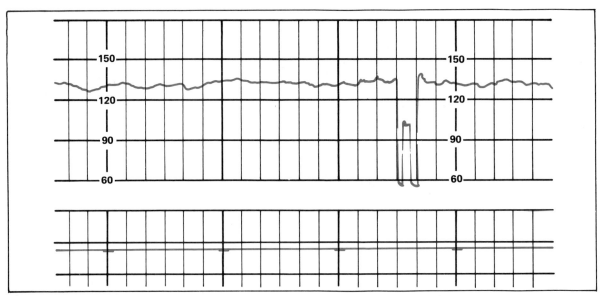

Figure 14-11

Nonreactive nonstress test reading. No accelerations, variability, or movement are present.

2. Nonreactive, figure 14-11. Any of the reactive conditions not met.

3. Suspicious, figure 14-12. Less than two accelerations, 15 beats per minute, last-ing 15 seconds with movement; or accelerations, but unassociated with movement.

4. Unsatisfactory. Recording inadequate for interpretation.

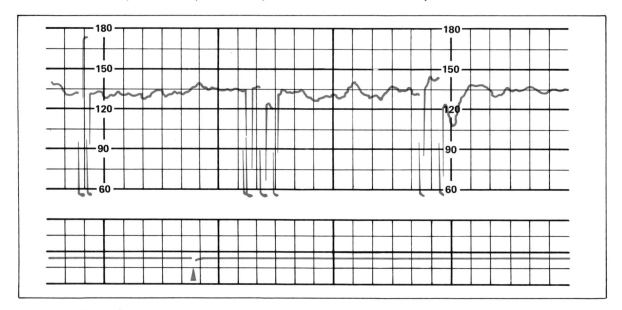

Figure 14-12

Suspicious nonstress test reading

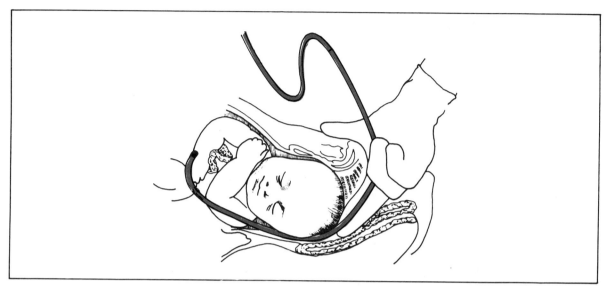

Figure 14-13

Insertion of the intrauterine catheter

INSERTION OF
INTRAUTERINE CATHETER

The intrauterine catheter is inserted by the physician. However, the nurse should be familiar with the procedure.

Purpose

An intrauterine catheter is inserted to determine pressure changes within the uterus by monitoring uterine contractions in order to assess fetal distress.

Equipment

- Sterile gloves and drape
- Cleansing solution
- Catheter insertion guide
- Catheter
- Catheter adapter
- Syringe containing 5 to 10 milliliters of distilled water
- Micropore tape

Procedure

1. Perform a sterile vaginal exam.
2. Place the middle and index fingers between the posterior cervix and the presenting part of the fetus.
3. Place the catheter insertion guide between the fingers.
4. Insert the catheter following the curvature of the pelvis. It must pass the presenting part of the fetus and enter the amniotic cavity, figure 14-13.
5. Lower the catheter insertion guide so that its front end moves behind the presenting part of the fetus. Amniotic fluid will flow out if it is positioned correctly.
6. Insert the perforated end of the catheter into the catheter insertion guide to the mark indicated on the catheter. The catheter may be lowered to check for amniotic fluid, if necessary.

7. Remove the insertion guide when the catheter is properly positioned.

8. Connect the catheter to the stopcock using the catheter adapter.

9. A syringe containing 4 to 5 milliliters of distilled water is connected to the catheter by way of the stopcock, figure 14-14. *CAUTION:* Never use normal saline in the catheter.

10. Flush the catheter with the distilled water to ensure there is no air in the catheter.

11. Turn off the stopcock.

12. Tape the catheter to the patient's thigh to avoid accidental displacements.

13. Place the transducer at a level even with the maternal xiphoid.

INTERNAL FETAL HEART MONITOR

Purpose

The purpose of this procedure is to assess fetal distress by monitoring the fetal heart rate with the use of an electrode attached to the presenting part of the fetus. The procedure is performed by a physician with nursing assistance.

Equipment

- Sterile gloves
- Leg plate coated with conductive gel
- Velcro strap
- Appropriate EKG electrode
- Drive tube
- Guide tube

Precautions

1. Clearly identify the fetal presenting part. Do not apply the electrode over the face or fontanels of the fetus.

2. When removing the electrode, do not pull it from the fetal skin.

3. Use sterile technique.

Preparation

1. Apply conductive gel to the metal surface on the back of the leg plate.

2. Place the leg plate on the inner upper aspect of the thigh.

3. Fasten leg plate with a Velcro strap.

Procedure

1. Unpack and remove ends of electrode wires from between the drive and guide tubes.

2. Retract the drive tube and electrode one inch inside the guide tube.

3. Do a vaginal examination and advance the guide tube between the examining fingers until it reaches the presenting part.

4. Hold the guide tube so that it is at a right angle to, and pressing firmly against, the presenting part.

5. Grasp the guide tube grip. Advance the drive tube and the electrode through the guide tube until the electrode reaches the fetus, figure 14-15.

6. Maintain pressure against the presenting part and rotate the drive tube clockwise until slight resistance is met.

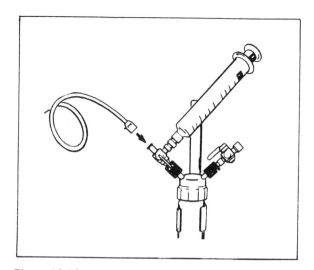

Figure 14-14

A syringe of distilled water is connected to the catheter.

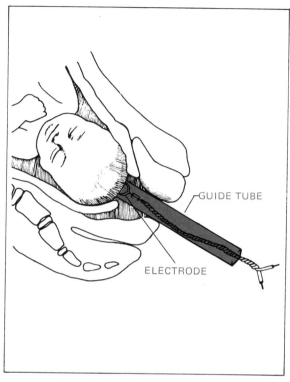

GUIDE TUBE

ELECTRODE

Figure 14-15

Attaching an electrode to the head of a fetus

7. Attachment is indicated by resistance to further rotation and recoil of the drive tube which usually occurs after one or two turns.

8. Release the locking device on the drive tube by slipping wires out of the slotted drive tube handle. Carefully slide the guide and drive tubes off the electrode wires.

9. Attach the other end of the electrode to the leg plate on the mother's thigh.

The strip chart and the rate meter on the monitor should show the instantaneous fetal heart rate. The patient's name, hospital number, position (of the presenting part), dilatation, date, onset time of monitoring, and reason for monitoring should be written on the recorded information. To remove the electrode, simply rotate the body or wires of the electrode counterclockwise. *CAUTION:* Do not pull the electrode from the fetal skin.

FETAL BLOOD SAMPLING

Fetal blood sampling is a method of determining fetal distress by analyzing a small sample of blood taken from the presenting part of the fetus. This can be done during the course of labor if the cervix is dilated enough to allow withdrawal of fetal blood into a capillary tube from a small puncture in the skin of the presenting part of the fetus. The fetal pH blood values normally decline during the intrapartum period from 7.30–7.35 to 7.20–7.25. It is recommended that delivery be accomplished immediately if two successive determinations are below 7.20.

Indications that a sample of fetal blood should be obtained for analysis include: (1) abnormal baseline fetal heart rate (under 120 or over 160);

(2) presence of late deceleration periodic heart rate pattern; (3) presence of severe variable deceleration periodic heart rate pattern; (4) loss of beat-to-beat heart rate variability; (5) inability to define type of deceleration pattern; (6) assessment of fetal glucose level, gases and other.

Before performing the procedure for obtaining the blood sample, informed consent of the mother, and ideally the father, must be obtained. The position and station of the fetus must be determined. The presenting part of the fetus must be at least to the −2 station; dilatation of the cervix must be at least 2 centimeters. If the procedure is done transvaginally the membranes must be ruptured.

Advantages of fetal blood sampling include:

- It prevents unnecessary intervention.
- It indicates a need for further evaluation when blood pH values are unsatisfactory and other clinical signs of distress are absent.
- It provides early diagnosis of acidosis thus preventing a number of neonatal difficulties.

The big disadvantage of the procedure is the actual obtaining of the blood sample which requires repeated vaginal examinations, careful sterile technique, and highly refined skills.

Purpose

The procedure is done to determine the status of the fetus during labor by analyzing a small sample of blood taken from the presenting part of the fetus. The procedure is usually performed by the physician, who is assisted by a nurse.

Equipment

- Sterile gloves
- Sterile tray with cover

- *Amnioscope* (device for looking inside the amniotic cavity)
- Light source for amnioscope
- Long-handled forceps for cotton balls
- Cotton balls or large, long swab
- Ethyl chloride/silicone ointment
- Handle for puncture blade
- Appropriate shallow, squared puncture blade (do NOT substitute)
- Long, heparinized capillary tube
- Transport tubing for capillary tube
- Magnetic stirring rod and magnet; sealing wax
- Ice tray

Procedure

1. Place the patient in stirrups in lithotomy position or on her side.
2. Perform a vaginal examination. This is done to determine (1) if the membranes have ruptured, (2) the assessibility of the presenting part, and (3) the size of amnioscope needed.
3. Insert amnioscope using the examining finger for guidance.
4. Attach the light source to the amnioscope and observe the presenting part.
5. Clean presenting part with a sterile cotton swab.
6. Apply ethyl chloride to the presenting part; remove any excess with sterile swab.
7. Apply silicone ointment to the area.
8. Puncture appropriate area with the fetal scalp blade.
9. Withdraw a sample of fetal blood from the puncture site with a heparinized capillary tube.

10. Mix the blood sample with a magnetic stirring rod in the capillary tube. Place the transport tubing in the ice tray.

11. Clean the puncture site with sterile cotton swabs. Apply gentle pressure for at least 90 seconds in order to stop the bleeding.

12. Observe the puncture site to determine if bleeding has stopped.

13. Analyze the blood sample immediately.

SUGGESTED ACTIVITIES

- Arrange to have a representative of a company that sells fetal monitors visit the class and demonstrate the use of fetal monitors.
- With the aid of the instructor, practice reading fetal monitor charts.
- Under the supervision of the instructor, arrange with the obstetrical unit of a local hospital to observe the attachment of a fetal electrode and/or the obtaining of a fetal blood sample.
- Make a chart indicating the type of fetal monitor, how it is applied, the condition that indicates its use, and the contraindications, if any.
- Define and indicate the significance of the following:
  - Early deceleration
  - Variable decelerations
  - Late decelerations
  - Prolonged decelerations

REVIEW

A. Multiple Choice. Select the best answer.

1. Slow heart rate of less than 120 beats per minute is fetal
   a. tachycardia
   b. acceleration
   c. bradycardia
   d. cardiac arrest

2. Information on how well the placenta is nourishing and supplying oxygen to the fetus is obtained by the
   a. phonotransducer
   b. uterine activity transducer
   c. intrauterine catheter
   d. oxytocin challenge test

3. Direct fetal monitoring can take place
   a. any time after 28 weeks gestation
   b. early in labor
   c. only after membranes have ruptured
   d. a and b

4. In order to obtain a fetal blood sample, the presenting part must be at least to the
   a. −2 station
   b. ischial spine
   c. +4 station
   d. ischial tuberosity

5. The phonotransducer is able to supply information on fetal heart rate by using
   a. recorded electrical impulses
   b. ultrasonic sound
   c. microphone amplification
   d. a gauge to record intrauterine pressure

6. Nervous system hypoxia may be indicated on the fetal monitor as
   a. excessive variability of heart rate
   b. minimal variability of heart rate
   c. heart rate of over 160 beats per minute
   d. heart rate of less than 120 beats per minute

7. The top half of the fetal monitor indicates
   a. fetal heart rate   c. pH of fetal blood
   b. uterine contractions   d. all of these

8. The purpose of the intrauterine catheter is to determine
   a. if meconium is present
   b. muscle tonus in the abdominal wall
   c. fetal heart rate
   d. pressure changes within the uterus

B. Match the descriptions in column I to the correct term in column II.

Column I	Column II
1. uterine contractions closer than every two minutes or prolonged contractions	a. acceleration
	b. amnioscope
	c. deceleration
2. rapid heart rate of more than 160 beats per minute	d. hyperstimulation
	e. loss of beat-to-beat variability
3. transient rise in fetal heart rate	f. fetal tachycardia
4. transient fall in fetal heart rate	
5. device for looking inside the amniotic cavity	
6. minimal variability of fetal heart rate baseline	

C. Briefly answer the following questions.

1. What is a transducer?

2. Name three types of external transducers used for fetal monitoring.

3. Explain the direct method of fetal monitoring. What are its limitations?

4. List five of the most important reasons for performing fetal monitoring.

5. Name three indications for fetal blood sampling.

6. Define acute fetal distress.

7. List three confirmations of fetal presentation or position and when they are possible.

UNIT 15

PAIN RELIEF FOR
LABOR AND DELIVERY

OBJECTIVES

- State the purpose of anesthesia.
- Distinguish between the anesthesias given during childbirth in terms of administration, desired effects, and untoward effects.
- Name the advantages of using regional rather than general anesthesia.

Although the modern philosophy of child-birth stresses the fact that it is a completely normal and natural process, there are occasions when anesthesia is needed. It must be understood that any drugs taken by the mother before delivery also affect the baby. Some drugs produce a sleepy and lethargic baby; other drugs have little effect on the baby. Since the chief objective is to deliver a healthy baby with as little discomfort as possible for the mother, the choice of medication is left to the obstetrician.

The labeling of drugs used in labor and delivery must include a list of the known short-term and long-term effects that the drug can have on the mother and the child. This information also must describe the effect the drug has on the duration of labor or delivery. The label also indicates whether forceps or other interventions or resuscitation of the newborn are likely to be needed. The effect the drug has on the later growth, development, and functional maturation of the child must also be indicated. Labeling must also include the effect the drug has on the mother's milk and how it can affect the nursing infant.

There is no drug that overcomes the discomfort of labor completely and yet is perfectly safe for both mother and baby. There are many drugs, however, that permit the patient to relax between contractions, thus conserving the patient's strength.

ANALGESIA

Analgesic drugs eliminate the sensation of pain and are generally used in the first stage of labor. These include sedatives, amnesics, narcotic analgesics, and inhalation agents.

Sedatives

Tranquilizers such as Vistaril, Phenergan, and Sparine are often used to relieve anxiety and to relax the patient. These drugs help to relieve tension without confusing the brain. They are particularly helpful for long labors if tension is building.

188

Barbiturates such as Seconal and Nembutal are given to sedate the mother and produce sleep. Barbiturates do not relieve pain. If it is suspected that the mother is in false labor, she may be given a barbiturate so she can go to sleep. However, barbiturates cross the placental barrier rapidly and are not handled well by the newborn. They are not used near the time of delivery.

Amnesics

Amnesic drugs may be used throughout labor to induce loss of memory of pain. Scopolamine is an amnesic that was used quite commonly in the past but is seldom used today. Scopolamine does not stop the pain sensation but it does alter thought processes. Women who receive this drug feel all of the pain sensations of labor but do not remember the pain later.

Narcotic Analgesics

Narcotic analgesics such as Demerol act to relieve pain. They also produce sedation and decrease anxiety. Narcotics have a depressant effect on neonatal respiration and so are not given close to the time of delivery. They also can have adverse side effects for the mother.

Inhalation Agents

Inhalation agents such as nitrous oxide, Trilene, or Penthrane can be used during the first stage of labor to produce an analgesic effect. The gas is inhaled during the contraction and makes the mother feel light-headed. It does not cause any significant respiratory depression or other side effects on the mother and baby and does not interfere with the uterine contractions or labor progress. It can be administered by the patient herself after an explanation of its purpose and use.

ANESTHESIA

Anesthesia relieves pain at specific sources. It may be used in both the first and second stages of labor, and during the episiotomy procedure and repair. Anesthesia can be administered as general anesthesia or regional anesthesia.

General Anesthesia

If used, general or inhalation anesthesia is usually administered in the second stage of labor. It affects the entire system of the patient and may be passed to the fetus through the placenta. Because it may cause toxic effects in the fetus, interfere with the normal establishment of the baby's respiration, and cause postpartum hemorrhage in the mother, it must be administered only by a skilled anesthetist. General anesthetics used are cyclopropane, ethylene, nitrous oxide, ether, chloroform, and thiopental (Pentothal); they are administered intravenously. General anesthesia is seldom used in a normal birth situation.

Regional Anesthesia

Regional anesthesia interrupts the pain pathway at a specific source. It is the safest method of anesthetizing a patient because it involves only a localized area. Regional anesthesia has little direct effect on the baby. It also is desirable for the mother as it causes no nausea or vomiting and it lets her be awake to help during the delivery. Examples of regional anesthesia procedures are paracervical block, caudal, lumbar epidural block, spinal, saddle block, pudendal block and local, figure 15-1.

Paracervical Block Anesthesia. This anesthesia can be administered to the patient in labor when only partial dilatation of the cervix has occurred. An anesthetic solution is injected into the region

TYPE	ADMINISTRATION SITE	AREA AFFECTED	MAY BE GIVEN AT	TAKES EFFECT IN	EFFECTS LAST FOR	COMMENTS
Para-cervical block	Into nerve trunks at both sides of cervix	Cervix and uterus	Dilatation of 4–9 cm	3–4 min	1–2 hr	Given by physician. May be repeated as needed. May cause slowing of fetal heart rate
Caudal block	Into caudal canal at base of sacrum	Below ribs to knees	Dilatation of greater than 5 cm	15–20 min	45 min–1 1/2 hr	Repeat dose may be administered through catheter placed in caudal canal. Given by an anesthesiologist. May cause a drop in maternal blood pressure, resulting in a drop in fetal heart rate. Diminishes urge to push
Lumbar epidural block	Lumbar spine region	Waist to knees	Dilatation of greater than 5 cm	10–15 min	45 min–1 1/2 hr	Same as for caudal block
Spinal block	Between 3rd and 4th lumbar vertebrae	Breast to toes	2nd stage of labor	3–5 min	1 1/2–2 hr	Often used for cesarean section. Possible drop in maternal blood pressure
Saddle block	Between 3rd and 4th lumbar vertebrae	Inner thighs, perineum, and buttocks	2nd stage of labor	3–5 min	1 1/2–2 hr	Used for discomfort during delivery or when forceps are indicated. Given by physician or anesthesiologist. Possible drop in maternal blood pressure
Pudendal block	Into pudendal nerve trunks via vagina	Vagina and perineum	2nd stage of labor	2–3 min	1 hr	Used for discomfort during delivery or when forceps are indicated. Used for episiotomy and repair. Fetal risks unknown.
Local infiltration	Perineum	Perineum	2nd or 3rd stage of labor	5 min	20 min	Used for episiotomy and/or its repair

Figure 15-1
Regional anesthetics

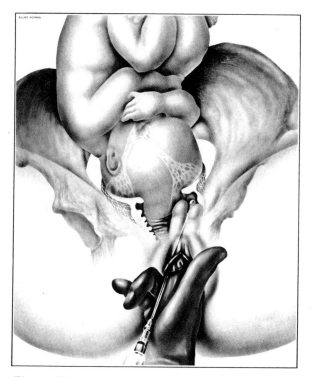

Figure 15-2

Paracervical block

around the cervix to reduce the pain caused by cervical dilatations. However, some obstetricians believe that this kind of anesthesia could have a depressing effect on the infant and may slow the rate of cervical dilatation.

Caudal Anesthesia. In caudal anesthesia, a local anesthetic drug is injected into the caudal space in the sacrum. The advantage of this form of anesthesia is that the mother is not able to feel the labor contractions. She must have careful nursing care. The nurse must time and evaluate the contractions by placing her hand on the patient's abdomen or by using a fetal monitor. The bladder must be kept empty, by catheterization if necessary, since the patient is not able to void spontaneously. The patient's blood pressure must be taken frequently. Caudal

anesthesia sometimes causes a drop in the mother's blood pressure which can have an adverse effect on the fetus.

The technique of caudal anesthesia, discovered in 1901, was first applied to childbirth in 1909. Use of the continuous technique was limited due to its reputed high rate of failure. However, with increased clinical experience, the failure rate has been considerably reduced. If properly administered, continuous caudal anesthesia is one of the safest techniques for both mother and fetus.

Anesthesia is begun when the patient is in *active labor;* that is, contractions are 45 seconds or more in duration at intervals of 2 to 3 minutes; cervical dilatation is 6 centimeters or more for primigravidas, 4 centimeters or more for multiparas. The patient is placed in a modified Sims' position. Caudal punctures are made with a thin wall, 18-gauge needle with stylet. Vinyl tubing is inserted into the caudal canal. Eight milliliters of the chosen drug — such as mepivacaine hydrochloride (Carbocaine) — is injected slowly through the vinyl tubing. The patient is then observed for signs of inadvertent spinal block. Five to ten minutes later, if the catheter appears to be in the correct position, a full dosage of 17 to 22 milliliters of the drug is injected.

Lumbar Epidural Block. An epidural block is much like the caudal anesthesia. It is performed by injecting a local anesthetic into the epidural space of the lumbar region; this blocks precisely the same anatomic area as the caudal block.

There are several advantages of a spinal epidural block over a caudal block. Less anesthetic is required and the onset of uterine pain relief is more rapid. There is less risk of infection and there is no risk of puncturing the maternal rectum or the head of the fetus.

Both caudal and epidural blocks eliminate the reflex urge to bear down during the second stage. If this becomes a problem, low forceps may be indicated to help in delivery.

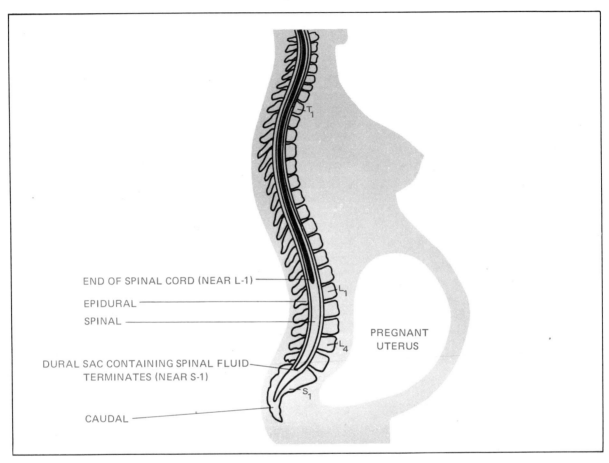

END OF SPINAL CORD (NEAR L-1)

EPIDURAL

SPINAL

DURAL SAC CONTAINING SPINAL FLUID TERMINATES (NEAR S-1)

CAUDAL

PREGNANT UTERUS

Figure 15-3

Injection sites for regional anesthesia in obstetrics

Spinal Anesthesia. The spinal anesthetic is injected into the spinal fluid. It is generally given after the cervix is fully dilated. The spinal is sometimes used for a mother who is extremely tired and cannot push any longer. It allows the doctor to use forceps to deliver the baby. The spinal can also relax a tense perineal floor. Spinal anesthesia can be given for a cesarean delivery.

The mother's blood pressure may be lowered after a spinal is given so she must be carefully monitored. To guard against possible headache, the patient is required to remain flat on her back for 4 to 8 hours after the anesthetic is given. The so-called spinal headache is caused because of leakage of spinal fluid through the puncture in the dura which causes pressure changes within the spinal cord. This problem has been lessened with the use of finer gauge needles in administration.

Saddle Block Anesthesia. Saddle block anesthesia is a form of low spinal anesthesia. It becomes effective within 2 to 3 minutes after administration and is of short duration. Therefore, it is necessary to time its administration properly; delivery should be anticipated within an hour or so following the onset of the anesthesia.

The drug is introduced into the lowest part of the spinal canal. It provides insensitivity to the area that would come in contact with a saddle if one were horseback riding; hence the name, *saddle block*. Headaches sometimes occur following anesthesia of this type, therefore, it is recommended that the patient be kept flat in bed 4 to 8 hours following delivery.

Pudendal Block Anesthesia. This anesthesia affects the area of the perineum and vagina. Procaine, Metycaine, or Xylocaine may be injected into the pudendal nerve trunk, numbing the birth canal and perineal area. It is used for episiotomy, delivery, and repair of the perineum. It relaxes the perineal muscles but the patient is still able to aid contractions by bearing down.

Local Anesthesia. Local anesthesia may be produced by injecting an anesthetic drug directly into the perineal area. This numbs the perineum in preparation for the episiotomy. It is administered just before the baby is born. If this injection is not given prior to birth, it is given after the baby is born so the repair of the episiotomy is painless. In many instances there is a natural anesthetic action produced by the pressure of the baby's presenting part against the perineum. When this happens a local anesthetic may not be necessary until after the birth when the natural anesthetic action is no longer in effect.

ABDOMINAL DECOMPRESSION

A method of relieving the pain of childbirth without anesthesia is called the *Emerson Birtheez method.* By touching a microswitch which she holds in her hand, the woman can turn on a negative-pressure Birtheez pump each

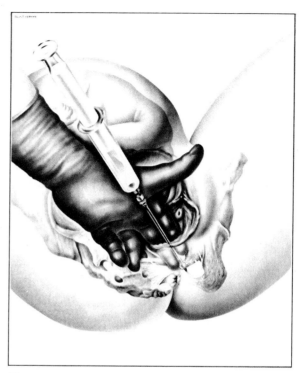

Figure 15-4

Pudendal block

time she feels a contraction start. The pump is connected to an airtight dome over the abdomen. As the pump quickly removes air from this dome, the mother's abdominal wall is lifted somewhat. This moves the abdominal wall out of the way of the uterus permitting contractions to take place more efficiently. There is less pain and the labor is shortened. One of the important benefits of this method is the ability of many patients to go through labor without anesthesia. The babies show no respiratory distress and begin to cry as soon as they are delivered.

Pain-relieving drugs may be necessary during the birth process, at least in small amounts. However, if a mother can help her child by using techniques that reduce the need of anesthesia to a minimum, it is worth the effort.

PREPARED CHILDBIRTH LABOR GUIDE • LAMAZE TECHNIQUES © Childbirth Education Association of Seattle

	Pre-Labor	Established Labor: Stage I: Effacement [%] & Dilatation of Cervix [cm]	Stage II	Stage III
	Softening of Cervix	Remember: Lie on side — Breathing: Deep Chest / Focal Point Accelerated / Effleurage Relax Transition	Birth of Baby	Delivery of placenta and immediate recovery

Dilatation scale: 1cm 2cm 3cm 4cm 5cm 6cm 7cm 8cm 9cm 10cm

Contraction timing:
- 35-40 sec / Rest 15-20 min
- 45-60 sec / Rest 3-5 min
- 60-70 sec / Rest 2-3 min
- 60-90 sec / Rest 2-3 min
- 60 sec / Rest 2-3 min

Pre-Labor — Softening of Cervix

Characteristic Signs:
- Nesting urge
- Premonitions
- Sense of exhilaration
- Braxton-Hicks contractions
- False labor
- Effacement

Activity:
- Prepare and pack for hospital and baby
- Mild exercise may relieve contractions
- Mild activity
- Rest and nap

Established Labor: Stage I (Accelerated)

Characteristic Signs:
- Bloody Show
- Contractions become longer, stronger and more frequent
- Membranes may rupture
- Possible back pain
- Excited, confident and talkative

Activity:
- Rest and nap if possible
- Breathing techniques (if necessary)
- Empty bladder every hour
- Analyze & time contractions
  - Call doctor
  - Enter hospital
  - Perineal shave/enema
  - Examinations

Reminders for Coach:
- Time contractions
- Remind her to relax
- Adjust physical environment as needed
- Follow her lead

Stage I (continued)

Signs:
- Feel discouraged
- Feel trapped
- Contractions may be difficult to handle during exams
- Doctor may rupture membranes (Labor will accelerate)
- Monitoring device may be in place

Activity:
- Remain alert, eyes open
- Try to anticipate contraction
- Wipe brow
- Chew ice, damp cloth or sponge
- Empty bladder
- Relax

Coach:
- Offer ice; do back massage/counter pressure for back pain; do effleurage; help with breathing techniques and relaxation
- Offer reassurance

Transition

Signs:
- Strong, irregular contractions
- Pressure on rectum
- Nausea
- Cramps in thighs or legs
- Sensitivity to touch
- Uncontrollable shaking
- Forgetfulness
- Drowsiness
- Irritability
- Urge to push
- Difficult to remain in control

Activity:
- Take each contraction individually
- Remember that this phase is intense but short
- Do not push without permission. Tell Doctor/Nurse immediately

Coach:
- Do not leave her alone
- Be alert to signs of transition
- Help with relaxation between contractions
- Ease back pain

Stage II — Birth of Baby

Events:
- Episiotomy
- Crowning
- Birth of head
- Birth of body

Activity:
- Relax perineum
- Push as directed
- Be prepared to pant during delivery of head

Stage III — Delivery of placenta and immediate recovery

Events:
- Possible uncontrollable shaking
- Possible injection to contract uterus
- Lull in contractions
- Episiotomy repair

Activity:
- Continue breathing patterns with contractions
- Push to deliver placenta
- Transfer of mother to recovery area
- Transfer of baby to nursery
- Uterine massage

Figure 15-5

Prepared childbirth labor guide

SUPPORTIVE NURSING CARE

Much discomfort from labor and delivery can also be alleviated by a supportive nursing approach. The fear-tension-pain syndrome plays a major role in childbirth. If the nurse can keep the laboring woman and her immediate support person well informed of what is happening to the body during the labor process, then the expectant mother's fear level will diminish. With less fear, there is less tension. Therefore, pain is more easily kept under control. The nurse can also reinforce the principle that the body works effectively in the birthing process. The female body is designed to give birth. If the nurse can establish increased confidence that the sensations being felt are normal, then she can greatly reduce the fear and pain perception.

Along with education, the nurse can also help the laboring woman to find a comfortable position. A frequent change of position usually is helpful. The woman may wish to walk during part of her labor. The use of heat and cold are also effective tools in decreasing pain. Cool or warm compresses to the face, neck or back may be comforting. Standing in a shower or sitting in a warm bath (if permitted) can enhance relaxation. Swabbing dry lips and giving sips of fluids or ice chips can also help. A back massage can be very effective in counteracting the pressure felt from a posterior positioned baby. A caring attitude from the nurse can do much to decrease the laboring woman's pain sensations.

If the woman and her support person have attended childbirth preparation classes, they can be encouraged to breathe in the suggested pattern, and to use the other concentration tools taught in class. If medication is medically necessary or desired, an explanation should be given. An informed consent should be obtained. If medication is designated, the woman should never be made to feel that she has in some way failed at childbirth. The goal of all health care providers should be a healthy outcome, and a joyous experience for the expectant parents.

ADMINISTRATION OF INTRAMUSCULAR MEDICATION

Purpose

The nurse should review the technique used and correct any poor technique. The nurse should also understand the seriousness of a mistake made in the administration of a drug. It is necessary to learn the drugs the nurse may administer, their actions, and contraindications.

Equipment

- Disposable needle and syringe
- Water for injection
- Cotton ball; alcohol
- Medications the nurse may administer: Methergin, Lorfan, Atropine, Pitocin, Vistaril, Sparine, Largon, Scopolamine, Vitamin K (Synkayvite)

CAUTION: Never give an intramuscular injection unless you have been taught and have permission to do so.

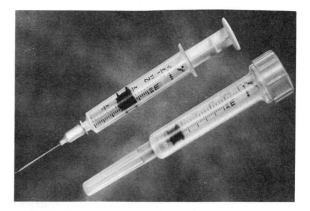

Figure 15-6

The monoject syringe and needle (Courtesy of Sherwood Medical Industries, Inc.)

Procedure

1. Check the doctor's order for medication. Note the medication ordered, the amount and the time to be given.
2. Remove the syringe from the wrapper.
3. Obtain and check the medication with the order. Open the ampule; observe sterile techniques.
4. Remove the cover from the needle. Be sure the size of the needle is correct.
5. Draw the medication into the syringe. Carefully re-cover the needle with the plastic shield.
6. Read the name of the medication from the bottle again and check it against the order.
7. Identify the patient. Call the patient by name and check her wristband. Explain the purpose of the procedure.
8. Expose the site of injection; cleanse the area with an alcohol sponge. Note the landmarks. Be sure nerves and blood vessels are avoided.

9. Pinch the skin and insert the needle into the skin with a quick motion. Pull up on the plunger to check if the needle is in a vein. (If blood appears, carefully withdraw the syringe, placing the alcohol sponge against the skin as you do so. Discard the medication and needle and repeat the procedure.)
10. Push the plunger slowly to inject the medication into the tissues.
11. Remove needle and syringe. Blot the site of injection with an alcohol sponge to check bleeding.
12. Discard the pieces in a plastic container designated for disposable syringes and needles.
13. Chart the medication. Note time, medication, site of injection, and any signs of reactions.
14. Check the patient for any adverse reaction every 15 minutes after administering the medication.

SUGGESTED ACTIVITIES

- Define psychoprophylaxis. Briefly describe its use in obstetrics.
- List at least three analgesics commonly used during the intrapartum period. Include indications and complications.
- Describe the procedures and list indications for and complications of the following modalities:
  - General anesthesia
  - Regional anesthesia
  - Spinal anesthesia
  - Local anesthesia

REVIEW

Multiple Choice. Select the best answer.

1. When saddle block anesthesia is used, the patient is kept flat in bed following delivery for
   a. 4 to 8 hours
   b. 3 to 4 hours
   c. 8 to 10 hours
   d. 12 to 24 hours

2. The mother's blood pressure must be taken frequently in
   a. caudal anesthesia
   b. paracervical block anesthesia
   c. pudendal block anesthesia
   d. saddle block anesthesia

3. Medications that relieve anxiety are called
   a. barbiturates   c. amnesics
   b. tranquilizers   d. narcotics

4. Medications that relieve pain, produce sedation, and decrease anxiety
   are called
   a. barbiturates   c. amnesics
   b. tranquilizers   d. narcotics

5. When medication is administered to reduce the pain caused by
   cervical dilatation, it is called
   a. pudendal block   c. caudal block
   b. paracervical block   d. epidural block

6. A caudal anesthetic is administered to a primigravida when the cervix
   has dilated
   a. 4 centimeters   c. 8 centimeters
   b. 6 centimeters   d. none of these

7. The anesthesia used for repair of the perineum is called
   a. pudendal block   c. lumbar epidural block
   b. paracervical block   d. none of these

UNIT 16

NURSING CARE IN DELIVERY

OBJECTIVES

After studying this unit, the student should be able to:

- List six indications of the second stage of labor.
- Describe nursing care during the second, third and fourth stages of labor.
- State how to prepare the patient for delivery.
- Explain the Apgar Scoring System.
- Describe the immediate care of the newborn.
- List six factors that influence parent-infant bonding.

While watching the progress of the patient in the first stage of labor, the nurse must be alert to the indications that the second stage of labor is beginning. The indications seen in most patients are:

- Rectal bulging during a contraction
- Urge to defecate or "bearing down" sensation
- Rapid dilatation of cervix within a few contractions
- Intense contractions which occur rapidly (one to two minutes apart lasting 60 to 90 seconds)
- Perspiration (beads of perspiration on upper lip)
- Nausea with emesis (occasionally)
- Sudden increase in show

- Rupture of bag of waters
- *Crowning* (appearance of the fetal scalp at the vulva), figure 16-1.

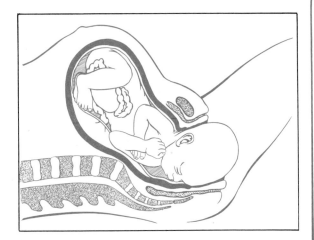

Figure 16-1
Crowning

The most critical time for the mother and baby, as well as an exceedingly busy one for the doctor and nurse, is the second stage of labor. The second stage of labor begins with the complete dilatation and effacement of the cervix and ends with the delivery of the baby.

PREPARING FOR DELIVERY

In some hospitals, women continue to be moved to a delivery room. However, many hospitals across the nation have adopted a family-centered concept. This includes leaving the laboring woman in the same bed surrounded by her support team. She delivers her baby without being moved to a different room. If a delivery room is to be used, there are some basic principles that underlie all common techniques. Procedure outlines are also followed for a cesarean birth.

Hand and Gown Technique

Since the delivery room is an operating room, all personnel are required to scrub their hands according to surgical technique. Sterile caps, masks, and gowns are worn by personnel at the delivery table; circulating personnel wear scrub suits or dresses, masks, and caps.

Delivery Room Setup

Before the patient is moved to the delivery room, it should be set up with the delivery table, sterile instrument table, sterile basins, and an infant warmer with resuscitation equipment for the baby. The sterile packs of linen and equipment should be in place and covered with sterile drapes. When everything is ready for delivery, the circulating nurse uncovers the sterile equipment taking great care not to contaminate it. Adequate preparation eliminates last minute hurry, confusion, and error.

ASSISTING DURING DELIVERY

There are many ways the mother can be made more comfortable during the second stage of labor, figure 16-2. Helping her to relax and at the same time to bear down with the contractions once the cervix is completely dilated helps to ease the delivery. It is futile to have the patient bear down before complete dilatation occurs; it is exhausting and could result in lacerating the cervix. The patient should be kept dry, clean, and as comfortable as possible. Two key concepts should guide the mother and her support team through the second stage of labor. One concept is the importance of not rushing. A woman should be encouraged to follow her own body signals, bearing down or pushing spontaneously as the urge demands. This allows the vaginal tissue to stretch open gently. The second concept is the effective use of different positions. The most common position in North America is semi-sitting with legs raised in stirrups, or with the feet in footrests or resting on the bed. If one position is uncomfortable or progress is slow, take advantage of the other positions that might use gravity to advantage or may aid progress and descent. As delivery approaches, a saddle block, local, or pudendal block may be given to numb the perineum.

POSITIONS FOR THE SECOND STAGE

Semi-Sitting

Advantages

1. Convenient for birth attendant
2. Easy position to maintain

Disadvantages

1. May aggravate hemorrhoids
2. May restrict secrum movement when more room is needed in the pelvis

Second Stage of Labor:	From complete dilatation of the cervix to the end of expulsion of the child (known as the "stage of expulsion"). It usually lasts 1 to 2 hours in the primipara; a few minutes to 1 hour in the multipara.	

PATIENT PROBLEM	NURSING INTERVENTION	RATIONALE
Desire to push; fear of soiling the bed	Explain to the patient and reassure her that this is unavoidable and acceptable at this stage.	The baby gives the mother a feeling of pressure in the rectum as it enters the birth canal. Mother must use her abdominal muscles to expel baby.
	Instruct her to bear down with each contraction until crowning, and then take short, quick breaths.	Mother should not push during crowning in order to avoid perineal lacerations and to allow the baby to be eased out slowly.
Leg cramps	Advise the patient to stretch her leg out forcibly, pulling her foot toward her knee.	Hyperflexion stretches the muscle and breaks the pain pathway.
	If persistent, hot towels may be applied to the affected area.	Heat will aid in muscle relaxation.
Dry lips	Apply oil or cold cream to lips.	Short, shallow breaths during labor tend to dry lips. Oil or cream will prevent cracking and will provide comfort to the patient.
Profuse perspiration	Apply cool cloth to forehead and hands.	Provides soothing comfort to mother during the hard work of labor.
Distended bladder	Assist the physician in catheterization.	A distended bladder impedes the progress of labor and causes the mother unnecessary discomfort.
Anxiety	Keep mother and father informed of the progress of labor and encourage and reassure them.	The more knowledge the mother has of what is happening within her body, the less fear and anxiety she will have. The same holds true for the father or "coach" who will be able to offer additional encouragement and reassurance if he is assured that labor is progressing as it should.
Urge to push during crowning	Encourage panting	Concentrating on proper breathing techniques should help the mother to resist the urge to push during crowning. This will help prevent perineal lacerations, allowing the baby to ease out of the birth canal.

Figure 16-2

Nursing care for discomfort during the second stage of labor (Adapted from Maternal and Child Health, Littlefield, Adams & Co.)

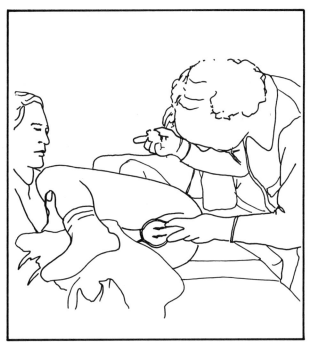

Figure 16-3

   3. May slow passage of head under pubic bone.

Side-Lying, Figure 16-3

Advantages
1. Gravity neutral
2. Useful to slow rapid labor
3. Pressure is off hemorrhoids

Disadvantages
1. May not be familiar to birth attendant assisting in delivery
2. Is unfavorable if you need to speed the second stage

Hands and Knees

Advantages
1. Helps assist rotation of an OP baby
2. May reduce backache

Disadvantage
1. Tiring for long periods

Lying on Back
With legs pulled back mother raises head to push.

Advantage
1. Pulling legs back and apart helps widen pelvic outlet

Disadvantages
1. Supine hypotension
2. Works against gravity

Squatting, Figure 16-4, A–F

Advantages
1. Takes advantage of gravity
2. Widens pelvic outlet to its maximum
3. Requires less bearing down effort
4. May enhance rotation and descent in a difficult birth
5. Helpful if an urge to push is not felt

Disadvantages
1. Difficult to get into position on a bed without squat-bar
2. Difficult for birth attendant to see perineum
3. May result in too rapid expulsion leading to perineal tears
4. May be uncomfortable

Supported Squat
Mother leans with back against support person who holds her under the arms and takes all her weight.

Advantages
1. Allows the pelvis to spread as baby descends
2. Gravity advantage

Disadvantages
1. Hard work for support person
2. Difficult for birth attendant to assist in birth.

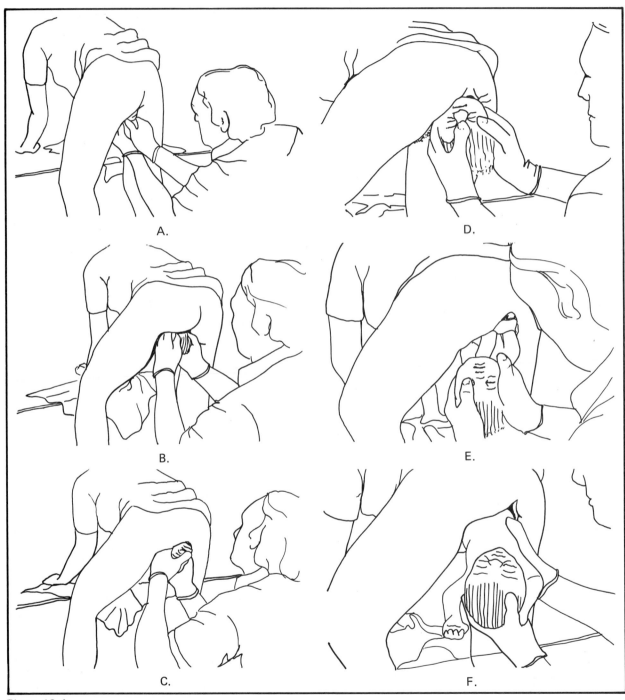

Figure 16-4

A) Within a short time the head has crowned, and delivery ensues. B) Delivery of the head is beginning. C) Complete delivery of the head. D) External rotation and restitution have occurred. E) The mother pushes slightly to facilitate delivery of the infant's body. F) Delivery of the infant's body.

Semi-Lithotomy

This back-lying position has head and shoulders elevated, legs in stirrups, and hips on edge of delivery table.

Advantages

1. Some gravity advantage
2. Mother able to see birth
3. Convenient for attendant
4. May be necessary for interventions

Disadvantages

1. Leg cramps are common
2. Restricts sacral movement
3. Possible supine hypotension

Lithotomy

Advantages

1. Convenient for attendant
2. May be necessary for interventions

Disadvantages

1. Works against gravity
2. Leg cramps are common
3. Difficult to view birth
4. Supine hypotension

After the anesthesia has taken effect and the perineum bulges, the doctor may perform an episiotomy. If so, this procedure is done just before the head of the baby is delivered. An episiotomy is an incision of the perineum made to facilitate delivery. A straight, clean surgical incision is made in lieu of the ragged perineal laceration which might otherwise occur. The direction of the episiotomy can be controlled. It spares the baby from prolonged pushing of its head against the perineum, thus shortening the second stage of labor. If the doctor does an episiotomy, the nurse adds a suture pack and a vaginal pack to the back table setup. The nurse assists the doctor and patient as needed during the actual delivery.

At birth, the infant takes his first breath and makes his first sound, a lusty cry. If he does not breath immediately, the doctor may take measures to stimulate the baby's cry by holding the head down and rubbing the baby's back or by flicking the soles of its feet. The respiratory system, which until now has been dormant, begins to function with this cry. The doctor wipes the mucus from the baby's mouth and checks its respiratory status. The cord is then clamped in two places — about 1 1/2 inches and 2 1/2 inches from the baby. When the doctor cuts the cord, the baby is physically separated from the mother. Figure 16-5 summarizes nursing care during the second stage of labor. After the cord has been cut and tied and the doctor has determined that there are no respiratory problems, the doctor may hand the newborn to the nurse, returning to the care of the mother.

The nurse can then wrap the newborn snugly to ensure warmth before handing it to the parents to facilitate bonding. Bonding is a gradually unfolding relationship which begins during pregnancy. It blossoms with the baby's birth as the parents and baby exchange messages and feelings through the meeting of their eyes, skin-to-skin contact, smell, and sound. The first few minutes and hours of life may be especially influential in the bonding process. During this period, the baby is alert and ready to respond to its environment. The mother and father are physically and emotionally attracted to their baby, and these reciprocal feelings may have long-lasting effects on the parent-child relationship.

The role of touch in maternal-infant bonding is fundamental. The mother may wish to have the newborn placed on her abdomen immediately after birth. To help maintain a warm temperature for the baby, the nurse may cover both mother and baby with a warm blanket. This permits skin-to-skin contact while helping the uterus to become firm through the stimulation of hormone release.

2nd Stage of Labor

- Keep the perineum cleansed.

- Place the patient's legs in stirrups when instructed to do so by the doctor.

- When the doctor is ready, coach the patient to take a couple of deep breaths as soon as the next contraction begins. Then with her breath held, head elevated, chin on chest, have her exert downward pressure exactly as though she were having a bowel movement. Effort should be as sustained as possible, with a quick breath taken every 6 to 12 seconds throughout the contraction. (This is to re-oxygenate the bloodstream and keep pushing at a maximum effort.)

- At this time, have the patient push with her flexed legs against the table or stirrups.

- Check fetal heart tones frequently.

- Relieve muscular cramps, if necessary. Leg cramps are common in the second stage of labor due to pressure exerted by the baby's head on certain nerves in the pelvis. These cramps are relieved by changing the position of the legs and forcing the foot upward with pressure on the knees.

- Note exact time of birth.

- Receive the baby from the doctor with a sterile towel.

- Complete the records and stay in the room until the doctor has finished.

- After the doctor has finished, clean the patient; apply perineal pads and change the patient's gown, if indicated.

- Re-extend the delivery table or birthing bed.

- Remove patient's legs from the stirrups, moving both legs at the same time.

- As soon as the delivery is completed, it is important that the delivery room be cleaned and made ready for the next delivery.

Figure 16-5

Nursing care during second stage of labor

The nurse may be asked to administer intramuscular oxytocic drugs to the mother according to the doctor's orders. This will increase uterine contractions and minimize bleeding. When the placenta is delivered, it is important that the nurse record the exact time of placental delivery. The placenta is disposed of according to hospital policy.

The nurse should then complete the records, staying in the room until the doctor has finished caring for the mother. Then, the nurse may clean the patient, apply perineal pads, and change the patient's gown, if needed.

The delivery table is then re-extended and both of the patient's legs are removed from the stirrups at the same time. As soon as the delivery is completed, it is important that the delivery room be cleaned up and made ready for the next delivery.

ALTERNATIVE BIRTHING METHODS

Avoiding unnecessary interference with normal birth will provide the best opportunity for parents to respond spontaneously to their baby. Parents must decide in advance about being together during labor and birth; giving birth in a labor room, birthing room, or delivery room; the mother's need for medication; breastfeeding immediately after delivery; sharing the first minutes and hours with their baby; rooming-in privileges, and allowing siblings to visit the new baby at the hospital. In hospitals that provide a wide range of alternatives, including homelike birthing rooms, Leboyer-type births, father-attended cesarean births, and family recovery rooms, parents can choose the birth experience that satisfies their needs.

Some areas offer a birthing center as an alternative to a hospital or home birth. Many alternative birth centers are located within a hospital. The physical set-up of the room differs from a standard labor room. The bed is larger, chairs and a dresser furnish the room, plants and pictures add decoration, and the standard equipment used for labor and delivery is stored away in cabinets until needed. The goal of the staff of an alternative birth center is to meet the individual needs of the woman during a safe, normal childbirth while monitoring the progress of her labor. Enemas, pubic shaving, I.V.'s, and electronic fetal monitoring are not routine procedures. The woman may choose the position that is most comfortable for delivery. The treatment of the newborn's eyes with either an antibiotic ointment or silver nitrate may be delayed for a short period so that the infant can have eye-to-eye contact with the mother and father. It should be mentioned, however, that women considered to be "high-risk" mothers should be in a hospital environment with the equipment and staff available to provide the best possible care for the mother and baby.

Leboyer Method

A recent approach to childbirth is the *Leboyer method* instituted by Dr. Frederick Leboyer. This method teaches the physician to maintain a gentle, controlled delivery of the child, taking into consideration the emotional and physiological needs of both child and mother. A constant awareness of the infant as a uniquely sensitive human being is stressed. Leboyer recommends that all unnecessary stimuli in the delivery room be minimized and that the delivery be conducted with soft lights and with the least amount of trauma to both mother and baby. The four areas that Dr. Leboyer feels most important are:

* Gentle, controlled delivery
* Avoidance of stress on the craniosacral axis
* Avoidance of overstimulating the newborn's *sensorium* (sensation center of the brain) or breathing
* Importance of the maternal-infant bond

IMMEDIATE CARE OF THE NEWBORN

Purpose

Immediate care is necessary in order to enhance the well-being of the newborn.

The goals of this examination are to assess the newborn's ability (a) to adapt to an extrauterine existence, (b) to detect obvious congenital anomalies, (c) to detect the effects of an adverse fetal environment and (d) to detect evidence of birth trauma. The placenta, membranes, and umbilical cord should be examined by the obstetrician before disposal.

Procedure

1. As soon as the baby is delivered, **record the exact time of birth.**
2. With a sterile towel, receive the baby from the doctor.
3. Rate the baby according to the Apgar Scoring System; record the score.
4. Wipe the baby dry and wrap it in a warm blanket. It is vital that the newborn be kept warm. The infant should be protected from thermal stress, preferably by use of a radiant warming device.
5. If the immediate condition of the mother and baby permit, take the baby to the head of the table for the mother and father to see and hold. This is an important time in the establishment of the parent-infant bond.
6. Place the baby in the heated incubator or crib, on its right side and with the head of the crib lowered; this promotes drainage of mucus.
7. Suction the baby with the bulb or a DeLee aspirator (mucous trap) to remove mucus or other secretions that may be present in the infant's mouth, nose, and pharynx. Positioning and suctioning

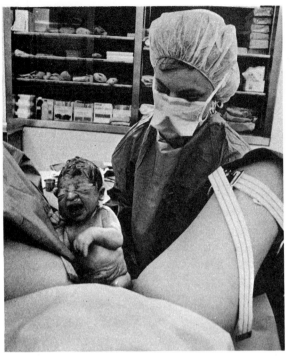

A — The baby is born

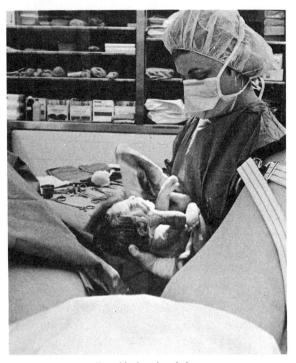

B — He is wiped dry

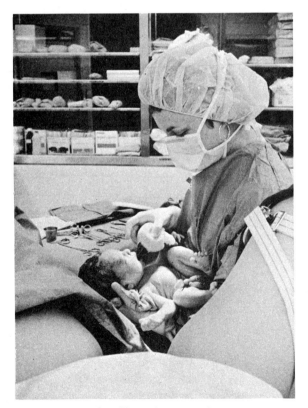

C — Mucus is removed

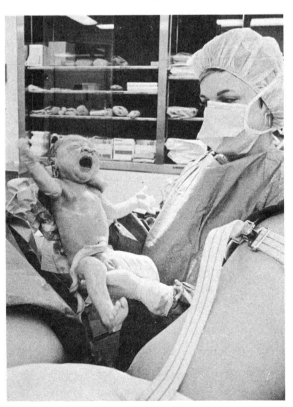

D — Assessment is made

Figure 16-6

The immediate postnatal period

are necessary so the infant does not aspirate this material.

CAUTION: If a bulb syringe is used, the bulb must be squeezed and all air expelled from the syringe before it is gently inserted. Otherwise, the material in the oropharynx will be forced into the bronchi and lungs when the bulb is collapsed. Gentle suction is provided as the bulb regains its original shape.

8. After respirations are sustained and resuscitation has been completed, an examination should be performed rapidly but gently. The order of the examination is usually (a) visual inspection, (b) auscultation of the chest, (c) palpation of head, clavicles, abdomen, and extremities and (d) manipulation of the infant by passing catheters through various orifices. This will give an immediate evaluation of the newborn to determine if any medical intervention is necessary.

A. Inspection

- Obvious malformation of head, for example, microcephaly, anencephaly, cleft lip or palate, malformed ears, and micrognathia (abnormal development of mandible). Also observe for excessive, frothy oral secretions that may suggest the presence of esophageal atresia.

- Neck. Goiters and cystic lymphangiomas may compromise the airway making immediate tracheal intubation necessary.

- Abdomen. Omphalocele is an anomaly. The intestines and sometimes the liver or spleen are present in a membrane-covered sac protruding through the base of the umbilicus. Gastroschisis is an anterior abdominal wall defect. (The eviserated organs should be covered with sterile gauze moistened with warm saline. Care must be taken to maintain the infant's body temperature and fluid balance). Absent abdominal muscles and abdominal masses can indicate tumors or cysts.

- Extremities and back. Absence and malformation of parts of the extremities may be obvious and may not be associated with other defects. Meningomyelocele, a defect in the closure of the neural tube, presents with a fluid-filled sac usually on the thoracolumbar spine. The anus may reveal absence of an anal opening. Genitalia, if ambiguous, may require endocrinologic consultation before the sex is determined.

- Skin. Vernix caseosa, a white cheesy substance, is normally present on the skin of pre-term infants. It is absent in post-term infants, and is only present in the skin folds of term infants. Cyanosis of the feet and hands can persist for some time after respirations have been adequately established. Pallor of the skin may indicate anemia, resulting from hemolysis or hemorrhage, or a state of shock with inadequate cardiac output. Yellow or staining of the skin, predominantly the nails, umbilical cord, and vernix, due to bile pigments from meconium stained amniotic fluid, suggest previous fetal distress. (Close observation for respiratory distress caused by meconium aspiration is indicated.) Generalized petechiae and ecchymosis may be present in congenital viral infections such as that with rubella. Petechiae over the head and neck are common in rapid or difficult deliveries. Premature babies bruise easily and ecchymosis may appear in areas where they have been firmly grasped during delivery.

- Respiratory tract. Signs of respiratory distress include: (a) tachypnea (greater than 50 breaths per minute), (b) chest wall and sternal retractions, (c) nasal flaring, and (d) grunting indicate a need for close immediate observation. Slow respiratory frequency (less than 30 breaths per minute), if shallow, suggests central nervous system depression.

- Urine and meconium. The passage of urine and meconium from the appropriate orifices indicate patency of the urethra and anus. This should be noted.

- Cry. Absence or weakness of crying should alert the observer to the possibility of central nervous system depression.

B. Auscultation of the Chest

- Cardiovascular System. The heart rate and rhythm should be noted. A rate of over 160 beats per minute or under 120 beats per minute usually indicates the need for diagnostic intervention.

- Respiratory System. Course rales usually disappear in the first hours of life. The presence of bowel sounds in the chest may indicate a diaphragmatic hernia. Unilateral absence of breath sounds suggest a pneumothorax diaphragmatic hernia or lobar emphysema.

C. Palpation

- The size and tenseness of the fontanelles and cranial sutures should be noted.

- Caput succendaneum, edema of the presenting part of the head, is boggy and usually crosses suture lines. Cephalhematomas usually do not cross suture lines and are slightly ballotable.

- A dry crackling sound over one of the clavicles can indicate a fracture.

- The liver is usually palpable in the newborn. However, obvious enlargement can suggest congenital viral infection or severe hemolytic disease.

- If a fracture during delivery is suspected, careful crepitation and displacement of the humerus should be done.

D. Manipulation

- Moro reflex is elicited by grasping the infant's hands, extending, and abducting the arms with just enough force to almost raise the head from the surface. Sudden release is normally accompanied by an embrase response. Absence of this reflex can indicate intracranial pathology. Asymmetry of the reflex suggests a fracture of the clavicle, the humerus, or a brachial plexus injury.

- Assess muscle tone by suspending the infant prone and passively flexing the extremities. If the infant is floppy, a spinal cord injury or CNS depression is suspected.

- It is unnecessary and traumatic to pass catheters through the nares routinely. If the infant is able to breathe when his mouth is closed, either spontaneously or by force, the nares are patent.

- If a catheter can be passed through the mouth and into the stomach, the esophagus is patent. This should be done, however, only if esophageal atresia or another anomaly is suspected. If aspiration from the stomach is greater than 20 to 30 ml. and is bile-stained, high-intestinal obstruction is suspected.

9. Gently wipe the infant's eyes. Instill two drops of one-percent silver nitrate solu-

tion in each eye (Crede treatment). Flush the eyes with normal saline or distilled water. An antibiotic ointment may be prescribed as an alternative to silver nitrate. This is usually less irritating to the eyes. This treatment protects the infant from any infectious organisms that may have been in the birth canal. It is required by law to prevent blindness caused by the gonococcus organism. If silver nitrate is not used in your nursing location, ophthalmic penicillin ointment can take its place as ordered by the physician.
CAUTION: The freshness and strength of the silver nitrate should be checked before instillation. If ophthalmic penicillin ointment is used, the excess ointment may be gently wiped away approximately 15 minutes after application.

10. Take the baby's temperature rectally, being careful not to chill the infant.

11. Fill out Identabands and attach to the infant. This *must* be done before mother and baby leave the delivery room. The Identabands are a wristband for the mother, and an ankleband and wristband for the baby. All three bands are printed with the same number. The mother's name, the doctor's name, the sex of the baby, and the date and time of birth are inserted into the bands. Some hospitals take footprints of the baby and fingerprints of the mother as a further identifying measure.

12. Complete the newborn record before the baby is taken to the nursery.

Apgar Scoring System

The newborn is carefully observed for any signs of respiratory or circulatory distress at all times. One method of assessing the infant involves the use of the *Apgar Scoring System,* figure 16-7. The infant's condition is evaluated at birth on five signs:

- Heart rate
- Respiratory effort
- Muscle tone
- Reflex irritability
- Color

Each sign is graded as 0, 1, or 2. A total of 10 is a perfect composite score.

To score the baby in one minute as the test demands, the nurse or physician evaluating the baby should wait 55 seconds after birth and then appraise the baby and enter the score. Once a nurse has observed a number of births, the scoring can almost be done at a glance. A baby who is pink all over, howling, and clenching its fists has a 10 score almost automatically. On the other hand, a baby who is quiet and limp probably scores 0 to 1. A zero-rated baby has better than a 50 percent chance of survival. A stillbirth has no score at all.

Resuscitation of the Newborn

The most important responsibility of the obstetrical nurse following a delivery is to observe the newborn closely and continuously for signs of respiratory or circulatory depression. Some infants who cry at birth subsequently develop *apnea* (temporary loss of breath) and may die unless appropriate resuscitative measures are taken. Therefore, the obstetrical nurse should observe a newborn continuously for at least 5 minutes after delivery and report any signs of depression to the obstetrician.

The responsibility for resuscitating a newborn rests with the anesthetist and obstetrician although the routine measures of aspiration of the mouth, nose, and pharynx; stimulation by flicking of the feet; and administration of oxygen (not under pressure) may be done by the nurse.

APGAR SCORING CHART			
SIGN	**0**	**1**	**2**
HEART RATE	Absent	Slow (below 100); (initiate resuscitation)	Good (over 100)
RESPIRATORY EFFORT	Absent (initiate resuscitation)	Weak cry; hypoventilation	Good strong cry; established respirations
MUSCLE TONE	Limp	Some flexion of extremities; weak or floppy resistance	Well flexed; strong resistance response
REFLEX RESPONSE	No Response	Grimace	Cough or sneeze
1. Response to catheter in nostril (tested after oropharynx is clear)			
2. Tangential foot slap	No Response	Grimace	Strong cry and withdrawal of foot
COLOR	Blue, pale	Body pink Extremities blue	Completely pink
Category Condition	0-3 poor, critical, severely depressed 4-6 moderately depressed 7-10 good		

Figure 16-7

The Apgar scoring system (Adapted from Nursing Inservice Aid No. 2, courtesy of Ross Laboratories, published with permission of Dr. Virginia Apgar.)

Resuscitation of the newborn infant in distress is discussed in greater depth in Unit 20.

THE THIRD STAGE OF LABOR

The third stage of labor begins after delivery of the baby and terminates with the discharge of the placenta. Nursing care given during the third stage of labor is shown in Figure 16-8. The nurse records the exact time the placenta is delivered. The mother is observed for hemorrhage and shock; the baby is observed for breathing, mucus, color, and cry.

The uterus is gently massaged to make it contract in order to expel the placenta, figure 16-9. The physician may order medications at this time to aid in stimulating contractions of the uterine muscles. When the placenta has been delivered and the uterus is emptied, the fundus of the uterus is gently massaged until it is hard.

After the doctor has inspected the placenta carefully to be sure no afterbirth remains in the birth canal, the nurse disposes of the placenta. Many hospitals now take part in *a placenta collection program.* The placenta is processed for the recovery and purification of *gamma globulin,* a serum used in the prevention and treatment of a variety of diseases. The umbilical cord may also be saved. (It has been used for femoral vein replacements.) The nurse puts the placenta in the container provided for it and places the container in the freezer supplied. The processing company picks it up.

3rd Stage of Labor

- Observe the mother for hemorrhage and shock.
- Observe the baby for breathing, mucus, color, and cry.
- Palpate and massage the uterus as directed by the physician immediately after delivery of the infant to stimulate it to contract in order to expel the placenta.
- When a sudden gush of blood is seen and the umbilical cord lengthens, apply gentle pressure on the patient's lower abdomen to assist in expulsion of the placenta.
- Hold a container just below the vaginal opening to receive the placenta.
- Check the mother's pulse and watch for signs of impending shock (rapid pulse and cold perspiration).
- Massage the uterus, if it relaxes. A relaxed uterus is evident in cases of profuse bleeding or *uterine atony* (lack of normal tone of the uterus).
- Check frequently for excessive bleeding; make sure the uterus remains firm.
- Give medications as directed.
- Apply perineal pads to the mother after delivery is completed.
- Dispose of placenta according to hospital policy.
- Remove patient via stretcher to recovery room.
- Finish notes on chart concerning time and type of delivery and exact time of placental delivery.

Figure 16-8

Nursing care during the third stage of labor

If the mother has had an episiotomy performed, it is repaired after delivery of the placenta. A round needle and continuous suture is used to close the vaginal mucosa and fourchet. This is followed by several interrupted sutures in the levator ani muscle and the fascia. A continuous suture is again picked up and used to unite the subcutaneous fascia. Finally, a running suture is continued upward as a subcuticular stitch. These sutures dissolve in about three weeks when the incision is healed.

Following delivery of the afterbirth, the mother must be observed closely for shock and hemorrhage. The average postpartum blood loss is 300 milliliters. If blood loss reaches 500 milliliters, it is considered a hemorrhage. Should this occur, grasp the uterus and massage it gently but firmly until it assumes a hardness. The fundus of the uterus lies just below the umbilicus as soon as delivery is complete.

THE FOURTH STAGE OF LABOR

The first few hours after delivery are vital to the well-being of the new mother. She should

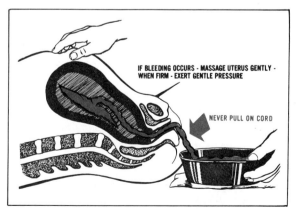

IF BLEEDING OCCURS - MASSAGE UTERUS GENTLY - WHEN FIRM - EXERT GENTLE PRESSURE

NEVER PULL ON CORD

Figure 16-9

Massaging the uterus aids in the delivery of the placenta

be closely observed for any adverse reactions, figure 16-10. Blood flow, pulse, temperature, and blood pressure should be checked every 15 to 20 minutes for possible hemorrhage, shock and infection. The fundus of the uterus should be checked for hardness and location. Check to be sure the patient is warm. Many women experience chill after giving birth. If the woman had an episiotomy, ice to the area during the fourth stage can often reduce swelling and thereby decrease the discomfort that may follow this procedure.

4th Stage of Labor

CHECK PATIENT FOR THE FOLLOWING:

- Vaginal drainage. If more than two sanitary napkins are saturated with bloody drainage during the first hour after delivery, there is excessive bleeding. The normal flow of vaginal blood within the first two hours after delivery is about two ounces. There should be no clots in the blood. If the blood flow increases, the uterus should be massaged until it becomes firm.

- Pulse. After delivery, there may be a slight drop in the pulse rate; it may be 60 to 80 beats per minute. A fast pulse may be a sign of shock or concealed hemorrhage. The nurse should notify the doctor immediately.

- Temperature. Slight rises in temperature may occur following delivery. In general, the temperature should remain within normal limits.

- Blood Pressure. The blood pressure should be taken frequently and noted. Any extreme variation should be reported. It is not uncommon for a new mother to complain of a headache. Lying flat may give relief.

- Fundus. The top of the uterus should be hard and firm. It should be located below the navel. If the fundus is soft or large, massage it gently with a circular motion until it is firm. Normally the uterus quickly responds to massage. Do not overmassage.

Figure 16-10

Nursing care during the fourth stage of labor

The nurse should keep a written record of all observations so that the physician may be informed of the progress and condition of the new mother.

If the baby's condition is good, many hospitals allow the baby to remain with the mother during this time. Many mothers wish to nurse their baby for a short time. The mother and father may feel like cuddling, holding, talking to, and getting to know their infant. Research has shown that the infant is in a heightened state of alertness and responsiveness in the first hours following birth. The infant may be intrigued with nuzzling or sucking at the breast, making eye contact with the parents and responding to verbal and touching contact. This reciprocal responsiveness is the first step in the parent-infant attachment called bonding. (See section on bonding in Unit 4.)

New techniques for measuring newborn behavior have been developed which show that newborn infants are much more discriminating and responsive than was previously realized. At birth, the alert newborn is attracted by a variety of visual, sound, and other stimuli. The infant is particularly intrigued by the eyes and other features of the human face. When the baby is in a state of quiet alertness, he or she will respond to these stimuli with behavior such as gazing, imitating, following with his or her eyes, and clinging. These reciprocal, synchronized responses between the newborn and its parents reinforce their developing relationship.

Many factors can influence the outcome of birth and the quality of the parent-infant bond. Among these factors are the parents' cultural and socioeconomic backgrounds, their personalities, their previous experiences with pregnancy, and their attitudes toward pregnancy and parenting, the birth process and the newborn, and any complications of the pregnancy or birth. The physical and mental health of the mother before and during pregnancy can affect the health

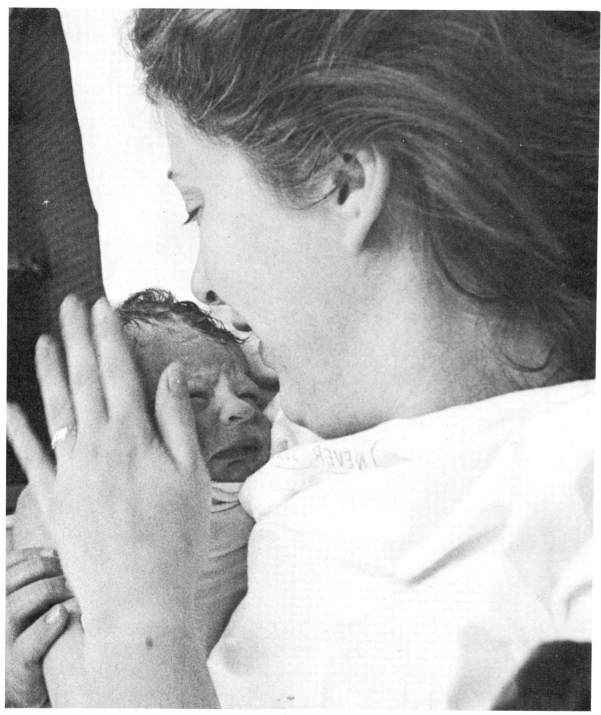

Figure 16-11
Mother greets her newborn child

and development of the fetus, as well as the capacity for the mother and baby to interact at birth. A positive childbirth experience appears to create in the mother and father an increased self-esteem and self-confidence that may foster parental bonding. The length of labor, the occurrence of a medical crisis during the birth, parental expectations for the birth experience, and the baby's sex and condition at birth are other factors that seem to influence early parent-infant bonding.

The nurse can be very helpful in facilitating the bonding process by pointing out and reinforcing the parents' perceptions of their baby's ability to interact with them. A father should be encouraged to touch, hold, and interact with his baby. Because early father-baby interactions may be basic to the development of a strong father-child relationship later in life, the nurse's support of the father's role in childbearing and child care after birth is essential. Mother, father, and baby are acutely sensitive to their surroundings and to each other immediately after birth. Therefore, the care, actions, comments, and attitudes of the hospital staff can profoundly influence the early establishment of the parent-infant bond.

SUGGESTED ACTIVITIES

- Describe the various positions for the second stage of labor. List the advantages and disadvantages of each.

- Identify components to be included in a newborn screening physical exam. Differentiate normal from abnormal findings.

- Describe and chart normal and abnormal physical findings in the neonate.

- Discuss the advantages and disadvantages of prepared childbirth. Discuss medicated versus nonmedicated labor and birth.

- Discuss the pros and cons of in-hospital birth versus out-of-hospital birth as they relate to:
  - Safety
  - Family-centered care
  - Sibling involvement
  - Immediate postpartum management

- Role play assisting with a delivery and immediate care of the newborn.

- Discuss the complications which may occur during the second stage of labor such as prolapsed cord, precipitate delivery, ruptured uterus, uterine inertia, severe dehydration of mother, drop in fetal heart tones or irregularities of tone, and premature separation of placenta. Investigate each complication and discuss the nursing care required for each.

REVIEW

A. Multiple Choice. Select the best answer.

1. The Apgar system of evaluating the newborn must first be done at
   a. one minute after delivery
   b. five minutes after delivery
   c. anytime before newborn is taken to the nursery
   d. within 24 hours after delivery

2. Placenta collection programs process the placenta for the recovery of
   a. red blood cells
   b. white blood cells
   c. hemoglobin
   d. gamma globulin

3. The purpose of an antibiotic ointment or one-percent silver nitrate being placed in the eyes of the newborn is to
   a. help the baby to see better
   b. prevent infection which may have been transmitted in passage through the birth canal
   c. prevent infection which may have been transmitted through the umbilical cord
   d. help prevent jaundice

4. When placing the patient's legs in stirrups, both legs must be lifted at the same time in order to prevent
   a. rupturing the membranes
   b. straining the patient's back
   c. straining the ligaments of the patient's pelvis
   d. blocking blood flow to the fetus

5. Leg cramps may be relieved by
   a. applying cold compresses to the legs
   b. stretching the leg out forcibly and pulling the foot toward the knee
   c. removing the legs from the stirrups momentarily
   d. giving pain-relieving medications

6. Nursing care during delivery includes
   a. coaching the patient
   b. checking fetal heart tones
   c. recording exact time of birth
   d. all of these

7. Immediate care of the newborn includes
   1. suctioning the mouth, nose and pharynx to remove mucus
   2. observing for signs of respiratory or circulatory distress
   3. instilling eye drops
   4. bathing the newborn
      a. 1 only
      b. 1, 2 and 3
      c. 2 and 4
      d. 1, 2, 3 and 4

8. During the fourth stage of labor, it is important for the nurse to monitor the mother's
   1. vaginal drainage
   2. pulse and blood pressure
   3. temperature
   4. firmness of fundus
      a. 2 and 3
      b. 4 only
      c. 1, 2 and 3
      d. 1, 2, 3 and 4

B. Briefly answer the following questions.

1. List six signs that indicate the second stage of labor is beginning.

2. Name the five signs scored in the Apgar Scoring System for evaluating the newborn.

3. List six factors that may influence parent-infant bonding.

4. Name the different positions a woman may use in the first stage of labor. Give one advantage and one disadvantage of each.

5. Write a complete examination of a healthy newborn in the delivery room. Include observations and the significance of the findings.

UNIT 17

COMPLICATIONS OF LABOR AND DELIVERY

OBJECTIVES

After studying this unit, the student should be able to:

- Differentiate between premature, prolonged, and precipitous labor.
- Identify complications caused by the forces, the passenger, and the passage.
- Describe three abnormal fetal positions.
- List four reasons for cesarean deliveries.
- Describe the care given if the mother is unconscious.

About 85 percent of all births are normal deliveries. However, some situations do occur that can threaten the life of both the mother and baby. Observation, reporting, technical skill, and physical and emotional supportive measures must all be carried out with a fine degree of competency.

PREMATURE LABOR

If labor begins three or more weeks before the expected date, it is termed premature labor. The baby born prematurely has not had sufficient time to develop and is quite small. Because the baby is small, medications that tend to depress the baby are avoided during labor. Since the small baby needs more protection than the full-term larger baby, forceps may be used to protect the head during delivery under suitable anesthesia.

If the baby is premature, special attention should be focused in four basic areas. The infant should be: (1) helped to breathe, (2) kept warm, (3) handled with care, and (4) protected from infection.

PRECIPITOUS LABOR

A precipitous labor is spontaneous labor that progresses very rapidly. A labor of this sort usually starts out almost immediately with very strong, frequent contractions. It can last anywhere from a few contractions to a couple of hours. Things are happening so fast that it is often very difficult for the mother to handle the contractions during a precipitous labor.

Any delivery should be gentle and controlled because it lessens the chance of cerebral trauma in the infant and vaginal lacerations in the mother. However, a gentle, controlled delivery may be

217

difficult with a precipitous labor. Doctors sometimes attempt to slow the progress of labor through the use of medication. The reasons for a precipitous labor and birth are not entirely understood. It is thought that the pelvic size and structure may have something to do with the chances for having a fast labor. If a woman has had one precipitous labor, her chances for another are very good.

PROLONGED LABOR

Occasionally, the nurse might observe that a woman is in labor for hours and hours without progress. There is obviously something wrong with the mechanism of labor. This is termed *dystocia* (difficult labor). The cause could be related to three factors: the forces, the passenger, or the passage.

Uterine Dysfunction (Forces)

A delay in any of the phases of labor is known as *uterine dysfunction*. This could be due to the poor quality of uterine contractions or to maternal exhaustion. The chief causes of uterine dysfunction are:

- Unwise use of analgesia
- Minor degrees of pelvic contraction
- Slight extension of the fetal head

Other contributing factors include overdistention of the uterus, maternal age, and rigidity of the cervix. Sometimes, the actual cause is unknown. The complications are unfortunate. Fetal injury or death are the most serious outcomes. For the mother, exhaustion and dehydration occur if labor goes on too long. Intervention can be effective in preventing these serious problems if good observation and support is given by the nurse

and the attending physician is kept notified of the patient's condition.

Abnormal Fetal Positions (Passenger)

Positions and presentations which are not normal often cause dystocia and subsequent complications. It is difficult for the child to move forward.

Persistent Occiput Posterior Positions. The occiput posterior position prolongs labor whenever the fetal head enters the pelvis with the occiput directed diagonally, posterior (in either the ROP or LOP position). Under these circumstances, the head must rotate through an arc of 135 degrees in the process of internal rotation instead of the normal 45 to 90 degree arc. With good contractions, adequate flexion and an average-sized baby, most of these infants spontaneously rotate through the 135 degree arc as soon as the head reaches the pelvic floor. However, the fetus may rotate only partially and be born with its face upward. It should be noted that the mother may experience a great deal of discomfort in her back as the baby's head presses against the sacrum during the rotation. Sacral counterpressure, back rubs, and frequent change of position from side to side can be helpful.

Breech. This occurs in about 3 percent of all term deliveries; the breech instead of the *vertex* (top of the head) presents at the pelvic outlet. There are three classifications of breech position:

- Complete: the buttocks and feet present and the knees are drawn up
- Footling: one or both feet present
- Frank: the buttocks present, the legs are extended up and are pressed against the abdomen and chest

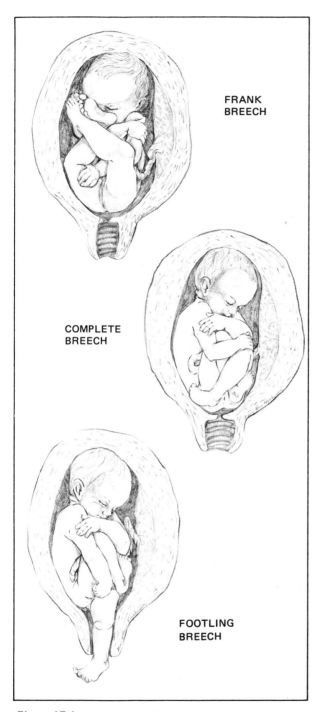

Figure 17-1

Types of breech presentations

FRANK
BREECH

COMPLETE
BREECH

FOOTLING
BREECH

In a breech position, the baby often passes meconium from its rectum after the rupture of the membranes. *Meconium* is a greenish black to light brown tarlike material. Upon seeing this substance coming from the birth canal, the nurse must be sure, in fact, that the baby is in the breech position. If the baby is in the vertex position, discharge of meconium is an indication of fetal distress.

The delivery of breech-positioned babies can be spontaneous and the outcome is generally good. Any danger comes from the trauma of delivery and the chance of a prolapsed cord. There is also serious risk if the head is not kept flexed, as it could extend and get caught on the symphysis and death could result. Many physicians today deliver a breech position baby by cesarean section because of these risks.

Shoulder, Face and Brow Presentations. In shoulder presentations the infant lies crosswise. This is a serious complication; it may cause a rupture of the uterus and put much more stress on the infant. This complication is seen in about 1 out of 200 cases. The physician will try to turn the baby by bringing one or both feet into the vagina. This altering of the fetal position in utero in order to facilitate delivery is known as *version*. More frequently, a cesarean section is necessary.

Face presentations are also seen about once in every 200 cases. The infant's face is often swollen and purplish due to birth trauma. Brow presentations are even more rare and are harder to deliver because the largest diameter of the baby's head is presenting.

Disproportion (Passage)

Cephalopelvic disproportion refers to the complication which arises when the infant's size is too large to pass through a small contracted pelvis at either the inlet, the midpelvis or the outlet. In these cases, the infant is usually delivered by cesarean section. A small pelvis is often detected during antepartal care and the woman can be given adequate mental preparation for the cesarean section.

About 1 in 100 babies are too large to pass through a pelvis which is normal in size. In such cases the baby generally weighs over 10 pounds. One of the common causes of an oversized baby is diabetes. Prolonged pregnancy can also be a factor.

MULTIPLE PREGNANCIES

When two or more embryos develop in the uterus at the same time, the condition is known as *multiple pregnancy*. The mother usually experiences greater discomforts and higher risks than the woman with a single pregnancy. A twin pregnancy is likely to cause more heaviness, lower abdominal pressure and backache. Premature labor, preeclampsia and postpartal hemorrhage are also more common.

At delivery, the nurse has the responsibility of supportive care and assisting the doctor. In multiple births, the infants are likely to be small and oxygen and resuscitative measures may be necessary. The care is similar to that of the premature infant. The nurse must realize that it may be difficult for the parents to adjust to the birth of more than one child, both emotionally and financially. Problems may also be compounded in feeding, especially if the mother wants to breast feed the babies. None of these problems is insurmountable but some parents may need an understanding person to help them over this initial adjustment period. A social worker or public health nurse can be called upon to give additional assistance in dealing with these problems.

CESAREAN SECTION

Under certain conditions, it is necessary that the baby be delivered through the abdominal wall by a process called *cesarean section*. The cesarean birth is becoming more common today. Approximately 10 to 20 percent of hospital births are cesarean deliveries, with the rate being even higher in medical centers treating high-risk mothers. There are numerous reasons for cesarean deliveries:

- Cephalopelvic disproportion
- Malpresentation
- Failure to progress
- Fetal distress
- Prolapsed cord
- Placenta previa
- Abruptio placenta
- Maternal disease (preeclampsia, diabetes, high blood pressure, acute case of Herpes genitalis)

In many hospitals, cesarean deliveries are performed in the operating room because it is considered major surgery. The setup is for major surgery and the obstetric technician or nurse acts as scrub nurse in such operations. The routine in preparation for delivery is similar to the usual procedure but the setup pack is different due to the special instruments used. If the operation is an elective one (not an emergency), the doctor may schedule it one to two weeks before the due date to avoid the beginning of spontaneous labor.

The majority of hospitals permit the father to remain with the mother during the procedure. He will be required to dress in a surgical scrub suit with cap, foot coverings, and mask. He will be asked not to touch any sterile trays or equipment. After the initial newborn evaluation, the father may hold his baby. The initial bonding process between the baby and his parents can begin while the surgical repair is completed.

The procedure takes about one to two hours, but it is often only 5 to 10 minutes after the surgery begins that the baby is born. Anesthesia is necessary for the procedure. Regional anesthesia, which allows the mother to be awake without feeling pain, is often used. A spinal anesthetic makes the mother very numb from the chest to the toes. However, some women report a sensation of tugging or pulling, shoulder pain, pressure, burning sensations, nausea, or shortness of breath during the surgery. A general anesthetic is occasionally used for cesareans when the anesthesiologist deems it necessary, or in an emergency situation.

There are two types of skin incisions for a cesarean birth. The midline incision is vertical between the navel and pubic bone. It allows for a quicker delivery in an emergency. The reasons for using this midline incision include: (1) the lower uterine segment cannot be exposed or entered safely because of the bladder; or a myoma occupies the lower uterus; or there is an invasive carcinoma of the cervix; (2) a large fetus is in a transverse lie, and the shoulder is impacted in the birth canal; (3) there is an anterior placenta previa implantation. The transverse skin incision or "bikini cut" is made horizontally just above the pubic bone. This type of incision is associated with less blood loss and reduced postpartum infection. After a lower segment transverse incision, a future vaginal birth is possible. Postoperative care of this patient is similar to that given any abdominal surgery patient. If the woman is given a general anesthetic and is unconscious, special care must be given after her delivery and repair.

Vaginal Birth After A Cesarean Section (VBAC)

It has been shown in various studies that a vaginal birth after a cesarean section will prove safe if the previous cesarean surgical incision was a low transverse incision. The issue that has prevented many physicians from allowing a vaginal birth following a cesarean section has been the fear of uterine rupture. In 1981, a review of over 8000 deliveries (reported in the literature) concluded that vaginal delivery not only was as safe as an elective repeat cesarean section but it was also in fact the preferred method of management in carefully selected patients.

Specific guidelines have been established by the American College of Obstetricians and Gynecologists (ACOG Newsletter 1982). They include the patient's acceptance and understanding of the risks and the benefits of both vaginal birth and repeat cesarean section. The woman should have undergone but one previous low transverse incision with no extension of the uterine incision. Finally, a judgment must be made as to whether or not the pelvis is adequate for the current pregnancy.

If a woman is going to attempt a trial of labor following a previous cesarean section, appropriate medical support must be available including (a) skilled nursing and (b) in-hospital obstetrician, pediatrician, and anesthesiologist. There should be an adequate blood bank promptly available. Electronic fetal heart rate monitoring is advisable during labor. There must also be an appropriately staffed operating room available.

PROLAPSED UMBILICAL CORD

If the umbilical cord can be seen beside the baby as it appears at the vaginal opening, or if the cord is seen coming out of the vaginal opening, it is called a prolapsed cord, figure 17-2. This is not a common complication; it happens only about once out of every 400 births. It is, however, a very serious complication because of the high infant death rate associated with it. The threat to the baby's life is caused by the cord being pressed between the baby and the mother's bony pelvis. This shuts off the baby's blood supply from the cord and, with it, the baby's oxygen supply. The baby quickly suffocates if immediate attention is not given. The mother's position should be changed to keep the baby from compressing the cord. The mother should be immediately put in a knee-chest position to keep the baby from compressing the cord. If the fetal heart monitor shows any signs of fetal distress, oxygen may need to be administered to

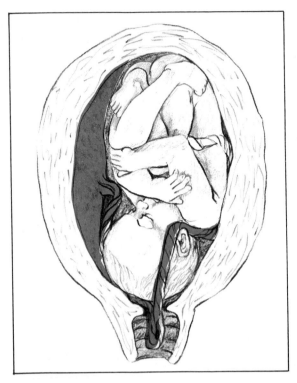

Figure 17-2

If the umbilical cord emerges before the baby, the baby's life is in danger because the cord is squeezed between the baby and the mother's bony pelvis. Note that part of the cord is under the right shoulder, shutting off the blood supply.

the mother. Pressure should be placed against the presenting part of the baby away from the cord. Medical assistance should be called for immediately.

Nuchal Cord

Immediately after the birth of the infant's head, the physician's fingers are passed along the occiput to the infant's neck in order to determine if a loop or more of umbilical cord encircles the neck. If the cord is coiled around the neck, it is gently drawn down and, if loose enough, slipped over the baby's head. This is done to prevent any interference with the baby's oxygen supply

as the shoulders are delivered. If the cord is too tightly coiled to permit this procedure, the cord is clamped and cut before the shoulders are delivered; the infant is extracted immediately and measures taken to avoid asphyxiation. If the cord is looped around the neck or body and is too short to allow the head to be delivered, a cesarean section is performed.

PLACENTA PREVIA

When the placenta covers or partially covers the cervix the condition is called placenta previa. As the cervix dilates, the placenta separates from the uterus, depriving the fetus of oxygen and causing painless bleeding in the mother. This condition is serious and usually indicates a cesarean birth.

PLACENTA ABRUPTIO

Abruptio placenta is the premature separation of the normally implanted placenta from the uterine wall. This may cause vaginal bleeding and can lead to decreased oxygen supply to the fetus. If the separation is more than 30 percent, the baby suffocates from lack of oxygen. Any abnormal bleeding during labor usually means the baby is born by cesarean section.

STILLBIRTH

If the baby does not breathe at birth and does not respond to resuscitative efforts, it is said to be *stillborn*. If a baby is stillborn or appears to be dying shortly after delivery, the parents should be asked if they want the baby baptized. It is important to give the mother the option of seeing and holding her stillborn infant. She needs as much emotional and psychological support as possible.

NURSING CARE

Giving good supportive care to a woman in labor demands much of the nurse. Observation, reporting, technical skill, physical and emotional supportive measures must all be carried out with a fine degree of competence. Yet, in a situation of added stress where the labor and delivery process is complicated, even more is demanded of the nurse. The importance of supportive care of the highest caliber cannot be emphasized enough.

CARE OF THE UNCONSCIOUS MOTHER

Purpose

Care involves protecting and observing the unconscious mother closely at all times to prevent postdelivery complications such as shock, hemorrhage, pneumonia, or injury.

Precautions

1. Never leave an unconscious patient alone.
2. Examine dressings and watch body openings for hemorrhage.
3. Be sure that air passages are kept open and that respiration is adequate.
4. Watch closely for symptoms of oncoming shock (pulse, respiration, blood pressure, perspiration).
5. Keep patient warm. Maintain quiet.
6. Be sure the room is warm and free from drafts.
7. Frequently check fundus for firmness.

Equipment

- Postdelivery bed
- Bedside table
- Sphygmomanometer and stethoscope
- Tongue blades
- Tissue wipes
- Emesis basin covered with towel
- Paper and pencil
- Suction machine, if patient has had a general anesthesia
- Oxygen setup
- I.V. standard

Procedure

1. When the patient returns to the ward or recovery room, roll the bed covers to the side of the bed away from the stretcher.
2. Give assistance in transferring the patient to the bed and cover the patient with the rolled covers.
3. Tuck in bed covers as soon as possible.
4. Obtain chart from anesthetist. Learn patient's condition, type of anesthetic given, drains used and parenteral solutions administered from anesthetist. Check the postdelivery orders carefully.
5. Check and record the following:
   - Rate and character of respirations
   - State of consciousness
   - Color and condition of skin
   - Rate and quality of pulse
   - Blood pressure
   - Amount of flow
   - Presence of packing
   - Firmness and position of fundus
   - Time of return from delivery room
6. Make patient comfortable. Place bedrails in position.
7. Carry out orders and record them.
8. Count and record pulse, respirations, and blood pressure every 15 minutes until stabilized. Count and record more frequently, if indicated.

9. If patient vomits:
   - Turn patient's head to one side, supporting the head and angle of the jaw with hands.
   - Clear air passage by suctioning, if necessary.
   - If air passage cannot be cleared immediately, obtain assistance of anesthetist.
   - If patient aspirates vomitus, suction and notify anesthetist and doctor immediately. Have oxygen ready to administer when air passages are clear.

10. Report immediately to charge nurse or doctor any signs of inadequate or obstructed respiration, shock, or hemorrhage, or any other untoward symptoms.

11. Remain with the patient as long as she is unconscious.

12. When the patient has fully reacted and is ready to be returned to her room, she should be accompanied by an R.N. or L.P.N. and one other person.

13. When the patient is settled in her unit she is checked by an R.N.; at the transfer of responsibility for the patient, the patient's condition is ascertained to the satisfaction of both nurses.

14. The delivery room nurse gives the report to one of the R.N.'s on the floor (to the charge nurse, if possible).

15. The recovery room notes are continued until the patient is returned to the ward. Detailed nurse's notes should be continued as long as the patient's condition indicates a need for detailed records.
    - Include all medications, treatment, blood and laboratory tests, and intravenous therapy while in the recovery room.
    - The first voiding should be noted.

SUGGESTED ACTIVITIES

- Investigate the problems which may arise in labor if the baby's head fails to rotate normally.
- Discuss the problems of a premature birth for both parents and the baby.
- Briefly describe the presentation and management of cord prolapse.
- Outline the rationale and the procedure for breech delivery.
- Describe clinical signs which reflect labor complications.
- Identify the causes of predisposing factors and management of third stage hemorrhage.

REVIEW

Multiple Choice. Select the best answer from the lettered items.

1. Premature labor is defined as labor that
   a. begins one week before the expected date
   b. begins three or more weeks before the expected date
   c. is spontaneous and progresses rapidly
   d. is of short duration

2. Precipitous labor is defined as
   a. labor lasting many hours without progress
   b. labor pains without dilatation of the cervix
   c. spontaneous labor that progresses very rapidly
   d. none of these

3. The term *uterine dysfunction* refers to a delay in any phase of labor. It may be caused by
   a. poor quality uterine contractions
   b. maternal exhaustion
   c. unwise use of analgesia
   d. all of these

4. The term *dystocia* means
   a. abnormal fetal position
   b. difficult labor
   c. disproportionate passage
   d. short labor

5. A frank breech birth is one in which
   a. the buttocks and feet present and the knees are drawn up
   b. one or both feet present
   c. the buttocks present, the legs are extended up and are pressed against the abdomen and chest
   d. the occiput is directed diagonally and posterior

6. When an infant's size is too large to pass through a small contracted pelvis at either the inlet, the midpelvis or the outlet, it is called
   a. face presentation
   b. breech presentation
   c. persistent occiput posterior position
   d. cephalopelvic disproportion

7. When the placenta covers or partially covers the cervix, the condition is known as
   a. placenta previa
   b. placenta abruptio
   c. prolapsed placenta
   d. malpositioned placenta

8. Which of the following precautions are taken when delivering a premature infant?
   1. Medication is used to sedate the mother due to the risk.
   2. Medications are avoided or used sparingly.
   3. Forceps may be used.
   4. No episiotomy is done.
   a. 1, 3 and 4   c. 3 and 4
   b. 2 and 3   d. 1, 2, 3 and 4

9. Some reasons for a cesarean section are
   1. cephalopelvic disproportion
   2. failure to progress
   3. prolapsed cord
   4. severe pain in the first stage of labor
      a. 1 and 3　　　　　　　c. 1, 2 and 3
      b. 2 and 3　　　　　　　d. 1, 2, 3 and 4

10. A woman having a cesarean section under regional anesthesia may feel
    1. a tugging or pulling sensation
    2. shortness of breath
    3. a burning sensation
    4. shoulder pain
       a. 1 only　　　　　　　c. 1, 2 and 3
       b. 2 and 3　　　　　　　d. 1, 2, 3 and 4

SECTION 3 LABOR AND DELIVERY

Self-Evaluation

A. Match the descriptive phrase in column I to the correct term in column II.

	Column I	Column II
m	1. normal fetal heart tones	a. Apgar Scoring System
o	2. taken and recorded every four hours during labor	b. blood pressure
b	3. taken and recorded every two hours during labor	c. cephalic presentation
c	4. fetal head enters the internal os for delivery	d. dilatation of cervix
j	5. long axis of the fetus parallels the long axis of the mother	e. engagement
e	6. presenting part fully enters the pelvis	f. frequency, duration, intensity
h	7. patient actively participates in labor	g. gamma globulin
g	8. serum processed from the placenta	h. hemorrhage
h	9. postpartum bleeding reaches 500 milliliters	i. identification
k	10. technique used to correct postpartum hemorrhage	j. longitudinal presentation
a	11. method of evaluating infant one minute after birth	k. massage uterus
d	12. characteristic which differentiates true labor from false labor	l. presentation and position
L	13. determined by abdominal palpation	m. 120–160 beats per minute
f	14. noted when recording contractions	n. second stage of labor
i	15. necessary before baby is removed from delivery room	o. TPR

B. Identification and Interpretation.

1. In the sketch at the right, draw the pelvic quadrants and identify each. List the six possible positions for a head presentation.

_____

_____

_____

_____

_____

_____

2. Observe the illustration. List the five stations shown. Identify the ischial spines by drawing a line across them. In the space below the illustration, name the station represented by the ischial spines. Explain the method of measuring degrees of advancement.

(A) _____

(B) _____

(C) _____

(D) _____

(E) _____

3. In the illustration below, name the process marked A and B. Define these processes and explain how they are determined.

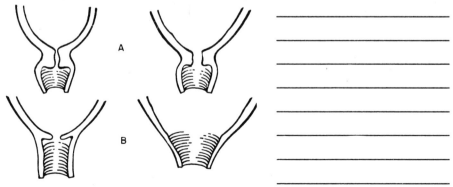

_____

_____

_____

_____

_____

_____

_____

_____

4. On the chart, indicate the proper nursing care for each discomfort or complication listed.

Stage of Labor	Discomfort or Complication	Nursing Care
First	1. Backache	1.
	2. Full bladder	2.
	3. Fear of anesthesia	3.
Second	1. Leg cramps	1.
	2. Profuse perspiration	2.
	3. Crowning	3.
Third	1. Soft uterus	1.
	2. Bleeding	2.

C. Briefly answer the following questions.

1. Define the four stages of labor.

2. List five signs of an abnormal condition in the patient in labor.

3. Why must the bladder be empty before a delivery?

4. Name four reasons for performing a vaginal examination.

5. List nine signs of the second stage of labor.

6. Outline the duties of the nurse regarding the newborn in the delivery room.

7. List two reasons for giving an enema in the first stage of labor.

8. What is *uterine dysfunction?* Name its chief causes.

9. What two conditions must the patient be observed for after delivery of the placenta?

10. Why is it necessary to be with the unconscious mother at all times?

11. Name three reasons why regional anesthesia is considered the safest method of anesthetizing a patient.

12. What causes "spinal headache" and how may it be prevented?

13. Name two fetal heart rate patterns that indicate acute fetal distress.

14. What are the two methods used for direct fetal monitoring?

UNIT 18

POSTPARTUM CARE

OBJECTIVES

After studying this unit, the student should be able to:

- Identify principles of nursing care during the postpartum period.
- Explain the process of involution.
- Identify complications which may occur during the puerperium.
- Cite causes for postpartum depression.
- State why sleep is an essential part of postpartum care.
- State measures of self-care for the patient.

The six-week period immediately following childbirth is called the *puerperium*. The term is taken from the latin words *puer,* meaning child, and *parare,* to bring forth. It takes about six weeks for the organs to return to their normal size and condition. This process is known as *involution.*

The principles of nursing care during the puerperium or postpartum period include:

- Promoting a revitalization of physical and emotional energy
- Encouraging normal involution of the reproductive organs
- Preventing infection of the reproductive and urinary systems
- Promoting rapid healing of tissue damaged during pregnancy and delivery
- Encouraging normal lactation or suppression of lactation with minimal discomfort

IMMEDIATE POSTPARTUM CARE

After the woman has delivered, she is encouraged to hold her infant, attempt to breast feed, if she chooses, and bond with her newborn. The father is also encouraged to participate in this process. The new family will stay together as a unit during this initial postpartum time. They should be supported as needed. She is usually both exhilarated and physically exhausted after

233

the birth of her baby. This first hour after delivery is known as the fourth stage of labor. The nurse should be knowledgeable of this stage.

The patient should be placed in the dorsal recumbent position and advised to lie quietly. Her pulse may drop, probably due to the lessening of arterial tension; the pulse rate may be from 60 to 80 beats per minute. A rapid pulse may be an indication of shock or concealed hemorrhage. Generally, the body temperature does not rise after delivery; however, it may rise to above 37.2°C (99°F) without ill effects. The pulse is the best guide to use in judging the significance of temperature.

A slow pulse with a slightly elevated temperature is not likely to indicate a complication. Nevertheless, the nurse should report any rise in temperature at once. The normal flow of vaginal blood within the first two hours after delivery is approximately two ounces. There are no clots at this time. If the discharge increases the nurse should massage the uterus. She should also check for a full or distended bladder. General hygienic care of the skin and mouth is essential to promote comfort and prevent odor. The patient should be encouraged to rest and sleep as much as possible. The diet is usually regular unless there have been complications.

It is not uncommon for the mother to experience a chill immediately after labor. This is usually caused by a nervous reaction — a disturbance of internal and external temperature due to the excessive perspiration which occurs during labor and ceases abruptly after delivery. A warm bed and the application of external heat help to avoid this reaction. The patient may also complain of a headache. A headache is an important symptom and must be reported because it indicates a change of pressure within the spinal column. The blood pressure should be taken and given in the report to the head nurse and doctor.

The Importance of Sleep

Rest and repair of body tissue require a recovery period of six weeks during which the mother must maintain normal sleep requirements. Fatigue, one of the earliest presumptive signs of pregnancy, shows the increased need for sleep because of increased metabolic requirements. In addition, the hard physical work of labor requires adequate energy reserves; restoration of this physical and emotional energy depletion can be secured through rest and sleep.

Although sleep is a psychophysiological phenomenon essential for maintaining both physical and emotional health, the exact metabolic or physiologic need has not been clearly explained. It is more crucial for emotional well-being than physical. When a person is deprived of sleep, psychological disturbances appear first and can be more disabling than physical manifestations. Chronic loss of sleep may lead to personality changes.

Sleeplessness in itself is not a disease; it is a symptom of another condition. There are many factors affecting a person's ability to sleep. Some reasons for sleeplessness are:

- excessive, prolonged or abnormal stimulation
- toxic substances
- muscular tension
- endocrine processes
- emotional states such as grief, anxiety, joy or fear

Sleeplessness in early pregnancy may be symptomatic of a thyroid condition. It is frequently the first warning of an impending emotional disorder. From what has been hypothesized about sleep deprivation and emotional disturbance, might there be some relationship between the two in the development of postpartum depression?

The nurse can be of great value if she understands the importance of sleep, what prevents sleep, and consequences of lack of sleep. From admission through delivery, the nurse should be alert for signs of undue excitement or apprehension and gear nursing care to provide maximum relaxation. These efforts will reduce fear, tension, and exhaustion. After delivery, if the mother is not ready for sleep — if she is excited, talkative, or hungry — the nurse should alleviate the cause and explain why sleep is so important, thus preparing the patient and her environment.

THE PROCESS OF INVOLUTION

Immediately after labor the uterus weighs about two pounds. It can be felt through the abdominal wall at the level of the umbilicus. Immediately after delivery it begins to return to its normal position, figure 18-1. Complete involution requires several weeks. By the time involution is complete, the uterus has shrunk so much that it lies entirely in the pelvis and it should weigh only a few ounces. The vaginal walls, the vulva, and all other tissues that became enlarged during pregnancy also undergo a process of involution. The abdominal walls recover from overstretching, but the striae usually remain.

Multiparas may be bothered by uncomfortable contractions of the uterus; these are known as *afterpains*. Afterpains may become more noticeable at the beginning of each breast feeding. They usually last only a few minutes. The contractions are useful because they keep the uterus free of clots and promote involution. Any severe afterpains should be reported to the doctor. If they are severe, an analgesic may be prescribed.

The uterine and vaginal discharge after delivery is called the *lochia*. It is red in color from

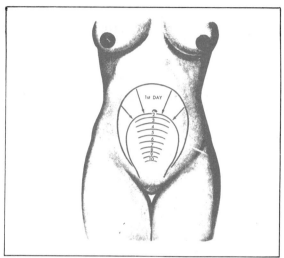

Figure 18-1

Changes in height of fundus during first ten days postpartum (Courtesy of Carnation Company)

the first to fourth day postpartum and is called *lochia rubra*. The discharge is referred to as *lochia serosa* when it changes to a dark brownish red and then to a yellowish brown from the fourth to fourteenth day. From the fourteenth day to the end of puerperium, the secretion is less profuse and whitish in color. It is called *lochia alba*.

The nurse must observe the patient carefully to make sure that involution and lactation are progressing normally. Many complications of the postpartum period can be avoided or prevented by early treatment. The nurse should daily check the following and report any unusual changes to the supervising nurse or physician.

- ✓ Fundus: firmness of fundus, fingerbreadths from umbilicus
- ✓ Lochia: amount and characteristics such as color and odor
- ✓ Episiotomy: clean, healing, irritated, inflamed

√ Breasts: soft, firm, engorged, painful
√ Nipples: erect, flat, inverted, cracked, painful

The Perineum

The procedures used for perineal care differ according to the policy of the individual hospital. The patient is instructed in the procedure. When the patient is allowed to take showers and have bathroom privileges she administers perineal care herself. The various procedures have the following characteristics in common:

- Perineal care is given during the bedbath or shower and after elimination.
- The soiled perineal pad is removed from front to back to prevent contamination.
- The perineum is cleansed from front to back to prevent contamination.
- After the perineum has been cleansed, the clean pad is applied from front to back.

Healing of the episiotomy may cause the patient some discomfort. Tissue surrounding the sutures may become edematous and cause pressure on the sutures. The doctor may order the application of an ice bag immediately following delivery to minimize the swelling. The doctor may order a topical or oral analgesic, the application of dry heat with a perineal lamp, or sitz baths for the relief of pain. Cleanliness and perineal care after each voiding are most important.

The Urinary System

During the puerperium, strain is put on the urinary system because the body is eliminating unusually large amounts of fluid to return to the normal fluid balance. The process of labor may have bruised the urethra and bladder and weakened the abdominal wall. Because of this, the patient may have difficulty voiding in spite of the increased necessity of voiding frequently. If ordinary means have not been effective within six hours after the delivery, the doctor may order catheterization. The nurse should be alert for signs of urinary retention and residual urine. A full bladder will keep the uterus from staying contracted and will displace it from the midline.

The Bowels

Constipation is a common problem during the puerperium. Loss of muscle tone following delivery and inactivity are predisposing causes. The doctor may order a mild laxative or an enema if the condition persists.

Recovering from a Cesarean Birth

A woman should be encouraged to get out of bed within twelve to twenty-four hours after her cesarean section. The nurse should aid the woman the first time, for she might be dizzy or light-headed. She should be encouraged to stand tall and move around. Movement helps alleviate gas pains and speeds recovery. Care should be taken to avoid wound infection. The incision should be inspected regularly for any signs of infection, and the patient should be instructed on how to identify problems. She should also be instructed on how to care for the wound site when she leaves the hospital. The usual stay is from three to six days. Postpartum changes are similar in both cesarean and vaginal births.

CONDITION OF THE BREASTS

The breasts change rapidly after delivery to prepare for the nourishment of the newborn. They secrete a small amount of colostrum during the first day postpartum. Colostrum provides the newborn with immune bodies and a large amount of vitamin A. It also acts as a laxative for the newborn. Milk is present on the second or third day postpartum, depending upon how early after birth the baby is allowed to nurse.

Engorgement

On the second or third day after delivery there is usually a rush of blood and lymph into the breasts. This is known as *engorgement*. Engorgement results from congestion and increased vascularity in the breasts as well as from accumulation of milk. It precedes true lactation and lasts about 48 hours. The breasts become swollen, hard and painful due to the increased blood and lymph supply.

If the mother decides not to nurse her baby, application of ice packs to each breast for at least an hour three or four times a day controls breast discomfort. The mother should wear a well-fitted bra that gives adequate support 24 hours a day. If the breasts are pendulous, a breast binder may be applied. The doctor may order a hormonal medication to inhibit milk production and an analgesic medication to relieve discomfort. Engorgement should subside in 24 to 48 hours. Occasionally, milk may reappear in the breasts in ten or twelve days, and the same treatment is indicated. Pills or hormone injections do not help at this time. If there is an area on either breast which becomes red, hot, and tender, the physician should be notified without delay.

If the mother is breast feeding her baby, she should not decrease nursing time as this only increases the discomfort from engorgement. Once the baby begins to nurse vigorously and regularly, engorgement seldom is a problem. The following steps may help relieve the discomfort of engorgement.

- The mother should express milk from the engorged breasts manually before nursing. In this way, the pain is lessened because the breasts become less full and softer. The baby is then able to more easily take the nipple and empty the breasts of still more milk.

- Both heat and ice packs may help relieve the discomfort of engorgement. Hot packs placed on the breasts or a hot shower

stimulates the breasts to leak milk. Ice packs on the breasts constrict the blood vessels and decrease engorgement. The mother may try either approach or both at different times.

- Massaging the breasts may help open any obstructed ducts that are causing the accumulation of milk. If breasts are too tender to massage, manual expression of milk from the breasts during a hot shower may help.

- A nursing bra that supports the breasts firmly but does not fit too tightly will make the mother more comfortable. A bra that is too tight can cut off circulation and actually causes plugged ducts.

Sore or Cracked Nipples

Some discomfort of the nipples is common when a woman first begins to nurse. The soreness usually disappears after the breasts become accustomed to nursing. The mother may express a small amount of milk from the breasts before nursing. This makes the milk flow more readily and the baby can nurse with less effort. Also, letting the baby nurse more often for shorter periods puts less strain on the sore nipples. The mother can offer the less sore nipple first so that the baby is less hungry by the time it nurses on the sore nipple. Nursing in different positions helps relieve the problem as it puts pressure on different parts of the nipple.

The breasts should be washed first during the daily shower to prevent contamination from other parts of the body. The nipple is washed first and the rest of the breast is cleansed by using circular motions upward from the nipple. Gentle handling and cleanliness are necessary to prevent cracks in the nipple and possible infection. Soap on the nipple area should be used sparingly and rinsed thoroughly as soap is drying to the skin and increases the risk of cracks in the nipple. Petroleum jelly, alcohol, or any other irritating substance should not be used on the nipples. Only a mild emollient cream such as lanolin should be used. The nipples should be kept clean and dry and exposed to the air as much as possible. Heat from an electric lamp (60-watt bulb) at a distance of at least 18 inches for 20 minutes two or three times a day will help heal sore nipples. Sore nipples should be examined by the physician.

Lumps

Lactating breasts are lumpy; the lumps may shift from day to day. The breasts may become especially lumpy if a woman goes too long between breast feedings. Breasts also may feel lumpy if engorgement is present. The nursing mother can be reassured that any lumps she may feel are most likely harmless. Examination of the breasts by a physician can allay the mother's concern.

Leaking

Leaking of milk from the breasts is a common problem at first for nursing mothers. However, leaking usually decreases as nursing is established. Generally, a woman feels a tingling in her breasts that signals that the rush of milk is imminent. If that sensation occurs when she is not ready to nurse, pressing the heels of her hands firmly against her breasts may check the flow of milk. The breasts also may begin to leak two or three hours after the last feeding without any warning signals. It may be necessary for the mother to wear breast pads if the nipples leak. Breast pads should be changed when they become damp and soiled. Some women do not tolerate continuous moisture around the nipple and should be cautioned not to wear plastic liners continually.

Sagging

Changes in the breasts take place as a result of pregnancy. Generally, the more weight gained during pregnancy, the more the breasts sag afterward. The firmness and contour of the breasts before and after pregnancy are influenced largely by heredity. Aging is the most common cause of sagging because it robs the skin of its elasticity. Sagging of the breasts is not caused by lactation.

Mastitis

Mastitis (inflammation of the breast) may occur during lactation. A duct becomes plugged, or the let-down is incomplete for a few feedings, or for some other reason the milk fails to flow from one section of a breast. *Stasis* (stoppage or slowing of normal flow of fluid) occurs, the milk backs up, the area becomes tender to touch or slightly reddened and infection begins to develop. It is important to get the affected area flowing again. The mother should be helped to relax so that her let-down reflex will function well. Hot compresses on the sore area and frequent nursing on the affected breast is often recommended.

The physician should be notified immediately and may order antibiotic therapy. Some physicians believe that the mother should stop nursing on the affected breast and continue to express milk from the breast manually or with a breast pump. Other physicians believe that it is necessary to stop nursing on the affected breast only if there is a purulent discharge from the nipple or an actual abscess. Not emptying the breast aggravates the backed-up milk problem and can make the situation worse. If antibiotic therapy is started immediately and the breasts are emptied regularly, mastitis can subside in a day or two.

COMPLICATIONS DURING THE PUERPERIUM

Some of the most common organisms which invade the reproductive system during the puerperium are streptococci, staphylococci, gonococci, pneumococci, and bacteria native to the bowel. In the nineteenth century, puerperal infection was commonly known as *childbed fever*.

Puerperal Infection

Puerperal infection, a term which refers to the infection of any part of the reproductive system after delivery, has been largely prevented in modern medicine by aseptic technique and effectively treated with antibiotic drugs.

Puerperal infection is suspected in any patient who is feverish during labor, delivery, or in the postpartum period. The symptoms vary according to the location and severity of the infection. Symptoms of local infection include a slight rise in temperature, edema, inflammation, and tenderness of the part affected. Indications of a severe infection are malaise, fever, chills, lower abdominal tenderness, faulty regression of the uterus and purulent lochia. It is important for the nurse to note the height of the fundus, characteristics of the lochia, and healing of the episiotomy so that medical attention can be given at the first sign of infection and proper isolation measures taken.

Treatment consists of the administration of antibiotic or sulfonamide drugs after the causative organism has been determined and comfort measures taken to relieve the symptoms of fever.

Puerperal Thrombosis (Thrombophlebitis)

A slowdown in circulation during the post-partum period may cause *thrombi* (blood clots) to form in the legs or pelvis. The inflammation of a vein which results in a blood clot is called *thrombophlebitis.* The most common site for this condition is the patient's legs. Signs of the condition may include a slight rise in temperature, swelling, areas of redness or whiteness (sometimes called "milk leg") of the leg or thigh, and pain. Pain or discomfort behind the knee or in the calf may be noted upon flexion of the foot when the leg is extended. This is known as a positive *Homans' sign.* The swelling may disappear after about two weeks, but it sometimes lasts for several months. The condition must be carefully treated. If a portion of a thrombus is dislodged into the circulation, it becomes an *embolus.* This embolus may be fatal if it is carried by the bloodstream into the heart or lungs, or into the brain.

To treat thrombophlebitis, the leg is elevated and a heat cradle is used to protect the leg from the irritation of bed linen and to apply dry heat. Anticoagulants are usually administered to lessen the danger of embolism. The patient usually remains in bed at least one week after the temperature has returned to normal.

Postpartal Hemorrhage

The average blood loss after giving birth is about 300 milliliters. *Postpartal hemorrhage* is bleeding in excess of 500 milliliters.

Uterine atony is the most common cause of postpartal hemorrhage. The uterus must stay contracted after delivery. Relaxation of the uterus allows the vessels in the uterus to bleed freely, particularly at the site of the placenta. Frequent massage of the uterus helps it to stay contracted. Also, oxytocics may be given to prevent uterine atony.

Laceration of the perineum, the vagina, or the cervix is sometimes the cause of postpartal hemorrhage. After delivery, the physician inspects the mother for any lacerations and makes repairs if any are present.

Retained placental fragments are an uncommon cause of postpartal hemorrhage. If the fragment is large, it will prevent the uterus from contracting, thereby causing hemorrhage shortly after expulsion of the placenta. If the retained fragments are small, hemorrhage may not occur until the fragments separate from the uterine wall leaving open blood vessels to cause hemorrhage. The placenta must be carefully inspected when it is expelled to be sure it is intact and no fragments are left within the uterus. If placental fragments are retained, they may be removed by dilatation and curettage.

Because of the risk of postpartal hemorrhage, the mother's vital signs should be monitored frequently (every 10 to 15 minutes) along with the quantity of blood loss for several hours after delivery.

Cystitis

Cystitis (inflammation of the bladder) is an occasional complication of the puerperium. If aseptic technique is carried out at all times and the bladder is emptied regularly and completely, inflammation can be avoided. Symptoms of cystitis are painful and frequent urination, pain over the bladder, and the presence of blood and pus in the urine upon microscopic examination. Diagnosis is made from a clean-catch specimen or a catheterized specimen.

The doctor usually orders one of the sulfonamide drugs. Fluids are forced. An indwelling catheter is ordered only if the patient cannot void.

POSTPARTUM DEPRESSION

It is not unusual for the mother to experience feelings of depression after her baby is born. Postpartum depression is caused by the physiological changes which are rapidly taking place, by exhaustion following the process of delivery, and by the fact that the long-awaited birth has occurred. After the delivery, the new mother may be doubtful of her ability to care for her baby. She may worry about the changes which may occur in the relationship between her partner and herself. The mother of a family may be uncertain of the reaction of the older children to the new baby.

The nurse may help the patient during this period by listening attentively, encouraging the patient to talk about her problems, and answering questions regarding daily health care. The nurse

should not attempt to give information of a medical nature, and she should not try to advise a troubled patient.

Mental or emotional illness may develop during the puerperium. The nurse should report to the physician any symptoms of insomnia, apathy, anorexia, delusions, feelings of anxiety or depression, and any dislike or repulsion toward the baby or her partner.

SELF-CARE INSTRUCTIONS

Under normal circumstances, most women leave the hospital two to five days after delivery. The woman is given a physical examination before discharge. She should also be given the opportunity to ask questions and discuss any problems or concerns that she may have. The mother is given instructions for her self-care at home during the puerperium and told to return to her obstetrician for a checkup within six weeks.

By the time the mother leaves the hospital, the lochia will be rapidly diminishing in amount and changing in color. Sometimes, because of excessive activity, the lochia may return to a red color for several days. Douching is not necessary, and in no case should it be started before the discharge stops or before at least three weeks postpartum. Consultation with her physician is recommended.

Resumption of Menses

The return of the menses after childbirth is quite variable and may take up to six months. The nursing mother may expect menses to reappear in two or three months, while nonnursing mothers usually start to menstruate in about six weeks. Many women do not menstruate while breast milk is their baby's sole supply of food. When formula or solid foods are used to supplement breast milk, menses may resume. This is because the mother's body produces less of the hormone, prolactin, when the baby sucks less often or less vigorously. As the amount of prolactin diminishes, its inhibitory effect on the ovaries decreases and ovulation and menses can develop. Some women do not resume their periods until their babies are completely weaned. However, some women begin menstruating even though they are breast feeding and their babies are receiving no other food.

The first menstrual period is often abnormal and profuse clots may be noted. It may stop and start again, but by the second period, it is usually quite normal. However, it may take a few months for a regular cycle to be re-established. It is possible for the cycle to differ somewhat in length from previous cycles.

Conception. The mother should realize that the possibility of conception exists at any time after childbirth, regardless of whether menses have recurred or not. She should not engage in sexual intercourse until the doctor indicates that it is permissible to do so. This is usually after the first checkup.

Lactation influences the return of menses and ovulation. During lactation, ovulation may be suppressed for as long as twelve to sixteen months. However, not all women maintain an anovulatory state during lactation and ovulation may start before menses. Therefore, it is not safe for a woman to assume that she cannot become pregnant just because she is not having her menstrual periods.

Breast Feeding During Menstruation. There is no reason why a woman should not nurse her baby while she is menstruating. Hormonal changes connected with the menstrual cycle may cause the milk supply to lessen temporarily. However, this is no problem if the mother allows the baby to nurse more frequently at this time.

Some infants may not nurse as well during menstruation and may tend to have more irritability at this time. This is a transient state and normal lactation will resume.

Personal Hygiene

The mother should continue the perineal care she learned in the hospital until after the episiotomy has healed. After bowel movements, as always, wiping should be directed upward and away from the vagina. After each bowel movement or urination, the mother should pour warm water from a clean pitcher or a peri bottle over the genitalia. She should then gently pat the area dry with cotton or facial quality tissue.

If the sutures continue to be uncomfortable, she may soak in a tub of warm water for 20 minutes and apply medication locally.

The mother should take a shower daily. For three to five days after delivery, her body may perspire more than usual as a means of ridding it of some fluids which were retained by the tissues during pregnancy.

Elimination

Hemorrhoids that appear for the first time in late pregnancy or as a result of delivery usually disappear. In the acute stage they respond well to cold witch hazel compresses and sitz baths. Occasionally, local medication may be ordered. The patient should avoid straining with stool. The mother should drink six or eight glasses of water a day. A stool softener, if prescribed by the physician, may be taken daily in the acute stages.

There may be a tendency towards constipation during the first few weeks postpartum. The condition usually responds to dietary measures

PARAMETER FOR ASSESSMENT	EXPECTED CHANGES	ABNORMAL FINDINGS	NURSING INTERVENTION
Pulse	May drop at first before returning to normal	Rapid pulse may indicate shock or hemorrhage.	Investigate cause. Report findings to the physician immediately.
Vaginal bleeding	Approximately 2 oz in the first 2 hr after delivery	Profuse bleeding Clots	Massage the uterus. Report finding to the physician.
Temperature	Mild elevation before returning to normal Patient may experience chill.	Elevation indicative of infection	Report to physician. Administer antibiotic, if ordered.
Blood pressure	Mild hypotension, after which BP returns to normal	Low blood pressure may indicate shock. High blood pressure may indicate preeclampsia.	Report to physician. Monitor blood pressure often.
Sleep	Mother will initially be excited and talkative before fatigue from labor and delivery efforts becomes evident.	Unable to relax in order to sleep	Explain the need for sleep. Prepare the patient and her environment in order to promote sleep.
Uterus	Gradual involution	Uterus fails to descend	Check involution each day. Remind the patient to empty her bladder regularly. Report findings.
Afterpains	Uterine contractions cause afterpains in the process of accomplishing involution. Pain increases with breast feeding.	Severe afterpain	Report findings to physician. An analgesic may be administered.
Perineum	Swollen and discolored; episiotomy healing	Infection indicated by pus Foul odor with lochia	Report findings to physician. Analgesics or antibiotics may be administered. Careful aseptic techniques Dry heat or Sitz baths to promote comfort

Figure 18-2

Postpartum nursing care

PARAMETER FOR ASSESSMENT	EXPECTED CHANGES	ABNORMAL FINDINGS	NURSING INTERVENTION
Bladder	Return to normal	Pain and frequent urgency, or an inability to urinate	Report findings to physician. Catheterize the patient prn. Force fluids. Obtain a urine culture. An antibiotic may be administered, if ordered.
Bowel	Normal function	Constipation	A mild laxative or enema may be administered, if ordered by the physician.
Breasts	Secrete colostrum until milk comes in	Breast becomes hot, red, or tender. Nipples become cracked and/or infected.	Apply heat or ice packs to affected breast. Teach mother how to massage breast. Report findings to physician if mastitis is suspected. An antibiotic may be administered, if ordered. Advise patient to use mild emollient cream on nipples. Apply dry heat to nipples. Instruct mother in use of nipple shield for nursing.
Postpartum depression	Possibility of mood swings	Severe depression	Listen attentively to patient. Encourage patient to talk about her problem. Report any severe symptoms such as insomnia, apathy, anorexia, delusions, or severe anxiety.

Figure 18-2 (Continued)

Sleep on your abdomen as much as possible. A small pillow may be placed under your breast to make you more comfortable.

Lie flat on your back. Breathe deeply with your abdomen six times. Raise your head a few times without moving any other part of your body. Attempt to touch your chest with your chin.

Lie on your back, stretch out your arms, then raise your arms up in front of you. Repeat six times.

Kneel with knees wide apart. Place shoulders and chest flat on floor. Do not let back sag. Draw up thighs. Stay in this position about five minutes every morning and night.

Lie flat on your back with arms at your side. Raise one leg (with knee straight) to halfway horizontal position. Then lower slowly. Do the same with the other leg. Then do the same with both legs.

Lie flat on your back with your arms crossed on your chest and your feet braced against the wall. Raise your head and shoulders slowly to a half-sitting position. Then slowly lower back to the floor. As your strength returns, raise yourself to a full sitting position.

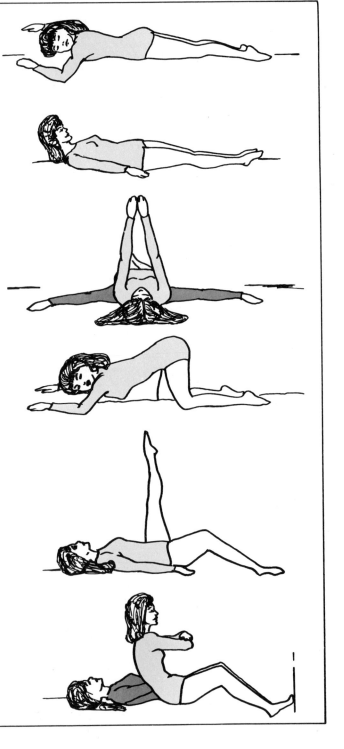

Figure 18-3

Postpartum exercises (Courtesy of the Maternity Center Association)

such as six to eight glasses of water daily; roughage such as celery, lettuce and greens; and adequate intake of citrus fruits, figs, dates, and prunes. A mild laxative may be ordered if necessary.

By the time the mother is discharged, the afterpains, if any, have usually disappeared. If they are still causing discomfort, they may be controlled by taking one or two aspirin tablets or acetaminophen every four hours as necessary.

Abdominal Support and Exercise

The abdominal support given by an ordinary girdle will make the mother feel more comfortable when she is on her feet. Exercise to improve the muscle tone of the abdominal musculature may be started two weeks postpartum, figure 18-3. The mother should begin her program of exercise gradually; the nurse should caution her about overexertion.

Diet

A sensible diet continues to be important. If less than 25 pounds was gained during pregnancy, the mother should not have a weight problem now. However, if she weighs more now than before she became pregnant, the only way to lose weight is by strict adherence to a reducing diet. If a diet is necessary, the physician prescribes the type of diet to be followed and supervises the mother's progress. If she is nursing her baby, she must increase the amount of calories in her diet as during pregnancy. She should drink the nutritional equivalent of one quart of milk daily and maintain a high-protein intake.

Activities

It is important to do things in moderation after the birth of a child. Usually it takes from six to eight weeks before a mother returns to her normal schedule of activity. Her return to normal is pro-

gressive; she begins to feel stronger day by day. Rest is extremely important. She should be encouraged to take naps during the day while her baby is sleeping. Strenuous work, heavy lifting, and excessive social activity should be avoided.

After the baby is a week or two old, there are no contraindications to travel except for possible overexertion and fatigue. If a long automobile trip is necessary, the mother is advised to get out of the car at frequent intervals and walk for several minutes to maintain adequate circulation.

POSTPARTUM CARE

The mother should return to the obstetrician within six weeks for a postpartum checkup. At this time she is examined and has the opportunity to discuss with the doctor any problems she may wish to bring up. Instruction in family planning may be given if the patient desires. The cervix is inspected. It is essential in terms of future health that the cervix be completely healed before discharge from medical care for this pregnancy.

If the effects of childbirth on the cervix require treatment, the patient is instructed to return regularly until full healing has occurred. The importance of complete healing cannot be overemphasized.

Discharge Planning

Discharge planning should include written instructions for observing and reporting signs and symptoms of complications, and the type of recovery to be expected. Also, date and time for follow-up appointment, and referrals to other community resources when appropriate should be given the mother.

When the patient is discharged, the obstetrician suggests that she have a yearly physical examination which includes a Papanicolaou smear for the detection of cancer of the cervix. These tests should be scheduled yearly.

ATTACHMENT AND BONDING

Attachment can be defined as an enduring affectional tie that one person forms to another specific individual. In 1972, Marshall Klaus and John Kennell performed a landmark study that provided the earliest evidence for the existence of a sensitive period in human maternal-infant bonding. Klaus and Kennell defined the sensitive period as the time "during which the parents' attachment to their infant blossoms. . . [and during which] complex interactions between mother and infant help lock them together." Between 1972 and 1982, seventeen additional studies were done on the effects of separating babies from their mothers directly after birth. Klaus and Kennell's initial findings corroborated that extra contact in the first several days led to more physical contact and affectionate displays between mothers and their infants. Several other studies tend to broaden the definition of bonding. Other factors affecting the process include: (a) the mother's economic status, (b) race, (c) housing, (d) education, (e) number of previous children and (f) age.

Marshall Klaus describes a bond as "a unique relationship between two people that is specific and endures through time." He considers fondling, kissing, cuddling, and prolonged gazing to be behaviors that indicate parental-newborn attachment. Klaus also divides the factors that produce a bond into two types: internal and external. Internal factors include not only how the mother and father were raised by their own parents but also the cultural influences as they were growing up. External factors, affecting a new mother's reaction to her newborn, include the way in which she is cared for during her pregnancy, labor, and delivery.

Nurses are in an ideal position to identify women at risk. These women are less likely to form maternal-fetal attachment. Prenatal care can then be altered according to these risks. These women may benefit from more frequent visits, focusing on the psychological rather than the physiologic changes. Providing extra support to the mother during labor and delivery, and encouraging extended contact in the immediate postpartum period, can be extremely helpful in promoting good maternal-infant attachment.

There are many reasons that parent-infant attachment is strengthened during the first thirty to sixty minutes of life. The labor stimulates a state of wakefulness and alertness in the baby that can last for several hours. During this time, the newborn is likely to become calm, begin observing, and sensing the new sounds, smells, sights, touches, and tastes around him or her. Klaus believes that the most important behavior during this time is touch. Studies show that new mothers instinctively begin by touching their baby's hands and feet. Then they stroke the baby's trunk. Often, the mother and baby lock eyes; they stare at one another. Finally, the mother begins talking to her baby, using both sounds and words in a special high-pitched voice.

Awareness of bonding-attachment has led to dramatic changes in the hospital environment. Klaus and Kennell's goal was to produce "conditions that are optimal for the development of parent-infant attachment in the first days of life." They recommend that during labor, the mother never be left alone. She should be attended constantly by someone giving guidance and reassurance.

Klaus and Kennell also advise that the mother and father be allowed at least fifteen to twenty minutes alone with their baby in a comfortable room after the birth. At this time, the mother should be encouraged to hold her baby naked against her bare chest even if she has decided not to breast feed. They also suggest that the baby be with the mother during the hospital stay either continuously or for long periods (minimum five hours a day). The mother should be the primary care provider for her infant, even if the baby requires an incubator for extra warmth,

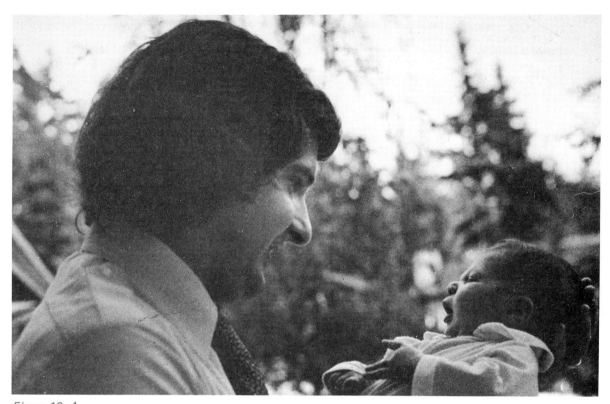

Figure 18-4

The father's role in the birth and development of his child is very important.

or is receiving ultraviolet treatment for neonatal jaundice.

If a newborn is very ill or is in intensive care, Klaus and Kennell recommend parents be allowed to visit the baby at any time, and they should be encouraged to touch and care for their infant. This contact and interaction will strengthen a mother's sense of confidence and give her a feeling of competence. A great deal of anxiety will be alleviated in this way during the first days she is alone with her baby at home.

Most of the research on bonding has involved mothers and their babies. Only a few studies focus on fathers. However, these studies also suggest that fathers, who have immediate contact with their newborn after birth, are more involved in the infant's care through the first

three months of life. It is also thought that these early bonding experiences extend beyond the newborn period. They affect the father-child relationship in later years.

With regard to breast feeding, Klaus and Kennell recommend total on-demand feeding. They also suggest fathers and siblings be encouraged to visit with mother and baby for long periods while they are in the hospital in order to strengthen intrafamily relationships.

In most hospitals, the father is at hand during the birth of the baby; in others, he is able to see the mother and child immediately after the delivery. The father is able to hold his baby and become acquainted with the newborn. Rooming-in helps to make obstetric care a family affair. By participating in the care of his child, the father is more likely to accept his new role and become aware of his unique position as a father.

The nurse and all other health personnel should consider both mother and father throughout the prenatal and postpartal period. Decisions regarding the pregnancy and plans for the new member of the family should be discussed with the mother and father. In addition, any questions regarding family planning can be presented and referrals can be made by the nurse.

SUGGESTED ACTIVITIES

Postpartum

- Practice applying a breast binder.
- Demonstrate postpartum exercises which improve abdominal muscle tone.
- Discuss the effect that lack of sleep can have on the body.
- Make a chart listing complications during the puerperium, their signs and symptoms, and nursing care to be given.
- Develop a plan to teach the patient about self-care during the postpartum period.
- Identify indications of and medical management of a retained placenta.

Attachment and Bonding

- List the variables that influence mother/infant interactions.
- List factors that enhance bonding.
- Describe observations of the mother with her baby that reflect the bonding process.
- Discuss the needs of the father during the immediate postpartum period.
- Identify the support measures that the nurse can provide to enhance the experience.

REVIEW

A. Item Selection. Principles of nursing care are listed with letters (a through e) followed by numbered statements. Read the statement and select the lettered principle which is demonstrated. Write the letter of the appropriate principle after each numbered statement.
   a. Encouraging normal involution of the reproductive organs
   b. Preventing infection of the reproductive and urinary systems
   c. Promoting rapid healing of tissue damaged during pregnancy and delivery

d. Encouraging normal lactation or suppression of lactation with minimal discomfort

e. Promoting a revitalization of physical and emotional energy

1. The application of dry heat and a topical analgesic to the perineal area
2. Fastidious care of the perineum during the daily shower and after each elimination
3. Preparing the patient and her environment to promote sleep
4. Application of a breast binder and administration of a hormonal medication
5. Massaging the uterus

B. Match the obstetrical terms in column I with the correct description in column II. Insert the appropriate letter before the term.

Column I	Column II
1. perineum	a. six-week period immediately following child-birth
2. embolus	
3. cystitis	b. discharge 4–14 days postpartum
4. puerperium	c. provides newborn with immune bodies and vitamin A
5. thrombophlebitis	
6. lochia alba	d. area between vulva and anus
7. mastitis	e. discharge 14 days to end of puerperium
8. engorgement	f. thrombus traveling in the circulatory system
9. lochia serosa	g. inflammation of a vein resulting in a blood clot
10. colostrum	h. return of organs to normal size and condition after delivery
11. lochia rubra	
12. involution	i. inflammation of the breast
13. stasis	j. filling of breasts with blood and lymph
14. afterpains	k. inflammation of bladder
	l. discharge 1–4 days postpartum
	m. uncomfortable uterine contractions during the puerperium
	n. stoppage or slowing of normal flow of fluid

C. Multiple Choice. Select the correct lettered answer.

1. Mrs. Jones tells her nurse that she is afraid of her baby and that she doubts she will be able to love the baby. The nurse should

1. ask Mrs. Jones what aspects of baby care she does not feel capable of handling and advise her
2. encourage Mrs. Jones to talk about her feelings and avoid giving her advice or criticizing her emotions
3. report the results of her conversation with Mrs. Jones to her attending physician
4. refuse to discuss these matters with Mrs. Jones

a. 1 and 2   c. 3 and 4
b. 4 only   d. 1, 2 and 3

2. A program of proper exercise
   1. helps the process of involution
   2. may be started two weeks postpartum with physician's permission
   3. improves the muscle tone of the abdomen
   4. is supplemented by lying on the abdomen while sleeping
      a. 1, 3 and 4   c. 2, 3 and 4
      b. 1, 2 and 3   d. 1, 2, 3 and 4

3. Recommended care of the perineum after discharge from the hospital includes
   1. wiping from front to back after each bowel movement and urination
   2. pouring warm water over the genitalia after bladder and bowel elimination
   3. changing the perineal pad frequently
   4. taking tub baths
      a. 1, 3 and 4   c. 1, 2 and 3
      b. 2, 3 and 4   d. 1, 2, 3 and 4

4. Some activities permitted during the first month postpartum are
   1. short-distance traveling
   2. marital relations
   3. heavy lifting
   4. mild exercise and light housework
      a. 1 only   c. 1, 2 and 4
      b. 1 and 4   d. 4 only

5. What must be completely healed before the patient is discharged from the doctor's care?
   a. Episiotomy   c. Cervix
   b. Uterus   d. Breasts

6. A Papanicolaou smear is a test for
   a. syphilis   c. cancer of the uterus
   b. cancer of the cervix   d. gonorrhea

7. Postpartum depression may occur in some women because of
   a. hormonal changes   c. physical exhaustion
   b. physiological changes   d. all of these

D. What should the nursing goal be for a patient in the postpartal period of her delivery? Use a care plan with short- and long-term goals.

UNIT 19

CHARACTERISTICS AND CARE OF THE NEONATE

OBJECTIVES

After studying this unit, the student should be able to:

- Differentiate between the characteristics of a full-term newborn and a premature infant.

- Identify standard nursing care for a full-term and a premature infant.

- Describe the steps involved in bathing the neonate.

- Describe four ways to properly hold a baby.

- State the purpose of gavage feeding.

The human baby is helpless at birth. Due to the force of gravity, activities which were possible in utero are now impossible. While in utero, the infant does not have to support its own weight or maintain its own balance as the amniotic fluid provides a weightless environment for the fetus. The fetus can turn around, move from side to side, and even do slow somersaults rather freely. The amniotic sac offers little resistance to the movements of the fetus yet it gives a sense of security by providing a point of contact in any direction when the fetus reaches out.

The newborn can perform only involuntary reflex responses. Impressive though the strength of the newborn's reflex grasp may be, it is far from the voluntary grasp the baby is capable of at four months of age or the determined holding-on that is achieved some time after that.

REFLEXES

Many of the newborn's reflexes help to ensure survival. Rooting, sucking, and swallowing are reflexes which enable the baby to obtain nourishment. Other reflexes help the newborn to relieve irritation or avoid unpleasant stimuli. Reflexes reflect the development of the newborn's nervous system. Some reflexes may also serve as the groundwork on which the baby begins the complicated business of learning the control of his or her body.

Moro or Startle Reflex. After birth, when the baby reaches out and does not find a point of contact it may have a feeling of falling into space. This produces a reaction known as the Moro reflex. The Moro reflex, also known as the startle reflex, is a defensive response of newborns. The infant tenses, throws its arms out in an embracing motion and cries loudly. This can occur when the infant is asleep or awake. By the fourth month, the baby is less easily startled and the response is less marked. By the sixth month the reflex disappears completely except in circumstances of extreme fright.

Galant Reaction. If the baby's back is stroked on one side while the baby is lying on its stomach, the whole trunk curves toward that side. This reaction disappears by the end of the second month.

Tonic Neck Reflex. This is a postural reflex in which the infant, when lying on its back, turns its head to one side and extends the arm and the leg on the side to which the head is turned at right angles from its body. The infant flexes the other leg and arm and may make a fist with both hands. This position has been called the infant's fencing position. It disappears around the fifth to sixth month.

Primary Standing. If supported upright on its feet, the infant stands, supporting some of its body weight. This ability disappears by the end of the second month.

Automatic Walking. When supported upright with some weight bearing, the infant's legs move reciprocally, imitating walking. This ability also disappears at the end of the second month.

Grasp Reflex. (Palmar) If a finger is placed on the palm of the infant's hand, the infant grasps firmly enough and holds on long enough to allow its body to be lifted. This strength diminishes rapidly and the reflex is gone by the end of the fourth month. The grasp then becomes conscious and purposeful. (Plantar) The feet exhibit the same reaction as the hands.

Although the infant cannot literally grasp with its feet, the infant's toes react to stimulation by trying to get hold of the object that is touching the sole of the foot or the toes. The reflex in the feet does not disappear until the eighth month.

Sucking Reflex. The newborn has the ability to grasp the nipple and areola area with its mouth, thus aiding the flow of milk. Sucking continues until the child can drink from a cup.

Rooting Reflex. The baby reacts to being touched on the cheek by turning its head in the direction of the touch in order to search for the nipple to feed. This reflex continues for as long as the baby is nursing.

Placing Reaction. When the baby's shins are placed against an edge, the baby steps upwards to place its feet on top of the surface. This reflex disappears at the end of the second month.

Protective Reflexes. Certain reflexes are absolutely essential to the infant's life; many of the reflexes are protective. Among the protective reflexes are the blinking reflex which is aroused when the infant is subjected to a bright light, and the reflexes of coughing and sneezing which clear the respiratory tract. The yawn reflex is, in a sense, protective, since the infant draws in an added supply of oxygen by yawning.

PHYSICAL APPEARANCE AND ACTIVITIES

A short neck, sloping shoulders, large rounded abdomen and narrow pelvis are all characteristics of the normal newborn, figure 19-1. The infant moves its arms and legs freely; the legs are often seen drawn up against the abdomen in the prenatal position. The hands are clenched and flail the air.

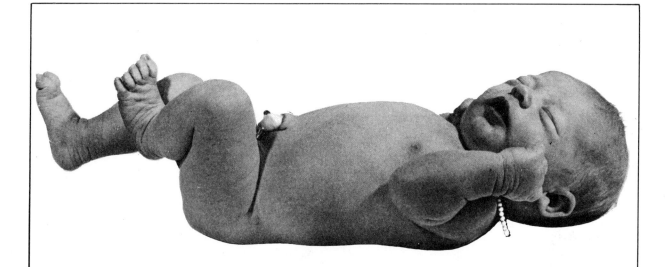

The feet look more complete than they are. Xray would show only one real bone at the heel. Other bones are now cartilage. Skin often loose and wrinkly.

Genitals of both sexes will seem large (especially scrotum) in comparison with the scale of, for example, the hands to adult size.

The trunk may startle you in some normal detail: short neck, small sloping shoulders, swollen breasts, large rounded abdomen, umbilical stump (future navel), slender, narrow pelvis and hips.

The skin is thin and dry. You may see veins through it. Fair skin may be rosy-red temporarily. Downy hair is not unusual. Some **vernix caseosa** (white, prenatal skin covering) remains.

Eyes appear dark blue, have a blank, staring expression. You may catch one or both turning or turned to crossed or wall-eyed position. Lids, characteristically, puffy.

Head usually strikes you as being too big for the body. It may be temporarily out of shape — lopsided or elongated — due to pressure before or during birth.

The legs are most often seen drawn up against the abdomen in pre-birth position. Extended legs measure shorter than you'd expect compared to the arms. The knees stay slightly bent and legs are more or less bowed.

Weight unless well above the average of 6 or 7 lbs. will not prepare you for how really tiny newborn is. Top to toe measure: anywhere between 18" to 21".

A deep flush spreads over the entire body if baby cries hard. Veins on head swell and throb. You will notice no tears as ducts do not function as yet.

The hands, if you open them out flat from their characteristic fist position, have: finely lined palms, tissue-paper thin nails, dry, loose fitting skin and deep bracelet creases at wrist.

The face will disappoint you unless you expect to see: pudgy cheeks, a broad flat nose with mere hint of a bridge, receding chin, undersized lower jaw.

On the skull you will see or feel the two most obvious soft spots or **fontanels**. One is above the brow, the other close to crown of head in back.

Figure 19-1

What a healthy newborn baby looks like (Courtesy of Baby Talk Magazine, Lew Merriam, photographer)

The healthy newborn has a lusty cry and within 24 hours has begun to suck, swallow, and move its lips. The skin may be covered with vernix caseosa although the skin itself is thin and dry. Veins may be seen through it; when the baby cries, a deep flush spreads over the entire body. Skin on the hands and feet is loose and wrinkled. Pinhead-sized white spots on the nose, cheeks or chin called *milia* may be present. These spots are caused by obstructed sweat and oil glands.

The breasts in both male and female neonates may be swollen due to maternal hormones they were exposed to prior to birth. Some babies even leak drops of milk from the breast nipples. This disappears without treatment. A slight milky or bloody vaginal discharge may be seen in female infants.

The infant reacts to light by blinking, frowning, or closing its eyes. The eyes are unfocused and since the baby cannot control eye movement, it may appear cross-eyed. The neonate reacts to loud or sudden sounds and wakes and sleeps without any apparent pattern. The neonate can taste and smell and is sensitive to heat and cold. Body temperature is between 36° and 37°C (97° and 99°F) by rectum. The baby sleeps from 16 to 20 hours a day, awakening when hungry or uncomfortable.

The normal full-term infant has pudgy cheeks, a broad, flat nose, receding chin, and puffy eyelids. Birth weight ranges from 5 1/2 to 10 pounds. The average weight for boys is 7 1/2 pounds; girls weigh a little less. The overall length is between 18 and 21 inches. The head seems too large for the body. The bones in the head have not grown together and soft spots (fontanels) can be felt. One fontanel is located above the brow and is called the anterior fontanel; the other is at the crown of the head near the back and is called the posterior fontanel. The anterior fontanel closes within 18 months; the posterior takes two to six months to close. A neonate's head circumference is usually about one to two inches larger than the chest circumference. This rule of measurement is referred to as the law of cephalocaudal disproportion.

The newborn looks surprisingly complete in contrast to its size. The hands, for example, resemble those of an adult with fingerprints, fingernails, and creases on the palms. The nurse soon learns that the newborn is a person in its own right and must be treated accordingly. The most important year in a baby's life is the first nine months in utero and the first three months after birth. During pregnancy all the baby's needs were supplied by the mother's body. After birth it is necessary to protect and nourish the baby as an independent individual.

The evaluation of the behavior of the newborn infant has concerned many in recent years. In the first half of the twentieth century, emphasis in developmental research was on the environment's effect in shaping the child. Many researchers now feel that the individuality of the infant may be a powerful influence in shaping the relationship the infant has with its caretakers. For this reason, behavior should be evaluated as early as possible. By three months, a great deal of important interaction has already occurred, and future patterns may already be set.

THE NEONATAL BEHAVIORAL ASSESSMENT SCALE

The behavior of the neonate is not the result of genetics alone. The intrauterine environment contributes to the physiological and psychological development. The fetus in utero is influenced by such things as nutrition, infection, hormones, and drugs. Evidence is rapidly accumulating to substantiate the fact that the behavior of the newborn is *phenotypic* at birth, not *genotypic;* that is, it is a combination of heredity and environment rather than heredity alone.

Dr. T. Berry Brazelton has developed an assessment scale for the purpose of "obtaining more exact knowledge of the developing neurological functions as early as possible and of the relationship of obstetrical complications to neurological abnormalities in later life."[1] Designed with the help of many researchers and colleagues over a span of twenty years, the resultant psychological scale assesses the infant's capabilities which may be relevant to its social relationships. Abnormal signs which are present in the early days or weeks may disappear to be followed by the appearance of abnormal functions months or years later. Documentation of the wide span of behaviors available to the neonate may reveal some predispositions to personality development. Although the Apgar scores of the infant's responsiveness immediately after delivery have proven to have a moderate predictive value for the future outcome of the infant's central nervous system, there must be clinical evaluation which reflects the neonate's future development.

New parents need guidelines for helping them evaluate the unfamiliar and unexpected situations that arise in the course of caring for a newborn. They need reassurance that "normal" includes a variety of behavior. This helps first time parents to relax and enjoy caring for their baby. The nurse is in a unique position to help parents focus in on their newborn's special personality. One way to help parents understand their baby's uniqueness is to teach them aspects of the Neonatal Behavioral Assessment Scale (NBAS). The scale contains 27 characteristics of newborns grouped into four categories: (a) irritability, (b) social responsiveness, (c) activity level and maturity of physical movements, and (d) response to stress. Every newborn scores differently. The baby's responses can reveal ways of approaching his or her care.

[1] T.B. Brazelton, W.B. Parker, B. Zuckerman, "Importance of Behavioral Assessment of the Neonate," *Current Problems in Pediatrics* 7:2 (December 1976):1–82.

State of Consciousness and Reaction Control

An important consideration throughout the tests is the infant's state of consciousness. This state depends on physiological variables within the sleep-awake cycle such as hunger, nutrition, degree of hydration, and time. The sleep states may be classified as (1) deep sleep with regular breathing, eyes closed, and no spontaneous activity except startles or jerky movements at quite regular intervals; and (2) light sleep. The awake states are categorized as (1) drowsy or semi-dozing; (2) alert, with bright look; (3) eyes open; and (4) crying.

The neonate is making a tremendous physiological readjustment to the extrauterine state and all of the baby's reactions must be viewed in this context. The fact that the neonate has any energy left over for periods of cognitive or affective responses is amazing. The neonate's reactions to all stimulation are dependent upon its ongoing state of consciousness; any interpretation of them must be made with this in mind. In addition, use of a particular state to maintain control of the neonate's reactions to environmental and internal stimuli is an important mechanism and reflects its potential for organization.

Further assessment of the infant's ability for self-organization is contained in the skills measuring the ability for self-quieting after aversive stimuli. This is contrasted to the infant's need for stimuli from the examiner to help quiet it. In the exam, a graded series of procedures (talking, hand on belly, restraint, holding and rocking) are designed to calm the infant. The scale results in an evaluation of control over interfering motor activity on the infant's part. In addition, the infant's responsiveness to animate and to inanimate stimulation is assessed. Examples of animate stimulation are cuddling and the voice and face of the examiner. Inanimate stimulation might include auditory, visual, and temperature changes (such as rattle and bell, red ball and white light, being uncovered). With these stimuli there is an attempt to elicit the infant's best performance in response to different kinds of stimulation.

The items on the scale are scored according to the infant's reactions and responses. Some are scored according to the infant's responses to specific stimuli; others, such as consolability and alertness are a result of continuous behavioral observations throughout the assessment. Most of the scales are set so that the midpoint is the norm. Since many infants lack coordination for 48 hours after delivery, the behavior on the third day must be taken as the expected mean.

The assessment itself usually takes between 20 and 30 minutes and involves about 30 different tests and maneuvers. It should begin with the infant asleep, covered and dressed, about midway between two feedings. The assessment includes the following procedures:

(1) Observe the infant for two minutes — note state
(2) Flashlight (3 to 10 times) through closed lids
(3) Rattle (3 to 10 times)
(4) Ball (3 to 10 times)
(5) Uncover infant
(6) Light pinprick (4 times)
(7) Ankle clonus
(8) Plantar grasp
(9) Babinski responses
(10) Undress infant
(11) Palmar grasp
(12) Passive movements and general tone
(13) Orientation, inanimate: visual and auditory
(14) Pull to sit
(15) Standing
(16) Walking
(17) Placing
(18) Incurvation
(19) Body tone across hand
(20) Crawling — prone responses
(21) Pick up and hold hand
(22) Glabella reflex
(23) Spin — tonic deviation and reflex
(24) Orientation, animate: visual, auditory, and visual and auditory
(25) Cloth on face
(26) Tonic neck reflex
(27) Moro reflex

As the nurse observes and records each assessment, it is then scored on a nine-point scale and 20 elicited reflexes each of which is recorded on a three-point scale. The midpoint is the norm The mean is related to the expected behavior of an average 7+. The Brazelton scale departs from many standard assessment procedures in that, in all but a few items, the infant score is based on the infant's best, not its average performance. Thus, particularly if the infant has responded poorly or not at all to a particular stimulation, the examiner should make every effort to verify that the infant is capable of a better response.

Of the four categories of behavior on the scale, *irritability* focuses on behaviors that frequently distress new parents. Parents of the irritable, fussy baby feel helpless; their attempts to calm and console their baby are ineffective. Using scale items in this category can help determine if the parents have a quiet and calm baby, a fairly well-organized baby, who gets upset only occasionally, or a very irritable baby, who by nature spends a lot of time crying. The evaluation cannot assess parents' skill at consoling their baby, but it can demonstrate what personality traits the baby brings to the situation. The point is to show parents that a baby's unique behavior and response to irritability is derived from the infant's personality, not their parents' abilities as parents.

Items on the scale that determine how quickly a baby gets use to a light or a noise help evaluate how the infant controls his or her own behavior. A flashlight is shone briefly in a baby's eyes ten times or a bell is rung four times. Many babies startle by these activities. Then they will gradually stop all eye and body movement as if they were unaware that anything is happening in their environment. Other babies seem to stop all responses to the bell or light; then they suddenly startle several more times. These types of babies may need some additional assistance to help them maintain calm, for example, a pat on the back for reassurance. Still other babies seem unable to tune out stimuli; in response to it, they get more and more upset. These babies need a lot of assistance from parents to calm down. It may be advisable for these babies to live in a quiet home where extra environmental stimuli is kept to a minimum.

One of the most satisfying aspects of a relationship with a baby is *social responsiveness.* The Brazelton Scale gives parents a good idea of how easily they can get a social response from their baby, how long the baby sustains the response, and whether the baby prefers auditory or visual interactions with people and things.

When a shiny object, like a ball, is moved in front of the baby's face slowly or a rattle is shaken out of sight, the baby may or may not follow the ball with his or her eyes or turn toward the rattle. A minimum response is for the baby to become still and alert. Sometimes parents have difficulty sustaining a response, or they have to work so hard to get a response that they stop trying. Parents can be taught to move the object more slowly and return it to the baby's line of vision, or to repeat the rattle sound. These exercises increase the opportunity for exchanges between parent and infant; they reveal how long a baby can sustain social interaction. They also increase the parents' insight into their baby's unique personality.

Consolability, another aspect of social responsiveness, is a measure of the infant's innate ability to calm down after fussiness. Babies quiet themselves by sucking on a fist or finger, or by looking at or listening to something of interest.

Consolability is particularly interesting to parents and can be assessed with the parents watching. Parents watch the crying baby for ten seconds and slowly introduce a small amount of consolation such as talking soothingly. If this is ineffective, parents can try gentle restraints, such as laying a hand on the baby's trunk or holding one or both arms. The next step is holding the baby, then rocking, then swaddling, or giving the infant a pacifier. These methods give parents a selection of strategies to quiet a baby who is fussy for no apparent reason. Some babies can calm themselves when they are fussing, but need help to stop crying. The benefit to parents is the discovery that consolability is not related to the effectiveness of their intervention, but rather to some internal process that the baby cannot yet control.

Activity level and physical responsiveness can be observed; these aspects will help parents learn whether they have an active, alert, or a passive, quiet baby. Parents learn their baby is unique, and cannot be changed or be molded to conform to expectations. Using information from the scale, parents may learn their baby may be happier in a large crib rather than a small cradle. Some babies prefer to be carried facing outward and to be visually stimulated instead of being carried on a shoulder.

The final category is *response to stress.* This includes physical changes such as startles, tremors of the chin and limbs, and changes in skin color. Some infants rarely startle; others startle for no apparent reason. If the baby demonstrates frequent startles and changes in skin color, parents can expect that the infant needs some restraint. Many parents do not know that babies normally have tremors; they mistakenly interpret them as shivers caused by cold.

The capabilities shown on the NBAS can give parents some idea of how a newborn contends with a new environment. In this way, nurses can teach parents and help influence the post-

258/SECTION 4 THE POSTPARTAL PERIOD

natal period. Even when the results are no longer valid, learning to observe and understand their child is a valuable parenting skill.

NOTE: For more specific reading about how to administer the NBAS, refer to T. Berry Brazelton, "Neonatal Behavioral Assessment Scale," *Clinic in Developmental Medicine,* no. 50, (1973).

CARE IN THE NURSERY

In many hospitals, infants remain with their mothers twenty-four hours a day. Evaluation of the newborn is performed in the mother's room. In some hospitals, newborns are taken to the nursery for evaluation. The baby's temperature is taken and recorded and it is weighed and measured. The passage of meconium and urine is also recorded. The cord clamp is checked and the baby is dressed in a shirt, diaper, and receiving blanket. The infant is placed in the Trendelenburg position in the bassinet with its head lower than the body. This allows mucus to drain out of the nose and mouth. The crib card, in the appropriate color, is filled out and placed on the baby's bassinet. The cord clamp may be removed after 24 hours if the cord has dried.

Within a few hours after birth, the pediatrician gives the baby a complete physical examination. The examination includes the: (1) head for fontanels; (2) mouth for *lingual frenum* (fold attaching underside of tongue to gum), *precocious dentition* (early eruption of teeth), cleft palate, and harelip; (3) heart; (4) lungs; (5) abdomen; (6) extremities; (7) genitalia; and (8) anus.

The pediatrician may order an injection of vitamin K be given to the newborn. In adults, normal bacteria within the intestines help produce vitamin K. The newborn's intestines are sterile at birth and cannot contribute to the production of the vitamin needed for blood clotting.

A PKU (phenylketonuria) test is performed before the baby is discharged from the nursery.

If the mother and baby are discharged from the hospital early, the mother should be instructed to return to the hospital nursery, or to her baby's physician's office for the PKU test. If taken before any source of protein has been ingested and absorbed by the baby, this test is invalid. Phenylketonuria results from a congenital defect in phenylalanine metabolism. It occurs in about 1 in every 10,000 births. The abnormal accumulation of phenylalanine prevents normal brain development. The diagnosis is made by a simple urine test for phenylketone bodies and/or by blood tests for phenylalanine. If this condition is detected early, damage can be prevented by a special diet for the newborn. (See disorders of the newborn.)

The nurse closely observes the infant for the following and notes the results of the observation on the infant's chart.

- color
    pallor (lack of color)
    cyanosis (bluish discoloration of skin)
    jaundice (yellowish discoloration of skin)
- respirations, apical pulse
- presence of excess mucus
- condition of the cord
- passage of urine and meconium

The baby's temperature is recorded every four hours unless the doctor orders a more frequent check.

The doctor or hospital policy determines the kind of bath care the newborn receives. Usually the newborn is given a sponge bath with water or a bacteriostatic agent until the cord has fallen off. During the bath the nurse observes the infant for irritation to the eyes, skin, and umbilical cord. The nurse weighs the infant and takes its rectal or axillary temperature after the bath.

Unless contraindicated by the condition of the mother or baby, the infant is fed by the mother in her room, on demand. Before taking the baby from the nursery bassinet, the bassinet card and Identabands are checked. Identification

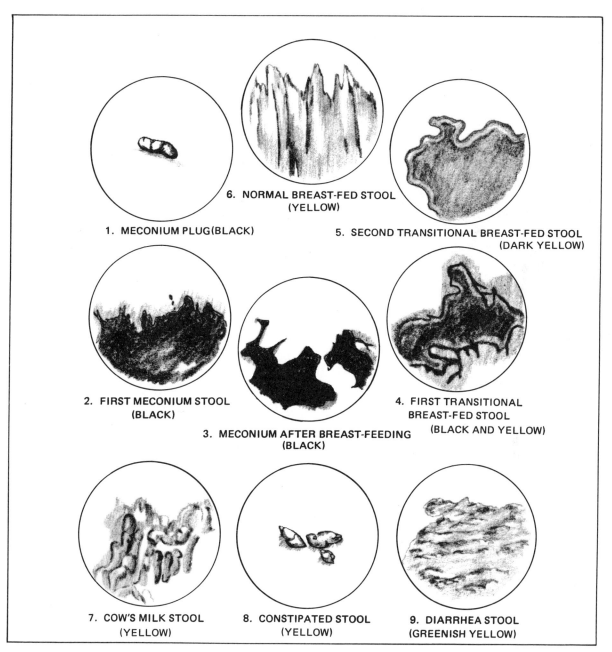

6. NORMAL BREAST-FED STOOL
(YELLOW)

1. MECONIUM PLUG(BLACK)

5. SECOND TRANSITIONAL BREAST-FED STOOL
(DARK YELLOW)

2. FIRST MECONIUM STOOL
(BLACK)

3. MECONIUM AFTER BREAST-FEEDING
(BLACK)

4. FIRST TRANSITIONAL
BREAST-FED STOOL
(BLACK AND YELLOW)

7. COW'S MILK STOOL
(YELLOW)

8. CONSTIPATED STOOL
(YELLOW)

9. DIARRHEA STOOL
(GREENISH YELLOW)

Figure 19-2

Infant stool cycle (Adapted from Clinical Education Aid No. 3, Ross Laboratories)

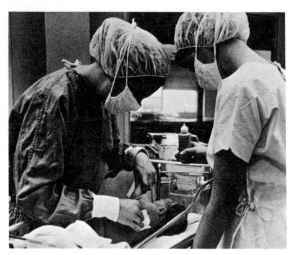

Figure 19-3

Mother observes a sponge bath in the nursery (Courtesy of Winthrop Laboratories)

of the mother and child is checked again in the mother's room. Also, if bottle feeding, the formula is checked to be sure it is the one prescribed for this particular child before the baby is taken to the mother's room for feeding. This is an excellent time for the nurse to instruct the mother in how to take care of her new baby and to answer any questions. If breast fed, the baby may be weighed before and after nursing.

FEEDING THE NEWBORN

Normal newborns, who are being bottle fed, can be started on feedings at the physician's discretion. This is usually within the first four to six hours. Should a newborn show clinical signs of hypoglycemia, a Dextrostix is indicated. If the Dextrostix reading is 25 milligrams or below, the physician must be notified. A follow-up blood sample is then drawn by heelstick and sent to the laboratory to be tested for blood sugar. Based on the result, the physician may begin feedings earlier than four hours.

If hypoglycemia is a possibility, Dextrostix testing should be done before each feeding until the infant's glucose level is stable and no clinical signs of hypoglycemia are present.

The first oral feeding offered is sterile water by nipple. Observation of the newborn's sucking, swallowing, and breathing coordination at this time is important. Enough sterile water needs to be consumed to determine if the esophagus is open. Should the infant choke, cough, or aspirate with this feeding, a feeding tube or DeLee mucous trap catheter may be passed through the mouth into the stomach to determine patency.

Once it has been determined that the infant is able to swallow without difficulty, the fluid intake may be changed to glucose water 5 percent by nipple. The amount taken is not as important as the infant's ability to suck and swallow and retain the feeding without difficulty.

Occasionally, an infant with abnormally fast breathing has some difficulty feeding. This must be taken into consideration and great care taken to ensure that the infant is breathing satisfactorily when being fed. Note any color changes in the infant during feeding.

Breast Feeding

Although milk is present in the breasts from the fifth or sixth month of pregnancy, high levels of hormones (progesterone and estrogen) prevent the milk from being released during the gestation period. At delivery, the levels of these hormones suddenly drop. This action triggers the production of large amounts of prolactin by the pituitary gland. The hormone, prolactin, is responsible for stimulating the mammary glands to produce milk.

During pregnancy and the first few days after delivery (before the milk is secreted) the breasts release colostrum. *Colostrum* is a thin, yellowish fluid composed chiefly of white blood cells and serum from the mother's blood. It is rich in antibodies, salt, protein, and fat. Colostrum also has a laxative effect and helps the newborn to expel the thick *meconium,* the substance in a neonate's intestinal tract.

About the third day after delivery, the breasts become warm, tender, and engorged with blood and lymph. The alveoli begin to function as a result of the prolactin, and a bluish-white milk replaces colostrum.

The success of giving an adequate supply of milk depends on the *let-down reflex.* As the infant sucks, the posterior pituitary releases oxytocin into the mother's system, causing the alveoli to contract. The milk flows into the main sinuses under the nipple and is released from the ducts in the nipple and areola of the breast.

Breast feeding is a natural function of the new mother. However, a positive and confident attitude is all-important to its success. The mother must be in a relaxed state while nursing or the let-down reflex is inhibited. Fear, pain, or other stresses release adrenalin through the body causing blood vessels to constrict; this prevents the hormone, oxytocin, from reaching the alveoli. (Oxytocin release may cause afterpains for a few minutes after nursing begins.) The nursing mother should be calm and relaxed. She may either sit or lie on her side in a comfortable position while nursing. The baby can be stimulated to take the nipple and areola into its mouth by tickling the lip with the nipple. Proper positioning of the baby is essential to successful breast feeding. The arm supporting the baby should be held at the side as if in a sling with the hand under the baby's buttocks. The infant should be elevated to the height of the breast, and then turned completely to face the mother, with abdomens touching. The other hand should support the breast with the thumb above and index finger below the areola, compressing it to make the nipple thrust out. The milk reservoirs are directly behind the nipple and they must be compressed by the baby's gums in order to release the milk, figure 19-4. The mother should

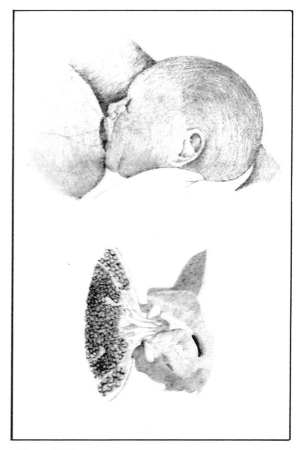

Figure 19-4

Proper position of infant's mouth on breast (Courtesy of Ross Laboratories)

be sure the baby's nasal passage is not obstructed by breast tissue so that the baby can breathe easily while nursing. To break suction when feeding is finished, the mother places her finger at the corner of the infant's mouth before removing the baby from the breast. The baby should not be pulled away from one breast so it can nurse from the other. When the baby takes a rest, the mother can alternate breasts.

Both breasts should be offered at each feeding as emptying the breasts stimulates milk production and prevents engorgement. The length of time the infant nurses varies widely from feeding to feeding and from infant to infant. Once a woman's milk supply is well established, a baby probably gets most of the milk from a breast in the first five to eight minutes. A woman may want to allow the infant this amount of time on the first breast and let the baby nurse on the second breast as long as desired. Infants continue to derive pleasure from the sucking and contact with their mothers long after their hunger has been satisfied. Twenty minutes overall is a good guideline if a mother wants to be sure her baby is getting enough milk.

Occasionally, it happens that a baby prefers one breast, perhaps because the baby is more comfortable on that side or because the milk flows more readily. The mother may try feeding first on the side the baby likes best so that the milk flows readily from the other breast when the baby uses it. She also can feed the baby at the second breast without changing the baby's position (by just moving the baby over). The mother may have to express the milk by hand from the nonpreferred breast for a while. The baby should begin to accept both breasts if the mother keeps trying.

The length of time at each breast will vary. It is advisable to allow the baby to nurse approximately five minutes each breast the first day; approximately 5–10 minutes each breast the second day; and approximately 10–15 minutes each breast the third day. More restrictive schedules can delay milk coming in as a result of decreased nipple stimulation. Also short feedings can prolong the engorgement period. This increases the likelihood of nipple trauma, if the baby has trouble latching-on to overfull breasts. Once the milk-producing cells have begun functioning, sucking and regular emptying of ducts in both breasts keep them producing milk for months or even years. The amount of milk produced is on a supply-and-demand system. The lactating cells of the alveoli replenish and produce the amount of milk the baby is demanding as it sucks and empties the ducts. To ensure an adequate supply of milk and to prevent the possibility of engorgement, both breasts must be emptied regularly. The last breast offered at a feeding should be the first breast given at the next feeding. The milk in the second breast is a mixture of *hindmilk* and *foremilk* and is of much higher caloric value. Hindmilk is stored in the alveoli and milk-producing cells of the breast. Foremilk is stored under the nipple and is not as rich in fats and calories.

Burping releases the air that may have been swallowed during the feeding. The baby should be burped frequently if on the breast, or burped every half-ounce if on the bottle. Otherwise, the baby will be uncomfortable and may burp spontaneously, regurgitating the entire feeding. Two methods of burping are shown in figure 19-5.

A mother may be uncertain about whether or not to wake her baby to feed it. If it has been longer than four hours since the last feeding or her breasts are full and uncomfortable, it is perfectly all right to wake the baby. Some mothers wake their babies to feed if they are trying to establish a more regular feeding schedule, especially if there is a pattern of long naps during the day and frequent feedings at night.

The gastric emptying time of breast milk in the infant is about one and one-half hours, so frequent feedings of breast-fed infants are warranted. The breast-feeding mother ideally uses the "demand" or unrestricted feeding schedule, offering her breast whenever her baby seems hungry, regardless of how long it has been since the last feeding. Frequent, demand feeding is important to establish and maintain a woman's milk supply.

Milk contains large amounts of water. Therefore, it is not necessary to give young infants additional water to drink. There is no harm in giving babies an occasional bottle of cooled boiled water to drink for comfort, particularly if they are crying between feedings, but it should not be given regularly.

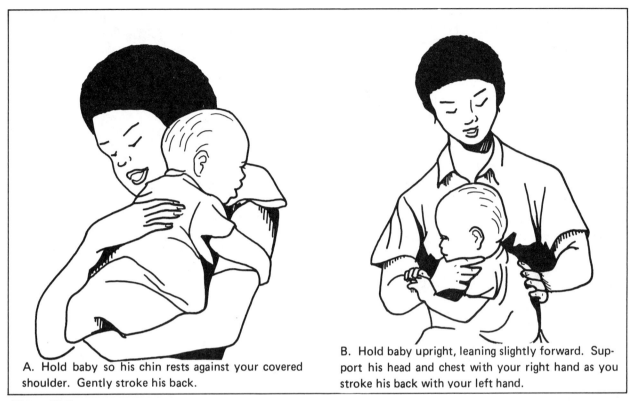

A. Hold baby so his chin rests against your covered shoulder. Gently stroke his back.

B. Hold baby upright, leaning slightly forward. Support his head and chest with your right hand as you stroke his back with your left hand.

Figure 19-5

Two methods of burping a baby

The nursing mother's diet has a direct effect on the quantity and quality of her milk and, therefore, should be closely supervised. An increase of fluid is also necessary. The mother's system uses up to 1000 calories a day to produce and give milk. The nursing mother should be counseled about taking any medication as some drugs cross into the milk supply. For example, some laxatives taken by the mother can produce loose stools in the baby. Certain foods also have a tendency to enter the milk supply; heavily spiced foods, chocolate, and caffeine can adversely affect some babies.

The level of estrogen and/or progesterone in birth control pills has been reduced so that it rarely affects milk production. Concern still exists because it is unknown if these hormones represent a carcinogenic risk to the nursing infant in later life.

If the woman becomes pregnant while still breast feeding, she can continue to breast feed the baby. Her milk supply may diminish after a few months of pregnancy because of the hormones produced during gestation. The quality of the milk, however, is not diminished and a pregnancy does not mean that a mother must wean her infant. It is possible to continue breast feeding during pregnancy right through to delivery and relactation. It does place additional emotional and physical demands on the mother. Especially demanding are the nutritional requirements of pregnancy and lactation together. For example, a woman would need 800 milligrams of calcium above her maintenance needs, as well as additional quantities of other essential nutrients to continue to breast feed while she is pregnant.

Breast feeding can be a positive, rewarding experience for both mother and baby. The closeness, both physical and emotional, begins a positive, strong bond between mother and baby. Good instruction and encouragement from the nurse in the beginning can help make breast feeding a successful experience. In addition, mother's milk is allergy-free, the right temperature, and always available.

BREASTFEEDING PROBLEM SOLVING

Checklist for Assessment and Intervention for Problems

Inadequate Milk Supply

- Offer both breasts at every feeding.
- Avoid supplementing or holding baby off.
- Do not take any medications unless you have checked with your doctor first.
- Allow baby to nurse as long as (s)he is interested.
- Recognize growth spurts with increased need to nurse (at around 2 weeks, 6 weeks, 3 months, and 5 months).
- Drink sufficient liquid (6–8 glasses daily); eat a good diet.
- Get plenty of rest; avoid exhaustion.
- Recognize that the breasts, even while breast feeding, eventually return to a more normal size.
- Breast feed 10–12 times a day in the early weeks.
- Learn proper technique for hand expression or use of breast pumps.

Sore Nipples

- Allow nipples to air after feeding.
- Watch for overuse or allergic response to ointments or creams.

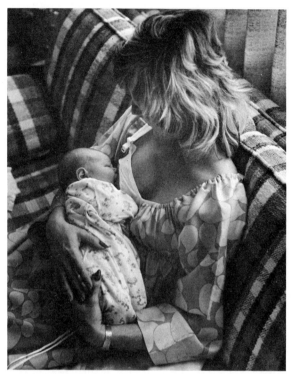

Figure 19-6
Breast feeding can be a positive, rewarding experience for both mother and baby.

- Position baby on areola (not just nipple); have baby face breast with body hugged close.
- Check nipples for thrush—if nipple soreness is persistent (long lasting), extreme soreness develops suddenly.
- Rotate positions at successive nursings to change pressure points.
- Begin breast feeding on least sore side.
- Wash nipples with water only. Avoid soaps and antiseptics.
- Use breast shields *without* plastic liners.
- Use a cylinder pump or electric pump. Avoid the "bicycle horn" pump.
- Bra should fit well, offering support, but not too tight.
- Nipple shield or bottle nipples may confuse baby's sucking response.

- If bra flap has adhered to nipple, moisten flap before pulling away.
- Offer areola by tickling baby's mouth to open *wide* (touch nipple to baby's bottom lip); pull baby very close with baby's abdomen against your skin.

Fussy Baby

- Be aware that most babies normally have a fussy period (common time 1–11 P.M.) Hold and rock the baby. It is fine to marathon nurse.
- Understand infant's need for closeness and contact. Baby carriers are great.
- Be aware that breast-fed babies nurse more often than bottle fed babies.
- Observe for possible illness in baby.
- Baby can sense if mother is overworked or under rested.
- Demand feeding works best. Because breast milk is easily digested, baby may need more frequent nursing.
- Evaluate your diet and eliminate possible allergens or foods that may produce gas (chocolate, cabbage, possibly cow's milk).
- Parent's emotional stress or crisis may affect baby's mood.
- Hold your baby frequently; offer various forms of stimulation.
- Decrease your coffee and cola intake.
- Avoid bathing baby while (s)he is fussy.
- Burp baby frequently during feeding.
- Allow baby to nurse as long as swallowing is heard.
- Baby may be fussy during menstrual period. (With total breast feeding, this usually does not resume before four months.) Milk production may be lessened due to hormones.

Cesarean Delivery. Breast feeding is just as desirable after a cesarean delivery as after any other delivery. If the mother has had a general anesthetic, or if her hospital is one that routinely places all babies born by cesarean delivery in a special-care nursery for 12 to 24 hours, she may need to wait until the baby's second day of life to begin breast feeding. Although intravenous fluids and other equipment may decrease the mother's mobility, the baby can be put to the breast with the help of the nurse. Postoperative medication should not pose a problem. Even if the mother must wait two or three days, she can start and maintain her milk supply by expressing milk or by using a breast pump. Her breast milk even can be collected and fed to the baby by the nursing staff.

The contractions of the uterus caused by the baby's nursing does not harm the mother's incision. With the help of a nurse, the mother can experiment to find the most comfortable position in which to feed her baby.

To protect the incision from the weight and wiggling of the baby, it is helpful while sitting to position the baby on a pillow placed on the mother's lap; to put the baby supported by pillows in a football hold at the mother's side; or the mother can lie on her side.

BREASTFEEDING PROBLEMS

Sore Nipples

Generally, the problem is a frequent one in the first 1 to 2 weeks of breast feeding. Possible causes follow:

- Infant is not properly put to breast; baby latches on to nipple at beginning of feeding instead of to the areola. Milk is obtained by gums compressing; the tongue strokes the milk reservoirs; the baby does not literally suck the nipple.
- Engorgement; infant is not able to grasp areola because of breast fullness. This is due to infrequent feedings or restricted nursing time.
- No variation in feeding positions; gums and tongue pressures are not distributed around entire nipple and areola surface.

- Slow let-down reflex; the infant nurses vigorously in an attempt to get milk.
- Prolonged feeding; greater than 15 minutes on the breast in the first few days.
- Frequent use of plastic lined disposable breast pads; they retain moisture and delay healing process.
- Improper technique in removing infant from breast; the suction is not broken; skin is stretched and traumatized as the infant tries to maintain a hold.
- Short, flat nipple; difficult for infant to latch onto breast, especially if engorgement is true.

Fallacy. Limiting the time at the breast to 2 minutes a side the first day, 3 minutes the second day, etc., is the best way to prevent sore nipples.

Fact. The converse is true. Many women do not get an adequate let-down in such a short period of time; the infant may nurse more vigorously, pull away, and make more frequent latching-on efforts. Limited sucking time and slow let-down can aggravate engorgement that further contributes to sore nipples.

Description. Amount of soreness may vary from slight to erosions and scabbing. Ongoing assessment should guide management.

Nursing Intervention.

1. Facilitate proper latching-on techniques by guiding the mother in shaping the nipple and waiting until the baby's mouth is open enough to take hold of the areola.
   - This decreases unproductive pressure and friction on the nipple.
2. Assist mother to relax and thus enhance a quicker let-down.
   - Infant can more quickly receive available milk and will satisfy hunger in less nursing time.

3. Break suction before removing baby from breast by inserting little finger into corner of the mouth and between gums, or by pulling down on the infant's chin.
   - To decrease trauma to nipple.
4. Offer guideline on amount of nursing time for first few days while nipples toughen up. This is approximately 5 to 10 min/breast/day 1; 10 to 15 min/breast/day 2; 15 to 20 min/breast/each day after.
   - Infant should not be allowed to dawdle at the breast during the early days of feeding, but they need adequate time to stimulate the let-down reflex and obtain available milk. Needs for time at the breast will vary with each mother-infant day.
5. Nurse more often but for shorter time periods. Ten minutes each breast every 1 to 2 hours is better for nipple integrity and milk production than 30 minutes each breast every 3 to 4 hours.
   - Less traumatic to nipples; more effective stimulation for milk production.
6. Air-dry nipples after each feeding for 15 to 20 minutes; leave bra flaps down between feedings when possible.
   - Exposure to air hastens healing; gentle friction with clothing will hasten toughening.
7. Apply thin layer of breast cream after air drying (Masse, A & D, Eucerin, Lanolin, or Vitamin E).
   - Soothing helps to prevent scab formation that may pull off with the next feeding, taking healthy tissue with them.
8. Rotate nursing positions (after mother has comfortably mastered one position); may want to practice at nonfeeding times.
   - To distribute pressure points around the entire areolar and nipple surfaces.

9. Determine where the sore spots are.
   - Will aid in selecting best alternative feeding position. Think of areola as a clock face; if sore spots are at 2 and 8, select a position that will put the tongue and gum pressure at 10 and 4.
10. Offer least sore nipple first.
    - The infant is better able to handle vigorous sucking activity that occurs at the start of a feeding.
11. Decrease sucking time on very sore nipples for a day (10 minutes or less); complete breast emptying by hand or pump expression.
    - May need to balance efforts of promoting healing by preventing milk stasis and encouraging milk production.
12. When the baby has finished with active, vigorous sucking activity, remove the infant from the breast.
    - Infant should not be allowed to meet all emotional sucking needs when nipples are sore. Suggest use of pacifier.
13. Apply warm, moistened tea bags to nipples, prior to air drying, for approximately 10 to 15 minutes. (Use real tea, not herbal varieties.)
    - Tannic acid has been found to help toughen nipples and promote healing.
14. Heat lamp treatment; have mother position herself approximately 16 to 20 inches away from an exposed 60-watt bulb for about 10 minutes. May need 1 to 3 treatments a day.
    - Heat promotes healing, increases blood supply, brings more O_2, and carries away dead cells, etc.
15. Last ditch measure; discontinue breastfeeding for one day. Hand or pump express and give milk in a bottle.
    - Use only for bad cases of fissuring, erosion, large scab formation and extreme pain.

16. Have mother check infant's mouth for white patches that will not rub off.
    - Infant may have thrush infection; this can infect mother's skin, causing soreness. Consult with physician if patches are present; mother and infant both need treatment.

Flat, Short Nipples

It is necessary to stimulate flat, short nipples to a more erect state to facilitate latching-on efforts and to lessen trauma. This is done by: 1) gentle manipulation, 2) a brief application of ice, and 3) milking the breasts for 1 hour before feeding. These actions help to stretch muscle/ligaments holding the nipple down.

Engorgement

Description. Fullness in breast(s) occurring when milk comes in; usually between the second and fifth day postpartum. It can vary from minimal to marked enlargement with accompanying hardness, soreness and aching, throbbing, low-grade fever and tight, shiny skin.

Causes.
- Increased fluid in breast
- Increased vascular and lymph supply
- Increased interstitial fluid
- Increased pressure from newly produced milk

Nursing Intervention.
1. Make sure that the mother knows that the acute phase of this problem will last 24 to 48 hours.
   - Knowing that the problem is short term is helpful to mothers. Problem dissipates as the milk supply and the baby's demand come into balance.
2. The main goal in management is to prevent or minimize the degree of engorgement.

- This is to spare the mother any unnecessary discomfort and to decrease the risk of plugged ducts, mastitis and sore nipples. It is also to facilitate the infant's latching-on efforts.
3. Management guidelines include shorter, more frequent nursing sessions around the clock as fullness begins to develop. The suggestion is given to feed approximately every 2 to 3 hours during the day and every 3 to 4 hours at night.
   - Frequent emptying helps to prevent the breasts from becoming over full. Night feedings are important.
4. Advise mother to take warm shower, or apply warm, wet towels to breast prior to nursing.
   - May stimulate a spontaneous let-down reflex with a subsequent reduction in breast tension.
5. Have mother gently hand express milk to soften the areola prior to nursing, with or without doing point #4.
   - The infant is better able to latch-on to the areola if it is softer and shapeable; results in less trauma to nipples. Also, sore nipples can inhibit a let-down, resulting in incomplete emptying; this aggravates engorgement.
6. Ice packs may be applied after and between feedings.
   - Cold will cause vasoconstriction and decrease breast tension.
7. A properly fitted bra is advisable.
   - It will offer support to overfull, heavy breasts. The bra must be big enough so as to not cause constriction; this could lead to plugged ducts and mastitis.
8. Avoid the use of glucose water supplements.
   - Will decrease infant's hunger/interest in frequent nursing at a time when

mother needs the infant's emptying help. It may also interfere with infant's imprinting on breast.

Plugged Breasts

Symptoms. Tender and/or red areas on breast.

Causes.

- Inadequate milk emptying; stasis of milk
- Going too long between feedings
- Wearing a bra that is too tight; this causes pressure points or constriction of portions of the breast.

Nursing Intervention.

1. Advise mother to feel for full or tender areas in the breast by using a circular motion. Follow with gentle stroking action in the direction of the nipple.
   - Early identification and management of plugged ducts will decrease the possibility of mastitis developing. To encourage milk flow, unplug involved ducts.
2. Apply a warm, wet towel or small hot water bottle to area.
   - Will enhance let-down reflex and emptying efforts. Increased circulation will aid in removal of dead cells, and destruction of bacteria.
3. Change feeding positions.
   - This will enhance emptying in affected areas by rotating the compression forces of the infant's tongue and gums.

Mastitis

Symptoms.

- Flu-like feeling, fever (101 to 104°F), aching, malaise, nausea and chills
- Red tender area not as localized as with plugged duct

- Large portion of breast may be erythematous, and streaking may be present
- Severe pain may occur

Description. This condition is a generalized soft tissue infection of the breast.

Nursing Intervention.

1. Consult with the physician when the above symptoms are present.
   - Antibiotic therapy is indicated. Neglect can lead to formation of necrosis and breast abscesses.
2. Advise mother to continue nursing on the affected side; increase frequency of feeding to twice the number of usual feedings.
   - Breast milk offers immunologic help to infant in order to deal with the involved organism; high acid content of the stomach will assist in destruction of the offending organism.
3. Allowing for pain threshold, suggest that the affected breast be offered first.
   - This maximizes emptying with infant's most vigorous sucking efforts. A mild analgesic 30 minutes before nursing may be helpful.
4. Advise mother to apply hot, wet compresses, followed by massage and hand expression.
   - Warmth will increase circulation to the breast, resulting in more O_2, enhance WBC and enzyme activity to destroy bacteria and dead cells.
5. An alternate approach to #4 is to use ice packs for 20 minutes or more.
   - Pain may be lessened with initial vasoconstriction, decreasing tension in the affected area. Prolonged application of ice will cause vasodilation with the same benefit as heat therapy.
6. Bed rest and increased fluids are advised.

- To facilitate the body's healing efforts.
7. Alternate feeding positions.
   - To facilitate emptying of all portions of the breast.
8. Nurse more frequently.
   - Frequent emptying prevents further/recurrent milk stasis.
9. Remove caked secretions on nipple by soaking prior to nursing.
   - To enhance maximum nipple duct patency; soaking will soften scab formation, allowing milk to flow more easily through softened covering.

Weaning. Weaning means transferring a baby from dependence on mother's milk to dependence on another form of nourishment. A mother can wean her breast-fed infant whenever she wants. Some mothers want to breast feed for a few weeks, others for more than a year. However long a baby is breast fed, the most important thing to remember about weaning is that it should be done gradually, if possible, for both the mother's and the infant's sake. Generally, replacing one breast feeding at a time with a substitute feeding is a good way to wean. When the infant is used to one substitute feeding, a second substitute feeding can be given after a few days. This process continues until the baby is no longer feeding at the breast.

Bottle Feeding

Both the nursing mother and the nonnursing mother should learn the techniques of bottle feeding. Supplementary bottles may be ordered by the pediatrician if the infant's need is greater than the mother's supply of milk. The nursing mother may want to give her baby an occasional bottle when her schedule does not allow her to breast feed.

On discharge from the hospital, the mother is given a set of instructions dealing with the formula. These instructions tell her the type of formula to use and how to prepare it. The baby may also be given one of the prepackaged commercial formula preparations on the advice of the doctor.

When bottle feeding the baby, care should be taken that the holes in the nipple are the proper size and that the nipple is full of milk to prevent the baby from swallowing air. After feeding, the baby should be placed on its stomach or on its right side. The newborn baby is able to raise its head so the mother should not be afraid that the baby might smother when lying on the stomach. If the baby is placed on the right side, the milk passes into the stomach since the stomach contour is to the right, thereby lessening the chance of aspiration. One or two ounces of water twice daily should be given in addition to the feedings. During hot weather, two or three ounces of water should be given twice daily. If the baby is constipated, an increase in the amount of water given daily will probably remedy the situation.

CARE OF THE PREMATURE INFANT

If the baby is born three or more weeks before the calculated date of birth (less than 37 weeks gestation), it is said to be premature or pre-term. Also, if the weight is less than 2500 grams (5 1/2 pounds) the newborn is designated premature. Weight is used to determine which babies require special care. The behavior and appearance of the infant are also considered in reaching the diagnosis of prematurity.

Although only 7 to 10 percent of all live births are premature, prematurity is the most frequent cause of death in infants. Premature birth may be caused by abnormal conditions in the mother, multiple pregnancies, or induced labor. The premature infant appears listless and inactive, weighs less than 5 1/2 pounds and is less than 18 inches in length. The fontanels are large and the *sutures* (lines of closure) are

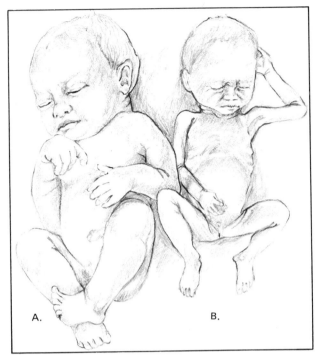

A. FULL-TERM BABY   B. PREMATURE BABY

Figure 19-7

The premature infant usually weighs under 2.5 kilograms (5 1/2 pounds). Because of lack of fat, the baby has thinner arms and legs, thinner cheeks and chin, a large head and large abdomen. The skin is loose and wrinkled and the baby looks old and anxious.

quite prominent. The cry is feeble and the sucking reflex is poor or absent. Features are sharp and angular; the skin is wrinkled because of the absence of subcutaneous fat, figure 19-7. The skin is dull red and covered with lanugo. Respirations are shallow and irregular. Body temperature is unstable and subnormal, frequently between 34 and 36°C (94 and 96°F). Since the blood vessels are frail, hemorrhage into the brain may occur. Many premature infants are unable to swallow and therefore require a great deal of care.

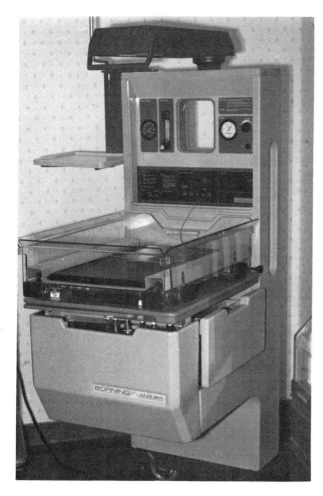

Figure 19-8

Care center supports neonatal assessments, monitoring hookups, and maintains infant body temperature. (Courtesy of Hill-Rom Corp.)

The survival of the premature infant depends on the skill, patience, judgment, and devotion of those giving nursing care. The basic principles to be observed in caring for the premature infant include:

- Maintenance of body temperature, figure 19-8
- Protection from infection
- Maintenance of airway and adequate oxygen intake

- Conservation of infant's energy
- Adequate fluid and calorie intake

Incubators are used to maintain the infant's body heat and to isolate the infant from sources of infection, figure 19-9. Incubators can be regulated to control heat and humidity and to administer oxygen. Some incubators such as the Isolette® have hand holes in each side which enable the nurse to care for the infant without removing the infant from the incubator.

The infant is placed in the incubator with the head of the bed lowered four to six inches to allow the mucus and secretions to drain from the throat. Suctioning equipment and oxygen should be available in case they are needed. Infants who remain in an incubator with an oxygen concentration greater than 40 percent for a prolonged period may develop blindness. Therefore, precautions must be taken to check the oxygen level frequently with an oxygen analyzer.

All babies weighing less than 2500 grams, those with cyanosis, babies having difficulty regulating body temperature, and infants who have respiratory difficulty require incubator care. In the incubator, the baby wears only a diaper; babies not in incubators are dressed in shirts and diapers and wrapped in blankets. Many babies may also wear stretchy cotton caps to prevent loss of heat from the head.

The temperature of the infant is taken every two to three hours until it has stabilized. Initially, the temperature is taken by rectum but in smaller infants it may be taken by axilla every three hours until the weight of 2500 grams is reached. As with the heavier infant, the temperature is then taken only twice a day after it has stabilized. The color, respiratory rhythm, and ease of breathing must be carefully checked at frequent intervals.

Babies weighing 1500 grams or more who can suck and swallow are fed in the usual manner

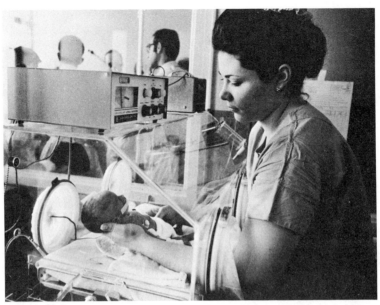

Figure 19-9

Caring for the premature infant in the Air-Shields® Isolette® infant incubator (Courtesy of Air-Shields, Inc.)

with bottle and soft nipple. Usually a 5-percent sugar solution is offered for four feedings on the second day of life. This is followed on the third day by an individually calculated formula. Since premature infants are susceptible to deficiency diseases, vitamins and iron are given after the seventh day.

The infant who has no sucking or swallowing reflexes may have to be fed by *gavage* (tube feeding) or medicine dropper, figure 19-9. The frequency and manner of feedings as well as the type and quantity of formula are prescribed by the physician.

To conserve the baby's energy, handling is kept to a minimum. The baby is left in bed for its bath, feedings, and examinations until weight increases to about 2000 grams. Weighing is done only twice a week unless the premature infant is in an incubator where trapeze-type scales can be used. If this is the case, the weight can be taken daily and the formula requirements calculated every 24 to 48 hours.

All personnel working in the premature nursery must be free of respiratory infections to protect the premature infant from infection. Routine checkups are given and the use of masks may be ordered. In addition, personnel are required to wear special uniforms, scrub their hands carefully, and wear gowns when handling the premature infant.

Gavage Feeding

Feeding by gavage is a method of providing nourishment when the infant is unable to suck or swallow or when it becomes too fatigued or has difficulty breathing while nipple feeding. Gavage feeding also is a means of administering oral medications.

A tube is placed through the infant's mouth or nose into the stomach. A syringe is attached to the tube and the formula or feeding is poured into the syringe. In a careful, controlled manner, the feeding is allowed to flow from the syringe into the infant's stomach. Care must be taken

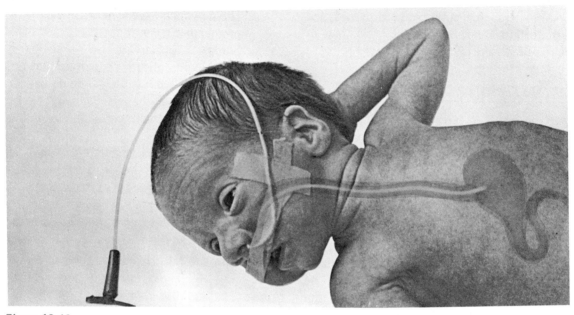

Figure 19-10

Plastic indwelling catheter inserted through nose will remain in place 3-4 days when taped as shown (Courtesy of Ross Laboratories)

to ensure that the tube is actually in the infant's stomach. Also, the nurse should be sure that no air is forced into the infant's stomach.

Intermittent gavage feeding is often preferred to indwelling gavage feedings. An indwelling tube may coil, knot, perforate the stomach and cause nasal airway obstruction, ulceration, irritation to the mucous membrane and nosebleed. If intermittent intubation is not well tolerated and an indwelling tube is used, the catheter should be size #3.5 or #5, taped securely to the skin and flushed with 1 to 2 milliliters of sterile water after every use. The catheter should be changed every 24 to 72 hours. No studies have been done to determine long-term effects of indwelling nasogastric tubes. Alternate nares should be used when the tube is changed and constant alertness to complications is stressed. When passing either an intermittent or indwelling catheter for feeding, observe the infant for brady-

cardia and apnea. Gavage feedings are usually increased in volume by one-milliliter increments every other feeding, depending on the amount of residual obtained prior to administering the feeding and the tolerance of the infant.

When the baby is matured enough to be fed by his or her mother, special feeding problems can still exist. Premature, small gestational age babies, hypoglycemic, dehydrated, sick babies can require supplementation. These babies do not suck long enough or strong enough to stimulate an adequate milk supply. They do not obtain enough calories and fluid without overtiring themselves. Mothers should be encouraged to express milk for supplementary use because of the benefits of breast milk, and the need to stimulate continued milk production. The use of a Lact-Aid or similar device is also recommended. Spoon, dropper, or an orthodontically correct nipple could also be used.

With the Lact-Aid, the breast receives additional stimulation for milk production and as a result the infant is not overfatigued in efforts to receive required caloric intake.

CARE OF THE INFANT AT HOME

Most new mothers are concerned about the proper skin care of the baby and the correct procedure for sterilizing the formula. These techniques may be demonstrated in the nursery before the mother and baby are discharged.

Bathing the Baby

A bath is given to the newborn with any mild castile soap, but it is recommended that a soap with cumulative antibacterial action be used. A small portable plastic tub may be used to bathe the baby. Placing a wash cloth on the inside bottom of the tub helps to prevent the baby from slipping during a tub bath. The tub should be set down in a convenient place which is secure and free from slippage; a rubber bath mat may be used under the tub.

- See procedure given later in this unit.

Care of the Umbilicus

The umbilicus should be washed off four times daily with ordinary rubbing alcohol until four days after the cord drops off. Some bleeding is common when the cord comes off. A large amount of blood or pus should be reported to the pediatrician.

Circumcision

Circumcision is a common minor operation in which the foreskin (prepuce) of the penis of the male baby is removed to facilitate cleaning and to prevent infection. There is no medical or legal reason for routine circumcision of the newborn; it is a matter of parental choice. Some facts the nurse may present for consideration are:

- It is a brief procedure
- The newborn experiences some pain because an anesthetic is not used
- Complications are rare
- Possible complications include bleeding and irritation of the head of the penis from the friction of wet diapers, followed by pain on urination and scarring of the urinary outlet
- There is a fee
- There is no evidence that circumcision prevents cancer of the penis or the prostate in the male, or cancer of the cervix in the female partner
- There is no evidence that circumcision or noncircumcision affects sexual performance

There are several procedures for performing the circumcision. The applied method is decided by the attending physician.

If the baby is circumcised, petroleum jelly applied to a gauze square is placed over the infant's penis for the first day in order to prevent the wound from sticking to the diaper. The wound usually heals in two or three days. The penis is gently cleansed with a moist cotton ball at bathtime. There is usually no need for additional care.

Diaper Care

Since urine contains alkali, the urine-soaked diaper is also alkaline. Improper washing of cloth diapers does not remove all of the alkali which accumulates. To prevent irritation to the skin, the alkali must be removed by a final rinse of a vinegar and water solution. The diapers are first rinsed in cold water, then washed with a mild soap such as Ivory or pure castile soap before the solution (1 tablespoon of white vinegar to 1 quart of water) is used to remove the alkali. Many persons use disposable diapers and discard them after they have been soiled. Careful cleansing of the baby's buttocks and genitalia after each diaper change, along with the use of alkali-free diapers, prevents uncomfortable diaper rash.

Tender Loving Care

Both the nurse and the mother should realize that the newborn infant reacts to the emotions of those who take care of it. The infant needs to be cuddled and loved just as it needs food, shelter, and rest. Understanding that the newborn reacts emotionally to people and situations is one reason that infants are fed *on demand* (when they are hungry) rather than on a rigid schedule. The mother should take advantage of bathing and feeding time to become acquainted with her new baby.

BODY SUPPORT FOR THE NEWBORN

At birth, the infant is not able to support itself and must depend on its caretakers for support. It is very comforting for a baby to be placed in the intrauterine (fetal) position with the arms and legs folded naturally against the body. It also gives the baby a sense of security to have a point of contact whenever it reaches out with its arms or legs. The main purpose for providing support, however, is safety; the baby must be protected from injury. For safety reasons, it is best to have two points of contact when holding and lifting a baby as even a newborn can be very wriggly.

Whenever a baby is carried or lifted, the head must be supported. The baby's head is larger and heavier than the rest of its body and the infant does not yet have control over its movements. Following are some common methods of lifting and holding a baby.

Lifting

Do not lift a baby by its arms. An infant lying on its back can be lifted easily and safely by the following methods.

1. Face the baby's side.

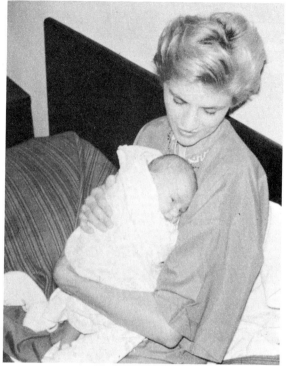

Figure 19-11

The infant needs to be cuddled and loved.

2. Slide one hand under the head and neck and grasp the baby's outer arm.

3. Support the baby's head with your forearm.

4. Slide the other hand under the baby's legs and grasp the thigh of the baby's outer leg. (Instead of grasping the baby's thigh, the feet could be grasped while holding one finger between the ankles, figure 19-12A.)

5. Gently lift the baby.

Another method which is often used is to lift the baby while facing its feet.

1. Face the baby's feet.

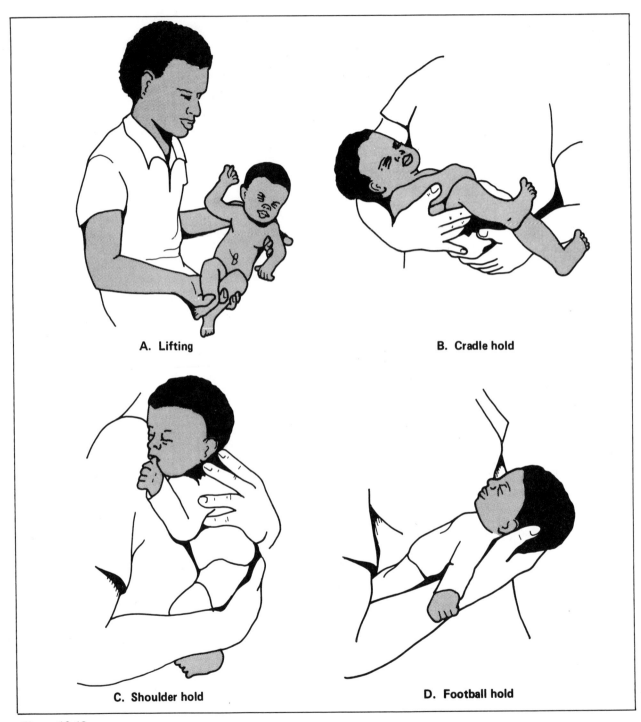

A. Lifting

B. Cradle hold

C. Shoulder hold

D. Football hold

Figure 19-12

Proper techniques for holding a baby (A–D)

2. Slightly lift the baby's legs and buttocks by grasping its feet with one hand. Place a finger between its ankles to keep the ankles separated.

3. With palm up, slide the other hand under the full length of the baby until the entire back and head are supported.

4. Gently lift the baby.

Cradle Hold

The cradle hold is one of the most common ways of holding an infant. A variation of it is usually used when feeding the baby.

1. Cradle the infant's head in the bend of your elbow.

2. Extend your forearm around the outside of the infant's body, figure 19-12B.

3. With the fingers of the same hand, grasp the infant's outer leg.

4. Place your other hand on the infant's buttocks for additional support.

Shoulder Hold

The shoulder hold requires two hands to properly support the baby's back. This hold can be used when burping the baby.

1. Place the infant in an upright position with its arms and legs against your chest, figure 19-12C.

2. Rest the infant's head against your shoulder.

3. Support the infant's back with your forearm, and its head with your hand.

4. Support the baby's buttocks with the palm of your other hand.

Football Hold

The football hold is a firm, secure hold that leaves one hand free to perform other duties. It is often used for rinsing the baby's head during the bath.

1. Place the baby's buttocks firmly between your hip and your elbow, figure 19-12D.

2. Support the baby's back with your forearm.

3. Support the baby's neck and head with your open hand.

All newborns have a need to be loved. As an infant learns of its environment mainly through tactile stimulation, cuddling the infant is one way of expressing love. The way an infant is held, touched, and fed greatly influences its outlook on life.

BATHING THE BABY

Purpose

The infant must be given proper skin care. The infant should also be provided comfort while being bathed, and the bath experience should contribute to a loving parent-child relationship.

Precautions

1. Always wash your hands thoroughly before starting the bath.

2. Never turn away or leave baby alone without being sure it is secure.

   If it is necessary to turn away or reach for something, keep one hand on the child to protect it from falling.

   If it is necessary to leave the room, pick up the child, wrap it in a blanket and place it in the crib, or carry the baby with you.

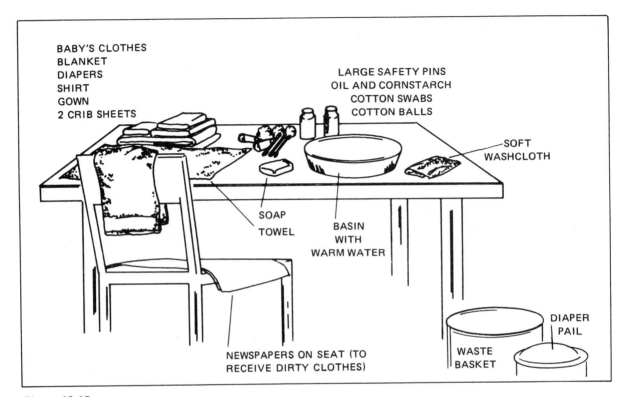

BABY'S CLOTHES
BLANKET
DIAPERS
SHIRT
GOWN
2 CRIB SHEETS

LARGE SAFETY PINS
OIL AND CORNSTARCH
COTTON SWABS
COTTON BALLS

SOFT
WASHCLOTH

SOAP
TOWEL

BASIN
WITH
WARM WATER

NEWSPAPERS ON SEAT (TO
RECEIVE DIRTY CLOTHES)

WASTE
BASKET

DIAPER
PAIL

Figure 19-13

A sturdy table can be set up for baby's bath

3. The room should be free from drafts. Temperature should be at least 22° to 24° Celsius (72° to 75° Fahrenheit).

4. Temperature of the bath water should never exceed 43°C (110°F). The general temperature range is 35° to 43°C (95° to 110°F). It may be slightly warmer for a sponge bath.

5. Avoid chilling the infant.

6. Avoid frightening the baby. The bath should be a pleasant experience.

7. Always wash face and head first. Use clean water and washcloth.

8. Never go back to the face after changing the diaper or washing the genitals.

9. Do not oversoap the baby. A soapy baby is slippery.

10. Use long, firm, smooth strokes.

11. Pat dry to protect the tender skin; never rub dry.

12. Report any unusual changes in the skin to the doctor or nurse.

Equipment

• Plastic tub, basin, or bathinette

• Bath mat or soft, thick towel

• 2 towels (or 1 towel and a bath mat)

• Mild baby soap

• Cotton swabs (for cord care)

- Cotton balls
- Container for waste (paper bag or waste-basket)
- Soft washcloth
- Baby oil (or cornstarch)
- Diaper pail
- Baby clothes (clean shirt, diapers, gown)
- Small, cotton receiving blanket
- Cribsheets (2)

Procedure

The first six steps are the same for a sponge bath or tub bath. Usually the newborn receives a sponge bath for the first few days.

1. Wash hands and assemble equipment. Test the temperature of the bath water. It should be 35° to 43°C (95° to 110°F) for a tub bath.
2. Pour warm water into the plastic tub or basin. There should be no more than three inches of water in the tub.
3. Strip the crib to the plastic mattress covering.
4. Place the tub in a convenient location. This may be on a table or set on the crib mattress.
5. Place a towel under the infant. Have a second towel ready to cover the infant.
6. Before undressing the baby, wash the baby's face, eyes, ears, and nostrils.
   a. Using a rotary motion in the tip of the nostril, clean the nostrils with a cotton ball which has been moistened and shaped into a pledget. DO NOT USE COTTON APPLICATORS. Use a clean pledget for each nostril.
   b. Moisten a cotton ball. Wipe each eye away from the *inner canthus* (angle of eye formed by the meeting of the upper and lower eyelids closest to nose); that is, toward the outer cheek. Use a clean cotton ball for each eye.
   c. Palm the facecloth. Wash the face with clear water. Start on the forehead and make a series of S's over and under the nose and chin. Be certain not to cover the nose and mouth at the same time or the child will be unable to breathe.
   d. Rinse the cloth and wash behind the ear and in the outer ear.
   e. Pat the skin dry. Rubbing irritates the skin. Be certain that the area behind each ear is clean and dry.

Sponge Bath

The procedure for a sponge bath differs from that of a tub bath although both start out the same way. After the face has been washed, the steps continue as follows:

1. Wash the infant's head with the specified solution and pat dry. If oil is used, be sure to remove any excess.
2. Remove the baby's shirt and diaper. If the diaper is soiled, fold the clean portion under the baby's buttocks and wash the genitals, thighs, and buttocks with cotton balls moistened with warm water. Wipe with a downward motion. Discard each cotton ball in a waste container.
3. Rinse and pat dry. Place soiled diaper in the diaper pail. Remove the baby's shirt.
4. Cover the baby with a towel.
5. Wash neck, arms, axillae, and abdomen with solution. Give special attention to the folds of the skin. Rinse and pat dry. Cover the baby.

6. Wash the lower extremities. Pay particular attention to folds of the thighs. Rinse and pat dry.

7. Turn the infant on its abdomen and wash the back and buttocks. Rinse and pat dry.

8. Turn the baby on its back. Be sure excess oils are removed and then dress the infant.

9. If talcum or oil is used, apply it first to your hands and then to the baby. Talcum powder tends to cake in the creases and causes irritation. Cornstarch may be used as it is not irritating.

SUGGESTED ACTIVITIES

- With another student, role play a nurse teaching a new mother how to hold her baby properly. Demonstrate lifting the baby, the cradle hold, the shoulder hold, and the football hold.
- Using a doll for the baby, practice giving the baby a sponge bath.
- Using a doll for the baby, practice giving the baby a tub bath. Use the football hold to rinse the baby's head.
- State how breast milk is formed.
- Discuss the advantages and disadvantages of breast feeding versus bottle feeding.
- Describe the ways a premature infant differs from a full-term infant.
- Describe the ways the nurse can use the Brazelton Neonatal Behavior Assessment Scale (NBAS) to help the parents recognize the "uniqueness" of their newborn.
- List four common problems frequently encountered in breast feeding. Describe the techniques to avoid or alleviate the problem.

REVIEW

A. Complete the following chart:

	Full-Term Newborn	Premature Infant
Size		
Cry		
Body shape		
Reflexes		
Skin tone		
Skin coating		

B. Multiple Choice. Choose the letter which indicates *all* of the correct phrases.

1. When the newborn is admitted to the nursery, it is
    1. given a tub bath
    2. placed in the Trendelenburg position
    3. weighed and measured
    4. given 2 ounces of formula
        a. 1, 2 and 3
        b. 1 and 4
        c. 2, 3 and 4
        d. 2 and 3

2. Standard nursing care for a premature infant includes
    1. placement in an incubator
    2. frequent checks of color and respiration
    3. minimal handling of the infant
    4. supplementary vitamins and iron
        a. 1, 2 and 3
        b. 1 and 2
        c. 1 and 3
        d. 1, 2, 3 and 4

3. The success or failure of breast feeding by a new mother may depend on
    1. the instruction and encouragement given by the nurse
    2. fear, pain, or other stresses
    3. size of breasts
    4. diet of mother
        a. 1 and 2
        b. 1, 2 and 4
        c. 2 and 3
        d. 1, 2, 3 and 4

4. When bathing the baby it is important to remember to
    1. wash the face and head first
    2. pat dry to protect tender skin
    3. sponge bathe until the navel is healed
    4. never leave the baby unattended
        a. 4 only
        b. 3 and 4
        c. 1, 3 and 4
        d. 1, 2, and 4

5. Gavage feeding is used when the baby
    1. cannot suck or swallow
    2. becomes too fatigued when nipple feeding
    3. has difficulty breathing while nipple feeding
    4. weighs less than 5 1/2 pounds
        a. 1 only
        b. 1 and 4
        c. 1 and 3
        d. 1, 2 and 3

6. Some facts a nurse may present to parents regarding circumcision are
   1. it is a brief procedure
   2. the newborn will not experience pain
   3. there is no evidence that circumcision prevents cancer
   4. complications are rare
   - a. 1 and 4
   - b. 1, 3 and 4
   - c. 1, 2 and 4
   - d. 1, 2, 3 and 4

7. A newborn is considered premature if it weighs less than
   - a. 3000 grams
   - b. 2500 grams
   - c. 4500 grams
   - d. 4000 grams

8. To break the oral suction of a nursing baby, the mother should
   - a. pull the baby away gently
   - b. squeeze the nipple together
   - c. place her finger at the corner of the baby's mouth
   - d. squeeze the baby's cheeks

9. When a baby's back is stroked on one side while the baby is lying on its stomach, the whole trunk curves toward that side. This reaction is called
   - a. tonic neck reflex
   - b. Moro reflex
   - c. placing reaction
   - d. Galant reaction

10. The rooting reflex is present for
    - a. the first six months
    - b. the first two months
    - c. as long as the baby is nursing
    - d. the first year

11. The anterior fontanel usually closes by
    - a. 6 months
    - b. 12 months
    - c. 26 months
    - d. 18 months

12. Frequently the pediatrician orders the newborn be given an injection of vitamin K. Vitamin K aids in
    - a. blood clotting
    - b. preventing jaundice
    - c. preventing the formation of phenylalanines
    - d. iron absorption

13. A baby can usually empty a breast of milk when nursing in about
    - a. 20 minutes
    - b. 5 to 8 minutes
    - c. 15 minutes
    - d. 3 minutes

14. When lifting and holding a baby always
    - a. support the baby's head
    - b. lift the baby by its arms
    - c. support the baby's back
    - d. place a finger between the baby's ankles to keep them separated

UNIT 20

DISORDERS OF THE NEONATE

OBJECTIVES

After studying this unit, the student should be able to:

- Name three causes for asphyxia neonatorum.
- Describe the signs of respiratory distress.
- Identify principles to follow when treating a newborn with breathing difficulty.
- State one disorder of the newborn for each of the eight body systems.
- State the cause and treatment for specific disorders of the newborn.

Becoming a parent is a major event, a turning point in life. This is particularly true for parents of a newborn with a disorder. Some parents can cope and adjust to the situation with increased maturity; others react with distress which leaves them emotionally drained. It is the responsibility of the health team to understand the psychodynamics that are taking place in both the parents and themselves. Only then can the situation be dealt with constructively and therapeutically.

ATTITUDES OF THE STAFF

The delivery of an infant with a disorder is difficult for the entire health team. The mother may sense this frustration and misinterpret it as hostility. She may feel sadness rather than the anticipated feeling of joy. All of this comes at a time when the mother may be physically and emotionally exhausted. The importance of the nurse's presence should never be underestimated. The mother needs to feel there is someone who understands. By simply holding the mother's hand or encouraging her to express her feelings, the nurse renders tremendous emotional support.

Realistic reassurance should be given to the mother and father. The parents need to feel that the child is accepted and treated like any other newborn, and that hospital personnel will give any assistance possible. The nurse can help to do this by cuddling the newborn and calling the infant by name. Also, the nurse can encourage the parents to talk about their feelings openly. The hospital staff should be careful not to offer the mother helpful platitudes such as "you can always have other children" or "don't feel so bad." This simply conveys a lack of understanding and empathy.

ETIOLOGY AND TREATMENT

Observation of the newborn is one of the nurse's most important duties both in the delivery room and in the nursery. Serious threats to the baby's health may be averted. Early treatment of congenital anomalies and diseases may be initiated when an alert nurse reports unusual signs and symptoms. These observations alert the physician or supervising nurse to the fact that a condition may exist for which medical attention is necessary.

Disorders of the newborn are acquired during development in the uterus (congenital), during the birth process, or as a result of medical conditions. Disorders may affect any one of the following body systems or may overlap and involve more than one system.

- Respiratory system
- Circulatory system
- Digestive system
- Nervous system
- Musculoskeletal system
- Endocrine system
- Genitourinary system
- Integumentary system

A few of the more commonly seen birth disorders of neonates are discussed in this unit. More comprehensive information may be obtained by referring to a text which deals with pediatrics.

The Respiratory System of the Newborn

The newborn's respirations are normally slightly irregular. They may vary from 40 to 60 per minute. If respirations have not begun within 30 seconds after birth, the condition may be called *asphyxia neonatorum* (imperfect breathing in the newborn). Failure of the infant to breathe spontaneously is usually due to one or a combination of three causes:

- Deprivation of oxygen (anoxia)
- Damage to brain tissue (cerebral injury)
- Unconscious state caused by drugs (narcosis)

Anoxia. Any interference with the function of the placenta or the umbilical cord which supplies oxygen to the baby puts the baby in grave danger of anoxia. A prolapsed cord, nuchal cord, premature separation of the placenta (placenta abruptio), or extremely severe uterine contractions could all produce intrauterine asphyxia. The child may literally suffocate while in the uterus because of the lack of oxygen.

Cerebral Injury. Cerebral injury is a common cause of apnea at birth when the delivery is particularly difficult. There may be brain hemorrhage that damages the respiratory center; other vital centers may also be injured. A disproportion between the size of the baby's head and the mother's pelvis can cause compression of the skull severe enough to cause damage to the brain.

Narcosis. A state of narcosis may be produced in the baby by analgesic and anesthetic drugs given to the mother during labor. Although the respirations may be sluggish at first, the infant usually does quite well when the effects of the medication have worn off.

Respiratory Distress Syndrome. Respiratory Distress Syndrome (RDS), also known as hyaline membrane disease, often occurs from minutes to several hours after birth. The reason why RDS occurs is unknown but it is thought to be due to a surfactant deficiency in the infant's system. The lack of this phospholipid inhibits the complete expansion of the alveoli in the lungs. As a result, the lungs lose their elasticity.

The main symptoms of RDS are cyanosis and *dyspnea* (difficult breathing). The disorder is more frequently found in premature infants and those born by cesarean section. Observation and recording of respiratory signs and symptoms are very important. Treatment consists of placing the infant in an incubator to meet the need for oxygen and maintenance of high humidity. Continuous positive airway pressure (C.P.A.P.) can be given to assist in ventilation. Antibiotics are often given along with intravenous feedings.

Signs of Respiratory Distress. The nurse should be alert to the following signs of respiratory distress which may be evident at birth or may develop several days later:

* Nasal flaring
* Excessive mucus
* Increase in rate of respirations accompanied by regular rhythm
* Increase in heartbeat (over 160 beats per minute)
* Retraction of chest wall upon inspiration (seesaw type of respiration)
* Expiratory grunt or feeble cry
* Cyanosis, except for hands and feet

Normally, the color of the newborn is slightly blue at the moment of birth because its lungs have not yet expanded. The skin becomes rosy pink as soon as breathing begins. The development of pallor and cyanosis should be reported immediately because they are signs of respiratory and/or circulatory difficulty.

There are five main principles to follow when treating a baby who does not breathe spontaneously at birth:

* Gentleness
* Warmth
* Positioning
* Removal of mucus
* Artificial respiration

Often the baby is in a state of shock and gentleness is essential in all procedures. Physical stimulation should be limited to rubbing the back or flicking the soles of the feet. The temperature of the room may also aggravate the state of shock so warmth to the baby must be provided. Excessive mucus should be reported immediately and emergency measures taken if necessary. Mucus may be removed with a suction catheter or with a bulb syringe. The baby should be placed in the Trendelenburg position with the head turned to one side. If the baby does not respond to these measures within 90 seconds after delivery, oxygen must be administered, and possibly external cardiac massage. Once the baby begins to breathe on its own, continued close observation is vital.

* See procedure for resuscitation of the newborn given later in this unit.

Silverman-Anderson Index. The Silverman-Anderson Index, figure 20-1, is designed to provide a continuous evaluation of the infant's respiratory status. Values are assigned to five criteria: chest lag, intercostal retraction, xiphoid retraction, nares dilatation, and expiratory grunt. A score of 0 (zero) indicates no respiratory distress; a score of 10 indicates severe respiratory distress.

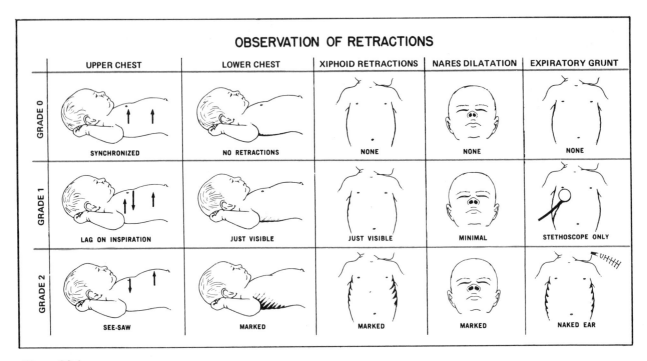

Figure 20-1

The Silverman-Anderson Index for the evaluation of respiratory status

Circulatory System of the Newborn

The heart, blood vessels, lymph vessels and lymph nodes make up the circulatory system. Blood is pumped to all body tissues. The circulating blood carries oxygen, nutrients, and chemicals to the cells of the body and takes away waste materials from the cells.

Jaundice. As the circulatory system adapts to extrauterine life, the newborn may develop jaundice. This normal characteristic which appears in some newborns is called *physiological jaundice.* It is caused by the liver's failure to cope with the increased breakdown of red blood cells no longer needed by the newborn. This causes increased amounts of *bilirubin* (a product of red blood cell destruction) to appear in the bloodstream, thus causing a yellowish tint to the skin. This type of jaundice becomes apparent between the third to fifth day of life and subsides around the eighth day; it has no medical significance. Jaundice can and frequently does occur in breast-fed babies due to a compound present in some mother's milk, which inhibits the breakdown of bilirubin.

Jaundice that appears before the third day of life should be promptly reported to the physician. Jaundice at this time could indicate the presence of a hemolytic disease such as erythroblastosis fetalis.

A blood test to determine the level of bilirubin is made in order to assess the degree of jaundice in the infant. The pediatrician may order *phototherapy* (the exposure of the infant to fluorescent blue light). The baby is placed unclothed under the light which helps to remove the yellow or jaundice from the skin. The nurse must protect the baby's eyes with a cover of soft bandage. The baby's body temperature should be carefully monitored and the infant should receive extra fluids.

Neonatal Hypoglycemia. The fetus derives glucose directly from maternal blood by a process of diffusion through the placenta. Glycogen is the stored source of glucose which is stored in the placenta as an additional source of fetal glucose. At 20 to 24 weeks gestation, the fetal liver becomes the major storage site for glycogen. The fetal heart and skeletal muscles are essential sources of energy. If the heart and skeletal muscles are defective, it lessens the infant's ability to withstand asphyxia. A direct relationship exists between the quantity of glucose stored at birth and the capacity to survive.

At birth, glycogen stored in the liver is normally twice the amount of adult concentrations. Glycogen stored in the heart is ten times as great; skeletal muscle stores are three to five times greater.

Increased energy is needed for breathing, temperature regulation, and muscle activity at birth. This increased energy output causes a sharp decline in glycogen stores. A low supply of glycogen is a serious threat to the infant. Blood sugar concentration reflects the release of glucose from the liver and the use of glucose by tissues. Use of glucose by tissues is abnormally increased by the metabolic response to cold stress, acidosis, and *hypoxia* (lack of sufficient oxygen in inspired air). Signs associated with low blood sugar include:

- apnea
- rapid and irregular respirations
- tachypnea
- tremors
- jitters and twitches
- convulsions
- lethargy
- coma
- abrupt pallor, cyanosis, grey shock
- sweating
- upward rolling of the eyes
- weak cry; high-pitched cry
- refusal to feed
- inability to regulate temperature

These signs should subside within five minutes if intravenous glucose is administered. If the signs do not subside, they are due to a cause other than hypoglycemia.

Normal blood sugar concentrations range from 30 to 125 milligrams per 100 milliliters in full-term infants weighing over 2500 grams, and from 20 to 100 milligrams per 100 milliliters in infants weighing less than 2500 grams. Untreated hypoglycemia in the infant may cause death.

Erythroblastosis Fetalis. The Rh factor caused by an Rh-negative woman giving birth to an Rh-positive baby may cause a disease technically known as *erythroblastosis fetalis.* In this condition the baby's red blood cells are destroyed, which is indicated by increased levels of bilirubin in the blood. Erythroblastosis fetalis is characterized by anemia, jaundice, enlargement of the liver and spleen and generalized edema of the newborn. If the anemia is severe enough, brain damage, heart failure or death can occur.

The treatment of this disorder consists of giving the infant frequent transfusions of Rh-negative blood during the first weeks of life. Phototherapy is a simple and safe method of treating mild hemolytic disease and greatly reduces the need for exchange transfusions. It is relatively ineffective, however, when serum

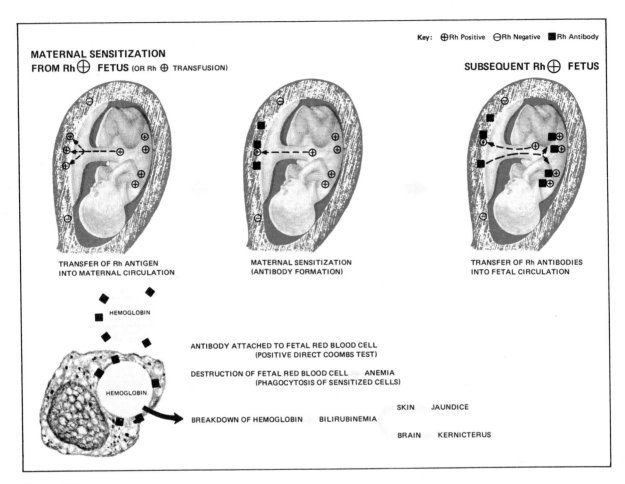

Key: ⊕ Rh Positive ⊖ Rh Negative ■ Rh Antibody

MATERNAL SENSITIZATION
FROM Rh ⊕ FETUS (OR Rh ⊕ TRANSFUSION)

SUBSEQUENT Rh ⊕ FETUS

TRANSFER OF Rh ANTIGEN
INTO MATERNAL CIRCULATION

MATERNAL SENSITIZATION
(ANTIBODY FORMATION)

TRANSFER OF Rh ANTIBODIES
INTO FETAL CIRCULATION

HEMOGLOBIN

ANTIBODY ATTACHED TO FETAL RED BLOOD CELL
(POSITIVE DIRECT COOMBS TEST)

DESTRUCTION OF FETAL RED BLOOD CELL   ANEMIA
(PHAGOCYTOSIS OF SENSITIZED CELLS)

HEMOGLOBIN

BREAKDOWN OF HEMOGLOBIN   BILIRUBINEMIA

SKIN   JAUNDICE

BRAIN   KERNICTERUS

Figure 20-2

Erythroblastosis fetalis (Adapted from Nursing Education Aid No. 9, Courtesy of Ross Laboratories)

bilirubin rises rapidly in severe cases. Photo-therapy is also helpful for infants with low birth weight, respiratory distress, acidosis, and sepsis. A specific gamma globulin, RhoGam, has made erythroblastosis fetalis rare in this day and age. RhoGam prevents an Rh negative mother from producing permanent Rh antibodies after aborting or delivering an Rh positive baby.

ABO Incompatibility. In ABO incompatibility, the etiologic process is much the same as in Rh incompatibility. The difficulty is caused by the presence of the naturally occurring antigen of the blood group A or B factors. Hemolytic disease due to A or B incompatibility is not usually anticipated unless there is a history of this problem among previous children in the family. The disease of the newborn is usually mild and may even pass unnoticed. It should be treated, however, if signs are well developed:

- mild jaundice during the first 36 hours of life

- enlargement of the liver and spleen

- central nervous system complications (rare)

• little or no edema

The treatment consists of phototherapy or an exchange transfusion using group O blood of appropriate Rh type if the infant's serum bilirubin level approaches 20 milligrams per 100 milliliters. The majority of affected infants need no treatment but should be watched carefully with special attention to respirations, pulse, temperature and increasing lethargy. The nurse should also watch for and report any increased jaundice, pigmentation of urine, edema, cyanosis, convulsions and any changes of the vital signs.

Digestive System of the Newborn

The digestive system is made up of all organs of the body which are involved in taking food and converting it into substances that the body may use and discarding those elements which are considered waste. The digestive system includes the mouth, teeth, pharynx, larynx and the alimentary or gastrointestinal tract (esophagus, stomach, intestines and other organs such as the liver, gallbladder, and pancreas).

Cleft Lip and Cleft Palate.   A *cleft lip* is a vertical cleft or split in the upper lip, figure 20-3. It is also known as *harelip.* A *cleft palate* is a fissure in the roof of the mouth forming a passageway between the mouth and nasal cavities.

Feeding is usually the most immediate problem. It is best accomplished by placing the infant in an upright position and directing the flow of milk against the side of the mouth. This decreases the amount of air swallowed. The baby should be bubbled or burped at frequent intervals. A variety of nipples may be tried including regular nipples with enlarged holes. Cleft palate nipples are also available. Breast feeding may be tried.

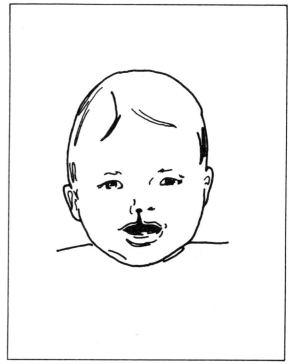

Figure 20-3
A complete cleft lip

Cleft lip and cleft palate can occur separately or together. Both conditions result from failure of the soft and/or bony tissues of the upper jaw and palate to unite during the eighth to twelfth weeks of gestation. Surgical repair is the usual course of action. Depending on the severity, the plan of treatment may be immediate or it may be delayed until the second year of life. The parents often require a great deal of support as this disorder can be quite disfiguring. Repair is generally successful; it is helpful if the parents know and understand this fact.

Thrush (Oral Moniliosis).   The organism which causes thrush is *candida* (monilia) *albicans* and is generally found in the vagina of the mother. *Thrush* is a fungus infection; spores grow on the delicate tissue of the mouth. An infant can be infected by improperly cleaned nipples or breast of the mother.

Thrush appears as pearly white, elevated lesions resembling milk curds. It is usually found on the tongue margin, inside the lips and cheeks, and on the hard palate. Prognosis with treatment is good and recovery usually takes place in three to four days. Nystatin or aqueous gentian violet (1 percent solution) or 1:1000 aqueous solution of Zephiran may be used in treating thrush.

Pyloric Stenosis. *Pyloric stenosis* is a common condition of the intestinal tract. There is an increase in the size of the circular musculature of the *pylorus* (the junction of the stomach and the small intestine). The musculature is greatly thickened. This mass constricts the opening of the pylorus; this impedes the emptying of the stomach.

The symptoms usually appear within two to four weeks. Vomiting is the initial symptom and may at first be mild, becoming more forceful until it is projectile. Since little of the feeding is retained, the baby is always hungry. There is failure to gain weight and the infant begins to appear starved. Little food passes through the pylorus; therefore bowel movements decrease in frequency and amount.

The signs of pyloric stenosis are dehydration, poor skin turgor, and an olive-shaped mass which can be felt in the right upper quadrant of the abdomen. Surgical intervention is usually necessary. If performed early enough, prognosis is excellent.

Umbilical Hernia. A *hernia* is a protrusion of part of an organ through the wall of the cavity in which it is normally contained. An *umbilical hernia* is caused by a weakness or incomplete closure of the umbilical ring allowing a portion of the small intestine or omentum to protrude.

Omentum is a double fold of peritoneum attached to the stomach which connects it to the abdominal viscera. The hernia is indicated by a soft swelling at the site of the umbilicus. The swelling may disappear when pressure is applied and reappear again when pressure is removed or when the baby cries. The condition often disappears by itself when the abdominal muscles become strengthened, usually when the child learns to stand or walk. It can also be surgically repaired after the first year of life.

Phenylketonuria. Normally, the liver produces an enzyme that acts on an amino acid called *phenylalanine;* the enzyme changes it to tyrosine. *Phenylketonuria* (PKU) is a metabolic disease caused by failure of the body to oxidize phenylalanine because of the missing or inadequate enzyme. Since the amino acid is unable to be broken down, it builds up in the blood and tissues causing damage to the brain. If left untreated, mental retardation usually results from phenylketonuria (PKU).

Treatment consists of early detection and dietary management restricting phenylalanine intake. Since phenylalanine makes up 5 percent of the protein factor in all foods, a low phenylalanine diet is a very restricted one. PKU disorders can be diagnosed from both blood and urine tests. Blood tests are done routinely on newborns in the hospital nursery about the third day. Urine tests are done about the second week. Retardation can be prevented with early detection and prompt treatment. Best results are obtained if treatment is started by the third week of life.

Colic and Diarrhea. Colic is most common during the first three to four months and is characterized by intestinal cramping due to accumulation of excessive gas. The infant may pass gas from the anus or belch it up from the stomach. The infant draws up its knees and cries loudly in pain. The exact cause of colic is unknown but it is felt that predisposing causes are excessive swallowing of air, too much excitement, too rapid feeding, or a tense mother who communicates this tenseness to the infant.

The treatment is to bubble the infant frequently, holding it upright to get rid of the air in the intestinal tract. Colic is not a serious condition and infants usually gain weight despite the periods of pain.

Diarrhea is a symptom of a variety of conditions which can be mild or severe. Faulty preparation of formula, overfeeding, an unbalanced diet (excessive sugar), and spoiled food may all cause diarrhea. A diagnosis is made from history and clinical evaluations. Weight loss and dehydration may follow. Treatment is usually a reduction in formula feedings in order to put less stress on the gastrointestinal tract. Fluid (5 percent glucose in saline solution) is increased and given orally every three to four hours until the diarrhea subsides.

Imperforate Anus. In the eighth week of embryonic life, a membrane which separates the rectum from the anus is usually absorbed leaving a continuous canal whose outlet is the anus. If this membrane is not absorbed, an imperforate anus results. A diagnosis is needed when the following symptoms appear:

- no anal opening is found upon examination
- no stool is passed
- later abdominal distention occurs

Obstruction in the male infant must be relieved at once for stool cannot be passed. In the female infant a fistula (opening) probably exits into the vagina or perineum. Surgical correction is necessary; the procedure depends on the anomaly.

Prognosis is good with early detection and surgical correction.

The Nervous System of the Newborn

All parts of the body are controlled and coordinated by the nervous system. The brain, spinal cord, and the nerves make up the nervous system. The sensory organs are part of this system also. They receive stimuli by sight, touch, taste, smell, and hearing. When impulses are transmitted to the brain through the sense organs, the body responds through action by the brain, spinal cord and nerves.

Spina Bifida. Spina bifida is a malformation of the spine in which the posterior portion of the laminae of the vertebrae fails to close. It can occur in any area of the spine but is most common in the lumbosacral region. This occurs in about 1 out of 1000 births.

There are three basic types of spina bifida:

1) Spina bifida occulta (defect only of the vertebrae)
2) Meningocele (meninges protrude through the opening of the spinal cavity), figure 20-4A
3) Meningomyelocele (spinal cord and meninges) protrude through the defect in the bony rings of the spinal canal, figure 20-4B

With spina bifida occulta, there is no need for treatment unless neurological symptoms show involvement of the spinal cord. Surgical correction is necessary with meningocele but prognosis is excellent. There is generally no evidence of weakness in the legs or lack of sphincter control.

With meningomyelocele, there may be anything from minimal weakness to a flaccid paralysis of the legs and absence of sensation in the feet. With surgical correction the neurological deficit can be improved. Therapy may further improve function as the nervous system matures.

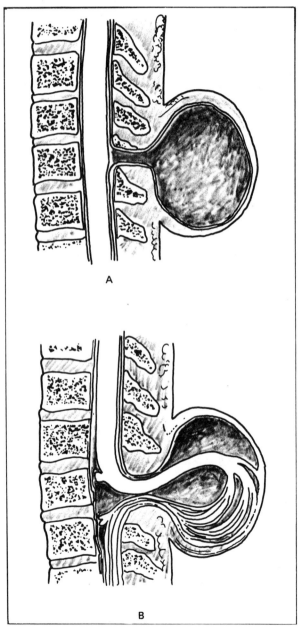

Figure 20-4

Two types of spina bifida. A) Spina bifida with meningocele. B) Spina bifida with meningomyelocele.

Nursing care in meningocele and meningomyelocele is mainly of a protective nature until surgery:

- Protect the bladder from infection by frequent emptying. This is done by applying firm, gentle pressure starting at the umbilical area and progressing downward.
- Protect the protruding sac from pressure.
- Protect the sac from dangers of infection from urine and feces.
- Protect the feet from deformity when the infant is placed on its abdomen. Ankles should be supported with foam rubber pads so that the toes do not rest on the bed.

Good general nursing care is vital for these babies as well as a caring attitude. Special consideration should also be given to the parents to help them understand this disorder.

The Alpha Fetoprotein screen, which is performed between the 15th and 20th weeks of gestation from maternal serum, will often indicate the presence of this neural tube defect. Early detection gives the parents a choice. They can continue with the pregnancy, knowing their newborn will need special attention at birth and can have permanent disabilities; or they can decide to terminate the pregnancy within the legal time restrictions. In either case, nursing support is needed to help a family understand the nature of a neural tube defect and all the possible outcomes.

Down's Syndrome. Down's syndrome is a congenital disorder that is characterized by irreparable brain and body damage. It is also known as *mongolism.* The true cause for this disorder is unknown. However, an abnormal chromosome count has been found to be present in the body cells of children afflicted with the disease. Mental retardation is often severe. Deformities are most often noticed in the skull and eyes. The eyes are set close together and slanted, the nose is flat, the tongue is large and usually protrudes from an open mouth. The head is

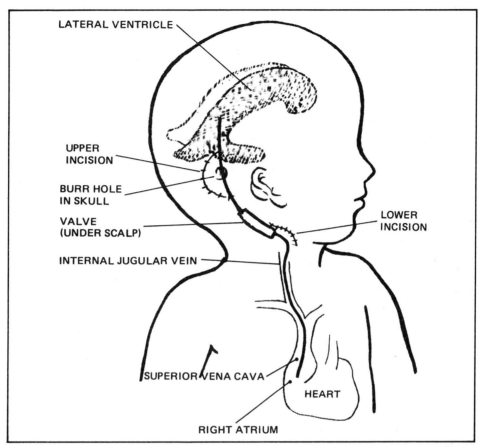

LATERAL VENTRICLE

UPPER
INCISION

BURR HOLE
IN SKULL

VALVE
(UNDER SCALP)

INTERNAL JUGULAR VEIN

LOWER
INCISION

SUPERIOR VENA CAVA

HEART

RIGHT ATRIUM

Figure 20-5

A ventriculoatrial shunt drains spinal fluid in a child with hydrocephalus.

small; the hands short and thick. Some of these children die early in lefe due to infection which their bodies cannot handle.

Hydrocephalus. Hydrocephalus is due to inadequate absorption of cerebrospinal fluid and an increase of fluid under some degree of pressure within the intracranial cavity.

The accumulation of fluid in the ventricles generally enlarges the infant's skull since the bones are not yet closed and will yield to pressure. Treatment should begin as soon as symptoms appear and before damage to the brain results. Several shunting procedures are now in use, figure 20-5. Prognosis is dependent on the promptness of treatment and the operation performed.

Facial Paralysis. Pressure of the forceps on the facial nerve may cause a temporary paralysis of the muscles on one side of the face. The mouth may be drawn to the other side; this is most noticeable when the baby cries. The condition usually disappears in a few days or even a few hours. The parents need assurance that this is a temporary condition. During initial feedings, sucking may be difficult for the infant. The mother needs support and patience in the feeding of her baby.

The Musculoskeletal System of the Newborn

The bones provide support and protection. Skeletal muscles are attached to the bones. Body movements are due to the action of these muscles. Some disorders of the newborn affect this system.

Torticollis. This condition is caused by the abnormal shortening of the sternocleidomastoid muscle. The neck is tilted to one side. Exercise or traction may be prescribed.

Erb's Palsy. The infant may suffer partial paralysis of the arm due to injury to the brachial plexus. The infant cannot raise its arm. Usually this injury is not permanent if it is caused by the delivery process.

Fractures. These may occur during delivery. The bones usually affected are the clavicle (collarbone), the humerus (upper arm) or the femur (thigh bone). The clavicle usually heals without treatment. Long bones sometimes need to be splinted; however, these fractures usually heal quickly.

Talipes (Clubfoot). The foot may turn inward, outward, downward, or upward. One or both feet may be involved, figure 20-6. Sometimes simple exercises, foot braces, special shoes, or casts may be used successfully. In other instances, surgery may be necessary.

Congenital Dislocated Hip. This condition is believed to be due to lack of embryonic development of the joint. However, the etiology is not clear. Most commonly, the dislocation occurs when the head of the femur does not entirely lie within the shallow *acetabulum* (socket of the pelvis). An observable sign is limitation in abduction of the hips (away from the body). Normally, when an infant is lying on its back with knees and hips flexed, the hip joint permits the femur to be abducted until the knee almost touches the table at a 90° angle. With dislocation, abduction on the affected side is limited to no more than 45°. Also, on the affected side the leg is shorter and there is a prominence of the soft tissue of the gluteal folds. Treatment

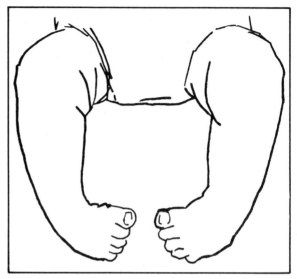

Figure 20-6

Anterior view of bilateral talipes equinovarus (Clubfoot).

should be started as soon as a diagnosis is made. The objective of treatment is to place the head of the femur within the acetabulum and to enlarge and deepen the socket by constant pressure. Ultimately, the dislocation is corrected.

The Endocrine System of the Newborn

Hormonal interactions take place while the fetus is in utero. Not only does the fetus have its own endocrine system but it is also receiving hormones produced by the mother. The placenta also secretes hormones. The mother secretes large amounts of estrogen during pregnancy. Also, those mothers who have endocrine disturbances such as diabetes and hyperthyroidism may affect the newborn's hormonal balance. The result may be a child with hypertrophy of the islands of Langerhans (from diabetic mothers) or congenital exophthalmic goiter (from mothers with hyperthyroidism). Other disorders of the newborn due to maternal hormones are less severe and usually are of a temporary nature.

Gynecomastia. This may affect both male and female infants. The breasts of the newborn enlarge and sometimes secrete tiny amounts of fluid. The breasts should not be squeezed as inflammation and infection may occur. The enlarged breasts return to normal without any special treatment.

Pigmentation. The genitals, nipples and a line on the lower portion of the abdomen (linea alba) may be darkened. These areas assume their normal color quite rapidly.

Infantile Menstruation. Since the female fetus has been getting uterine estrogen, the sudden withdrawal may bring about a tiny menstrual flow. The mother should be reassured and told that it is no cause for concern. Usually it ceases in a day or two. *CAUTION:* If blood loss is considerable, hemorrhagic disease may be present.

The Genitourinary System of the Newborn

The kidneys, ureters, bladder, and the urethra make up the urinary system. The external sex organs and related inner structures which are concerned with the production of new individuals make up the reproductive system. The genitourinary system is related to both reproduction and urination.

Malformations of the Urinary Tract. It is important to record the time, description, and kind of urine flow of every newborn. Although little urine is voided in the first two days, ample water should be given to handle the needs for hydration and excretion of wastes. Malformations may lead to death if they are obstructive as renal failure can occur. Abnormalities of the ureters, double kidneys, and double pelves on one or both kidneys cause no harm in themselves but may lead to renal infections and problems of the urinary tract.

Exstrophy of the Bladder. The interior of the bladder lies completely exposed through an abdominal opening. Infection takes place often but can usually be treated by the use of antibiotics. Surgery must be done to remedy this disorder. However, there is always the danger of kidney damage which results from inadequate drainage and infection.

Pseudohermaphroditism. When a newborn has the external sex organs of one sex and the gonads of the other sex it is said to be intersexual. Female pseudohermaphrodites have female internal organs but the enlarged clitoris and the fused labia of the external organs resemble a penis and scrotum. The male pseudohermaphrodite has testes but they are usually in the abdomen. The external genitals may be feminine. There are no ovaries.

Hermaphroditism. When an infant has the gonads and genitals of both sexes, the child is a hermaphrodite. This condition is rare. Treatment consists of removing the gonads of one sex.

Undescended Testicle. The testes fail to descend into the scrotum. Usually only one testicle has not descended. If the testicle descends spontaneously, it usually does this during the first year. Otherwise, surgery is indicated.

Hypospadias. The urethra terminates on the under side of the penis. Since the child will not be able to direct his urinary stream, he will be subject to embarrassment and ridicule if the situation is not corrected. Less common is the condition called epispadias; the urethra opens on the upper surface of the penis. This is sometimes associated with exstrophy of the bladder. Both are correctable by surgery.

The Integumentary System of the Newborn

The integumentary or skin system includes the epidermis and its appendages: hair, nails, sweat glands, oil glands and the corium layer, which is sometimes referred to as the true skin. The newborn may have skin disorders which range from a mild irritation to the more severe infection.

Miliaria Rubra. This is another name for prickly heat or heat rash. The sweat pores are blocked so the sweat seeps into the epidermis or dermis. Overdressing the baby should be avoided. Light powdering of the skin with cornstarch may be helpful.

Chafing. The skin may become quite inflamed in the folds of the skin. Prevention should be practiced by keeping the area dry and clean. Creases such as those in the neck, groin and buttocks require hygiene. The rubbing together of the skin areas gives rise to friction, and the skin may become quite inflamed and irritated.

Caput Succedaneum. The soft tissues of the scalp may become swollen as a result of the delivery. Fluid collects under the scalp on top of the skull. After a few days, the fluid is absorbed.

Cephalohematoma. This differs from caput succedaneum in that the fluid is bloody and collects under the covering layer of a skull bone and is located within the bone structure. Although it is disfiguring, the condition requires no treatment. The fluid is absorbed in a few days.

Impetigo. This serious skin infection is caused by staphylococcal organisms. Lesions appear on the body; when ruptured, they spread to other areas. It is a contagious skin disorder; the condition can spread quickly unless strict isolation of the infant is carried out. An antibacterial soap, usually hexachlorophene, is used. Ointments and systemic penicillin may be ordered by the physician.

INCIDENCE OF BIRTH ANOMALIES

The majority of babies born are perfectly formed, mature, healthy babies. However, a small percent are born with a disease or defect. With modern technology and advanced medical science, many diseases and deformities that once caused death can now be cured or greatly lessened.

RESUSCITATION OF THE NEWBORN

Purpose

The purpose of resuscitation is to establish or re-establish regular breathing patterns in the infant.

Precautions

1. Keep the baby warm. Keeping the baby warm minimizes oxygen demands while resuscitation is in progress. The infant's temperature should be maintained at 36.5° to 37°C (98° to 98.6°F) axilla.

2. Quickly establish an open airway. Ten to fifteen seconds of gentle suctioning with a bulb syringe or DeLee mucous trap is all that is usually needed. Delay in clearing the airway can result in brain damage.

3. Suction the oropharynx before the nose. If the nose is suctioned first, the infant may aspirate mucus or amniotic fluid.

Equipment

- Radiant heat source
- Bulb syringe or DeLee mucous trap
- Oxygen tank and liter gauge
- Oxygen tubing
- Infant oxygen mask
- Pen-Lon valve bag
- Ambu bag
- Wall suction tubing
- Suction catheters #8 and #6.5
- Bottle of sterile water
- Laryngoscope with two blades
- Portex blue-line endotracheal tubes #3.0, #3.5, #2.5
- Stylette
- Clean scissors
- Connector adaptor
- Closed system bag with water manometer
- Stethoscope

Procedure

1. Briefly flick the infant's feet or rub its back gently.
2. If breathing does not begin immediately, give 5 positive pressure breaths of oxygen-enriched air by mask.
3. Maintain the first 5 inspirations for 4 to 5 seconds at a water pressure of 30 centimeters on the manometer. Use this high pressure for the first few breaths only to clear excess fetal lung liquid and to open collapsed alveoli.
4. Check for chest movement and breath sounds.
5. If breathing does not start, suction and/or intubate.
6. If breathing begins, heart rate, color, and tone should improve immediately.
7. If breathing does not start, continue bag breathing at a rate of 40 per minute with water pressures that do not exceed 20 to 25 centimeters.
8. Check the infant's apical pulse.
9. If the apical pulse is below 100 beats per minute and falling in spite of assisted ventilation, initiate cardiac massage.

Cardiac Massage

10. To give cardiac massage, place one hand under the baby's back.
11. With the tips of the index and middle fingers of the other hand, depress the midsternum about 1/2 to 3/4 inch.
12. Gently but forcibly do this at a rate of 80 to 100 compressions per minute (a little more than once per second). Do not push too hard as this could cause injury to the infant.
13. Ventilate once after every 5 compressions. Do not interrupt the compressions while ventilating, but avoid compressing the chest and giving breath at the same time.

If the Apgar score is less than 6 at 3 to 5 minutes of age, the infant may need to be transferred to the intensive care unit. Resuscitation must continue during transport to the unit.

SUGGESTED ACTIVITIES

- Discuss the possible causes of birth defects. Draw on your personal experiences and talk about emotions involved.

- Write a report on how you think you would react when assisting in the birth of a severely deformed infant. Determine ways to overcome any negative feelings you may have.

- With another classmate, role play a nurse presenting a baby with a birth defect to the mother for the first time. Be prepared to offer acceptance and encouragement. Encourage the "mother" to talk about her feelings. Exchange roles and play the mother while another student plays the nurse.

- Research the causes for mental retardation. Present a paper or talk on one of the causes.

- Contact community resources for information about prenatal clinics. Make arrangements to attend one and discuss your observations with the class.

REVIEW

A. Multiple Choice. Select the best answer.

1. A metabolic disease caused by failure of the body to oxidize a certain amino acid is
   - a. erythroblastosis fetalis
   - b. hyaline membrane disease
   - c. narcosis
   - d. phenylketonuria

2. Jaundice that appears before the third day of life
   - a. has no medical significance
   - b. is called physiological jaundice
   - c. may indicate a hemolytic disease
   - d. is to be expected in all infants

3. The color of the normal newborn at the moment of birth is
   - a. rosy pink
   - b. slightly blue
   - c. pale white
   - d. slightly yellow

4. Temporary paralysis of the muscles on one side of the face can be caused by
   - a. pressure of forceps on the facial nerve
   - b. severe uterine contractions
   - c. analgesic drugs given the mother during labor
   - d. disproportion of the baby's head size and mother's pelvis

5. Mental retardation can be caused by
   a. phenylketonuria
   b. narcosis
   c. candida albicans
   d. pyloric stenosis

6. Meningomyelocele is a condition in which
   a. a vertebrae is defective
   b. the meninges protrude through the opening of the spinal cavity
   c. the spinal cord and meninges protrude through the defect in the bony rings of the spinal canal
   d. the posterior portion of the laminae of the vertebrae fails to close

7. Erb's Palsy is defined as
   a. an abnormal shortening of the sternocleidomastoid muscle
   b. partial paralysis of the arm due to injury to the brachial plexus
   c. temporary paralysis of the muscles on one side of the face
   d. one or both feet may turn inward, outward, downward or upward

8. A condition which can affect both male and female infants where the breasts enlarge and sometimes secrete tiny amounts of fluid is known as
   a. congenital exophthalmic goiter
   b. linea alba
   c. pseudohermaphroditism
   d. gynecomastia

9. The principles to follow when treating a baby who does not breathe spontaneously at birth are
   1. gentleness and warmth
   2. proper positioning
   3. removal of mucus
   4. artificial respiration
   a. 1, 2 and 3
   b. 2 and 3
   c. 3 and 4
   d. 1, 2, 3 and 4

10. Intrauterine asphyxia could be caused by
    1. prolapsed cord
    2. placenta abruptio
    3. omentum
    4. extremely severe uterine contractions
    a. 1 and 3
    b. 1, 2 and 4
    c. 1 and 2
    d. 1, 2, 3 and 4

B. Match the terms in column II with the descriptions in column I.

Column I

1. unconscious state caused by drugs h
2. deprivation of oxygen a
3. fissure in the roof of the mouth d
4. product of red blood cell destruction c
5. exposure to fluorescent blue light j
6. vertical split in upper lip f
7. an amino acid i
8. imperfect breathing in the newborn b
9. Respiratory Distress Syndrome g
10. difficult breathing e

Column II

a. anoxia
b. asphyxia neonatorum
c. bilirubin
d. cleft palate
e. dyspnea
f. harelip
g. hyaline membrane disease
h. narcosis
i. phenylalanine
j. phototherapy

C. Briefly answer the following questions.

1. List five signs of respiratory distress.

Increased heart rate
flared nostrils
grunting sounds
Seesaw diaphgm

2. What is the treatment for erythroblastosis fetalis?

Transfusion of RH Neg. Blood. (p. 287)

UNIT 21

FAMILY PLANNING

OBJECTIVES

After studying this unit, the student should be able to:

- List three areas which make demands on the new father.
- Explain why the new father should be included in plans for the new baby.
- Explain the various methods of birth control, their actions and limitations.
- Describe two sterilization procedures.

THE FAMILY UNIT

Pregnancy is a family affair. It is a biological event and an emotional experience beginning with a relationship between two people which develops into a new relationship between them and their offspring. Both the expectant mother and the father have a tremendous investment in the pregnancy. The expectant father is facing new financial, emotional and social demands.

THE FATHER'S ROLE

Usually, involved fatherhood begins during the prenatal period. At that time, well-planned instruction prepares the father for meaningful participation in the labor and delivery room. However, it should not be restricted to the mechanics of labor and the immediate environment of the hospital. Social pressures exerted on the father show up in his relationships with male friends, close members of the extended family, and with people at work. Therefore, he needs to understand the psychological changes taking place within himself and the pregnant woman. A person's attitude toward fatherhood and its responsibilities has its roots in early childhood and the interpersonal family relationships. How a new father feels affects the kind of influence and support he is able to give throughout the pregnancy. His feelings also determine the kind of relationship he is able to establish with his child when the baby is born.

Pregnancy is a time of increasing dependence in which the woman may experience a great need to be protected. Support, acceptance, and understanding are extremely important. If the father understands that *somatic* (body) changes of the mother may bring about withdrawal from him and a concentration on herself and the child, his anxiety is less marked. He needs to know that these changes are temporary and normal; they are not the result of something he has or has not done.

The expectant father should share the entire experience. Being prepared helps relieve any feelings of inadequacy in his supportive role. He needs to understand pregnancy and labor and how he can participate effectively in the birth of his child. Whenever plans are being made for the care of the mother and child, the father should be included. If he is helped to understand how vital his role is during the neonatal period, he is better able to meet the responsibilities of the postpartum period and beyond. A readiness to assist with household chores is not the only demonstration of cooperation and love. Of even more importance is the willingness to give encouragement and support. This provides the foundation upon which the parent-child relationship is built.

FAMILY PLANNING

Nurses have an ideal opportunity to discuss family planning with the parents. Since this is an integral part of comprehensive maternity care, counseling in contraception is appropriate. If the new mother used a method of contraception before pregnancy, it must be re-evaluated in view of the physical changes of childbearing. The patient's freedom to choose requires a knowledge of the choices. It is the responsibility of every nurse to be aware of all methods of contraception so that the method selected is acceptable to both husband and wife. The nursing mother should be counseled that the reproductive organs will soon return to the menstrual cycle and ovulation can occur at regular intervals. This means that breast feeding is not a dependable means of contraception and that she could become pregnant again.

Although birth control is an important element in preventive medicine, it is profoundly objectionable to many persons. Individual views must be fully respected, whether expressed by patients, nurses, or physicians. When the personal convictions of the physician and/or nurse prevent providing medical supervision and information on family planning, referrals should be made. Whenever there are clearly defined conditions in which the health of a woman may be jeopardized by pregnancy, it is generally recognized by the medical profession that contraceptive measures are proper medical practice.

METHODS OF BIRTH CONTROL

A summary of the various methods and devices used for family planning is given in figure 21-1. The student should study this chart carefully.

The changing public attitude toward family planning and a deepening concern about rising population have coincided with the introduction and use of two very effective contraceptives. The plastic intrauterine devices and the oral contraceptive pills possess a high success rate. Before 1960, contraceptives had a failure rate between 10 and 50 percent.

Oral Contraceptives

The birth control pill is believed to be 99.7 percent effective. It was introduced in 1960 and is taken by a large number of women regularly to prevent pregnancy. The principle of the oral contraceptive is that it provides a synthesis of two natural hormones, estrogen and progesterone, which mimic the action of the body's own hormones. Each pill contains both synthetic hormones which together effectively prevent ovulation or release of any ovum from either ovary during the time the pills are taken. Since no ovum is available to be fertilized, pregnancy cannot be achieved.

Although oral contraceptives are more popular than the intrauterine devices, they are also controversial. Three possible serious complications of the hormonal contraceptives known as The Pill are:

- *thromboembolic* disease (blocking of a blood vessel by an embolus)

Method or Device	Description	Action and Limitations	Contraindications, Side Effects, and Adverse Effects
Contraception			
The Pill	Oral tablet containing hormones (estrogen, progestin) taken as directed	Action: Suppresses ovulation; stimulates growth of endometrium	Contraindications: family history of breast or cervical cancer, diabetes; personal history of circulatory problems Adverse effects: blood and circulatory problems such as thrombophlebitis Side effects: nausea, weight gain, headaches, depression
Intrauterine Device (IUD)	Small object in shape of ring, loop, coil, or bow made of plastic or stainless steel. It is inserted in the uterus by a physician	Action: Action not completely known; disturbs uterine motility	Contraindications: spontaneous expulsion; insertion difficult in nulliparas Adverse effects: uterine perforation, pelvic inflammatory disease (PID) Side effects: pain, bleeding, vaginal discharge
Diaphragm/ Jelly	Occlusive vaginal diaphragm made of rubber used with spermicidal jelly	Action: Immobilizes and kills sperm; provides mechanical barrier Limitations: Possibility of displacement during intercourse; poor fit reduces effectiveness	None
Condom	Thin sheath made of rubber or similar material placed over penis before intercourse	Action: prevents sperm from entering vagina Limitations: may tear or slip off during intercourse	None
Spermicidal Foams	Chemical products inserted in vagina with applicator	Action: Coats vaginal walls and cervix; provides mechanical barrier; spermicide Limitation: not reliable	None
Rhythm	Woman takes temperature every morning before getting out of bed to establish pattern of ovulation. Temperature rises 3 successive days after ovulation	Action: Avoids conception by abstaining from intercourse for 3 days before and after estimated date of ovulation Limitation: restricts marital relations	Contraindications: irregular menstrual cycle
Sterilization			
Female: Hysterectomy Tubal ligation	Surgical procedure Surgical procedure	Excision of uterus Fallopian tubes tied and severed either by laparoscopy or 3- to 4-inch incision in lower abdomen	None None
Male: Vasectomy	Surgical procedure	½-inch incision on each side of scrotum; vas deferens cut and tied	None

Figure 21-1
Methods of family planning

- carcinoma of the breast and uterus
- metabolic disturbances

Investigations have shown that the risk of thrombophlebitis is increased about four to seven times in users of oral contraceptives. Scientific data have correlated the occurrence of thromboembolic disease directly with the dose of estrogen in the medication. The new lower hormonal dose pills have decreased the incidence of thromboembolic problems significantly among pill users. It has also been demonstrated that estrogen administered in the proper amount for the proper time may be *carcinogenic* (cancer producing). However, this information is still inconclusive and studies are still being made. Hormonal contraceptives produce numerous effects on several organs such as the liver, thyroid gland, and adrenal glands. They also produce changes in the salt and water metabolism and occasionally induce hypertension.

The non-contraceptive benefits of the pill have been widely under-published. It has a protective effect not only against menstrual disorders, ectopic pregnancy, benign breast disease, dysmenorrhea, anemia, and ovarian cysts but also offers protection against cancer of the ovary and endometrium. These positive effects have been overshadowed by publicity about the occurrence of heart attack, stroke, thromboembolism, liver tumors, and deep vein thrombosis. There is presently no valid evidence that oral contraceptives cause breast cancer.

There are approximately five pill-related deaths per 100,000 users per year. Most of these are among either pill users 40 years or older or pill users 35 years or older who smoke. Maternal mortality from obstetric causes is about 10 per 100,000 births. Maternal mortality from all causes is nearly twice this rate. The mortality risk from driving a car is 19 per 100,000 drivers per year and from smoking a pack of cigarettes a day, 500 per 100,000 smokers. The birth control pill is clearly safer than many daily risks that women are subjected to during their reproductive life.

The Intrauterine Device(IUD)

The intrauterine device (IUD) is a plastic coil, ring, loop or shield which is inserted into the uterus. No one knows exactly how the IUD works. It may prevent a fertilized egg from implanting in the wall of the uterus or it may cause muscular movements which force the egg into the uterus before it is ready to be implanted.

The intrauterine device is less of a health hazard than oral contraceptives; however, protection against pregnancy is not as good. Also, there are side effects in about 20 percent of the women

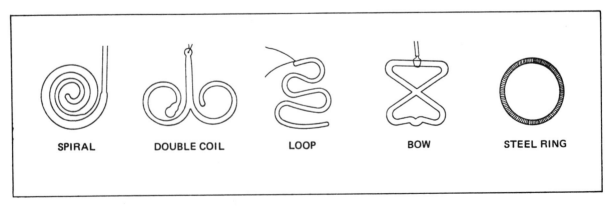

SPIRAL DOUBLE COIL LOOP BOW STEEL RING

Figure 21-2

Types of intrauterine devices

using IUDs. The uterus may expel the device, or there may be pain, bleeding, and vaginal discharge. Serious complications are rare, although the risks include pelvic infection and perforation of the uterus. Insertion of the device is difficult in women who have never had children. The IUD is inserted by a physician during or immediately following a menstrual period.

Many IUD manufacturers have recently recalled all their devices. This is due to increased litigation from health problems that were thought to be directly caused by the contraceptive device. These health problems include PID, which could lead to future fertility problems.

The Diaphragm

A diaphragm is a soft, dome-shaped device that is inserted into the vagina so that it covers the cervix. In this position, it keeps sperm from entering the uterus. It is used with a contraceptive cream or jelly placed inside the curve of the diaphragm and around its edge. This device may be inserted no more than two hours before intercourse and it must be left in place at least eight hours afterwards. Used correctly, this method is about 95 percent effective and is completely safe.

The Cervical Cap

In April 1988, the FDA approved the Prentif cervical cap as an effective and safe method of contraception. The cervical cap looks like a large rubber thimble with a soft latex dome and a firm rim. With a small amount of spermicide placed in the dome, the cap is fitted over the cervix. It stays firmly in place by gripping the cervix and forming a strong suction. The cap itself provides a physical barrier to sperm while the spermicide affords an additional chemical barrier.

Because it is smaller than the diaphragm, the Prentif cap has several advantages. It is more comfortable than the diaphragm and can be left

in place for several days. The cap stays snugly on the cervix, requiring no additional spermicidal cream or jelly. Consequently it is less messy. Like the diaphragm, the cervical cap must be left in place for eight hours after the last intercourse to be effective. Used correctly, this method proved to be 80 to 98 percent effective in 90 study sites nationwide since cervical cap research began in 1977.

Natural Family Planning

The *rhythm method* is based on the fact that conception occurs near the time of ovulation. Ovulation occurs about fourteen days before the beginning of a menstrual period. In a regular monthly cycle of twenty-eight days, this means that the fertile period is from about the tenth to the nineteenth day after the beginning of the menstrual period; sexual intercourse is avoided for those days.

When using the *basal temperature method* the woman measures her body temperature every morning after at least six hours of sleep, figure 21-3. The temperature during the first part of the menstrual cycle will be lower. This is followed by a slight temperature drop near the middle of the cycle. The midcycle temperature drop is about the time of ovulation. One or two days after ovulation, the body temperature rises slightly and it remains 3/10 to 1 degree higher until the beginning of menstruation. Starting from the day of temperature rise and allowing two to three safety days, conception should no longer be possible. This method is often used in conjunction with the rhythm method.

The *ovulation method* was developed by two physicians, John and Evelyn Billings. This method is based on the changes that occur in the cervical mucus during the menstrual cycle and the action of the mucus on sperm. This method can be used by women with irregular cycles. It relies upon observing and understanding vaginal secretions. Clear slippery mucus that appears at the time of ovulation is thought to keep the sperm alive and potent and also facilitates their progress through the vagina and cervix and penetration of the ovum. When vaginal secretions are clear, the couple avoids intercourse or takes additional precautions to avoid pregnancy.

Coitus Interruptus

Coitus interruptus is an interruption of sexual intercourse. The man withdraws his penis from the woman's vagina before ejaculation of seminal fluid. This method is very unreliable. There are active sperm in the seminal fluid which is in pre-ejaculate fluid.

The Condom

The *condom* is a rubber sheath which may be put on the erect penis before intercourse to prevent sperm from entering the vagina.

Condoms used carefully each and every time are thought to be 98 percent effective in preventing pregnancy. The actual user rate, however,

1. Enter the date of the month in the space provided on the graph.

2. Place a thermometer under the tongue for at least two minutes upon awakening each morning and before getting out of bed. Do this every morning even during menstruation. Do not eat, drink or smoke before taking the temperature.

3. Record the temperature reading on the graph by placing a dot in the proper place.

4. Indicate days of coitus (intercourse) by placing an arrow in the appropriate space.

5. The first day of the menstrual flow is the start of a cycle. Indicate each day of flow by shading the appropriate square on the graph.

6. Note any obvious reasons for temperature variation (such as medications, infection, colds, indigestion, etc.) on the graph above the reading for that day.

7. Some women may have a slight pain in the lower abdomen when ovulation occurs. If this is noticed, indicate the day it occurred on the graph.

8. Start a new cycle on another graph.

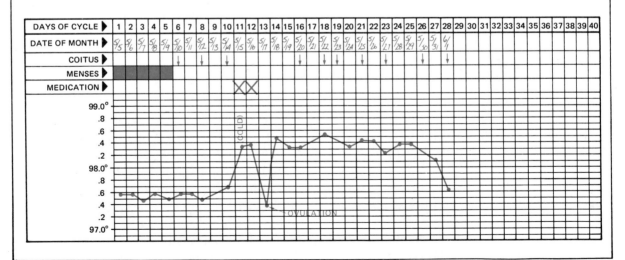

Figure 21-3

Basal temperature chart and instructions

TYPE	THEORETICAL FAILURE RATE (%)	ACTUAL FAILURE RATE (%)
Oral contraceptives (Pill)	0.1%	0.7%
IUD	1.9%	2.8%
Condom	2.6%	17%
Diaphragm	2.5%	18%
Withdrawal	16%	23%
Rhythm	14%	40%
Spermicides	3%	18%
Sponge	12%	20%
None	80%	

Source: F.D.A. statistics

Figure 21-4

Effectiveness of contraceptive methods

is about 90 percent. Condoms are used as a protection against many sexually transmitted diseases such as chlamydia and gonorrhea. They can also offer some protection against herpes and AIDS.

Spermicidals

Spermicidals (foams, tablets, creams, jellies, or suppositories) introduced into the vagina ten to fifteen minutes before intercourse produce a reaction destructive to spermatozoa. The reliability of contraception varies greatly in this method. It is important to avoid using a douche or a tampon for at least 4–6 hours after intercourse if spermicides are used; they both displace spermicides and remove protection.

The contraceptive sponge contains spermicide; it requires no prescription. It is inserted like the diaphragm; however, it can stay in place and remain effective for 24 hours.

STERILIZATION

After a couple have had their desired number of children, some men and women request *sterilization* (process of making conception impossible). The sterilization procedure for men is called a bilateral *vasectomy* and for women, a *tubal ligation*. The vas deferens is excised in the male; the fallopian tubes are cut and tied off in the female. The procedures are irreversible; that is, there is no certainty that an effort to restore fertility will be successful. However, experimental procedures are currently under way for temporary sterilization.

SUGGESTED ACTIVITIES

- Evaluate the *impact* of the following on the patient's choice of contraception: (a) oral contraceptive, (b) diaphragm, (c) natural family planning, (d) condoms, and (e) sterilization
  - Sexual activity pattern and habits
  - Reproductive life span

— Age
— Access to medical care
— Ability to pay for contraception
— Medical history
— Health

• Define what is meant by fertility awareness. Demonstrate the ability to instruct a patient on fertility awareness.

REVIEW

Multiple Choice. Select the best answer(s).

1. Use of The Pill is contraindicated for women who have
   1. a family history of breast or cervical cancer
   2. a personal history of circulatory problems
   3. never borne children
   4. a family history of diabetes
      a. 3 and 4   c. 2 only
      b. 1, 2 and 4   d. 1 and 4

2. Side effects of the IUD include
   1. pain
   2. vaginal discharge, bleeding
   3. nausea, headaches
   4. depression
      a. 3 and 4   c. 1 and 2
      b. 1, 2 and 3   d. 1, 2, 3 and 4

3. Spermicidal substances act by
   1. providing a mechanical barrier
   2. destroying sperm
   3. suppressing ovulation
   4. stimulating growth of the vaginal lining
      a. 3 only   c. 1, 2 and 4
      b. 1 and 2   d. 2 only

4. The IUD is a contraceptive device which
   1. is not suitable for nulliparas
   2. is made of fine grade rubber
   3. provides better protection than The Pill
   4. is less of a health risk than The Pill
      a. 1 and 4   c. 4 only
      b. 1 only   d. 1, 2, 3 and 4

5. The sterilization procedure for the male is
   a. tubal ligation   c. spermicide
   b. bilateral vasectomy d. all of these

6. A soft, dome-shaped device that is inserted into the vagina to prevent pregnancy is called a
   a. steel ring   c. condom
   b. diaphragm   d. spermicide

7. The side effects of a diaphragm include
   a. thromboembolic disease   c. metabolic disturbances
   b. carcinoma   d. none

8. The effectiveness of the ovulation method depends upon
   1. regular menstrual cycles
   2. observing and understanding vaginal secretions
   3. temperature changes
   4. using additional contraceptive measures
   a. 2 only   c. all of these
   b. 2 and 3   d. 1 and 2

9. Demands made upon the expectant father include
   a. financial demands   c. social demands
   b. emotional demands   d. all of these

Self-Evaluation

A. Multiple-multiple Choice. Select the best answer from the lettered selections which follow the items.

1. Treatment for a nonnursing mother with breast engorgement includes
   1. ice packs three or four times a day
   2. application of a breast binder
   3. analgesic drugs
   4. wearing a well-fitted brassiere
       a. 1 and 4   c. 1, 3 and 4
       b. 2 only   d. 1, 2, 3 and 4

2. Proper bathing of a newborn consists of
   1. sponge bath until the umbilicus has healed
   2. washing the infant's head before it is undressed
   3. water temperature of 85°F
   4. using a mild castile soap
       a. 1 and 2   c. 2 and 4
       b. 3 and 4   d. 1, 2, 3 and 4

3. An infant is considered to be premature if it
   1. weighs less than 2500 grams
   2. is born before 37 weeks gestation
   3. has a low Apgar score
   4. is slightly yellow in color
       a. 1 and 4   c. 3 and 4
       b. 1 and 2   d. 3 only

4. After childbirth, conception cannot occur again until
   1. the mother stops breast feeding
   2. menstruation resumes
   3. the end of the puerperium
   4. involution has been completed
       a. 2 and 3   c. none
       b. 2 and 4   d. 1, 2, 3 and 4

5. A congenital disorder characterized by irreparable brain and body damage is
   1. Down's syndrome
   2. PKU
   3. narcosis
   4. Respiratory Distress Syndrome
       a. 1 only   c. 1 and 3
       b. 1 and 2   d. 4 only

6. Physiological jaundice is
   1. caused by the liver's failure to cope with the breakdown of white blood cells
   2. a normal characteristic which appears in some newborns
   3. caused by increased amounts of bilirubin in the bloodstream
   4. an indication of erythroblastosis fetalis
       a. 1 only
       b. 2 and 3
       c. 4 only
       d. 1, 2 and 3

7. A normal full-term infant
   1. is between 18 and 21 inches long
   2. weighs between 5 1/2 and 10 pounds
   3. can taste and smell
   4. has thin, dry skin
       a. 2 and 3
       b. 2, 3 and 4
       c. 1 and 2
       d. 1, 2, 3 and 4

8. Care of the umbilicus includes
   1. changing the bandage twice daily
   2. cleaning with alcohol four times daily
   3. a daily tub bath to keep umbilicus soft
   4. continuing care for 4 days after the cord drops off
       a. 1 and 2
       b. 1 and 3
       c. 2 and 4
       d. 1, 2, 3 and 4

9. Adequate sleep for the mother following delivery is necessary in order to
   1. restore physical energy depleted during labor
   2. restore emotional energy depleted during labor
   3. give the body a chance to repair body tissue
   4. prevent psychological disturbances
       a. 1 only
       b. 1 and 3
       c. 1, 2 and 3
       d. 1, 2, 3 and 4

10. The nurse should instruct the mother in self-care which includes
    1. washing her breasts first when taking a shower
    2. applying clean perineal pads from back to front
    3. refraining from tub baths until 4 weeks postpartum
    4. proper exercise to improve abdominal muscle tone
        a. 1 and 4
        b. 3 and 4
        c. 1, 2 and 4
        d. 1, 2, 3 and 4

B. Briefly answer the following questions.

   1. a. Name three principles of nursing care for the premature infant.

      b. Give one example of how each principle can be demonstrated in the premature nursery.

2. What measures may be taken to ensure rapid healing of the episiotomy after delivery?

3. Name three signs of respiratory distress in the newborn.

4. What is the difference between contraception and sterilization?

C. Match the terms in column II to the correct description in column I.

Column I	Column II
1. located above the forehead and at the crown of the head	a. asphyxia neonatorum
2. return of organs to their normal state after childbirth	b. embolus
3. six-week period following childbirth	c. fontanels
4. dislodged blood clot that travels in the bloodstream	d. involution
5. a common emotional reaction following childbirth	e. let-down reflex
6. release of oxytocin causing alveoli of the breast to contract releasing milk into the main sinuses under the nipple	f. lochia
7. imperfect breathing in the newborn	g. circumcision
8. removal of the foreskin from the penis	h. postpartum depression
9. uterine and vaginal discharge after delivery	i. puerperium
10. reflex of infant to take the nipple into its mouth when gently stroked on the cheek nearest the mother's breast	j. rooting reflex

APPENDIX

TEMPERATURE CONVERSIONS FROM FAHRENHEIT TO CELSIUS (METRIC)

The metric system is gradually replacing other systems of measurement. In order to convert Fahrenheit temperatures, the following formula may be applied: (1) Subtract 32 from the Fahrenheit reading. (2) Multiply the result by 5/9.

The following chart may be used for quick reference.

°F	°C	°F	°C	°F	°C	°F	°C
70	21.1	117	47.2	160	71.1	197.6	92
71	21.7	118	47.8	161	71.7	198	92.2
72	22.2	119	48.3	161.6	72	199	92.8
73	22.8	120	48.9	162	72.2	199.4	93
74	23.3	121	49.4	163	72.8	200	93.3
75	23.9	122	50	163.4	73	201	93.9
76	24.4	123	50.6	164	73.3	201.2	94
77	25	124	51.1	165	73.9	202	94.4
78	25.6	125	51.7	165.2	74	203	95
79	26.1	126	52.2	166	74.4	204	95.6
80	26.7	127	52.8	167	75	204.8	96
81	27.2	128	53.3	168	75.6	205	96.1
82	27.8	129	53.9	168.8	76	206	96.7
83	28.3	129.2	54	169	76.1	206.6	97
84	28.9	130	54.4	170	76.7	207	97.2
85	29.4	131	55	170.6	77	208	97.8
86	30	132	55.6	171	77.2	208.4	98
87	30.6	132.8	56	172	77.8	209	98.3
88	31.1	133	56.1	172.4	78	210	98.9
89	31.7	134	56.7	173	78.3	211	99.4
90	32.2	135	57.2	174	78.9	212	100
91	32.8	136	57.8	174.2	79	213	100.6
92	33.3	136.4	58	175	79.4	214	101.1
93	33.9	137	58.3	176	80	215	101.7
94	34.4	138	58.9	177	80.6	215.6	102
95	35	139	59.4	177.8	81	216	102.2
96	35.6	140	60	178	81.1	217	102.8
96.8	36	141	60.6	179	81.7	218	103.3
97	36.1	141.8	61	179.6	82	219	103.9
98	36.7	142	61.1	180	82.2	219.2	104
98.6	37	143	61.7	181	82.8	220	104.4
99	37.2	144	62.2	181.4	83	221	105
100	37.8	145	62.8	182	83.3	225	107.2
100.4	38	145.4	63	183.2	84	230	110
101	38.3	146	63.3	184	84.4	235	112.8
102	38.9	147	63.9	185	85	239	115
102.2	39	147.2	64	186	85.6	240	115.6
103	39.4	148	64.4	186.8	86	245	118.3
104	40	149	65	187	86.1	248	120
105	40.6	150	65.6	188	86.7	250	121.1
105.8	41	150.8	66	188.6	87	255	123.9
106	41.1	151	66.1	189	87.2	257	125
107	41.7	152	66.7	190	87.8	260	126.7
107.6	42	152.6	67	190.4	88	265	129.4
108	42.2	153	67.2	191	88.3	266	130
109	42.8	154	67.8	192	88.9	270	132.2
110	43.3	154.4	68	192.2	89	275	135
111	43.9	155	68.3	193	89.4	280	137.8
112	44.4	156	68.9	194	90	284	140
113	45	156.2	69	195	90.6	285	140.6
114	45.6	157	69.4	195.8	91	290	143.3
115	46.1	158	70	196	91.1	295	146.1
116	46.7	159	70.6	197	91.7	300	148.9
116.6	47	159.8	71				

SUGGESTED CLINICAL RECORD

PRACTICAL APPLICATION	Initial of Supervisor
A. Admission to the Labor Room	
1. Records	☐☐☐☐
2. Clothing Care	☐☐☐☐
3. Vitamin K Injection	☐☐☐☐
4. Signature on Delivery Permit	☐☐☐☐
5. Prep	☐☐☐☐
6. Enema	☐☐☐☐
7. Fetal Heart Tones	☐☐☐☐
8. History	☐☐☐☐
B. Vaginal Examination	
1. Dilatation of Cervix	☐☐☐☐
2. Station	☐☐☐☐
3. Effacement of Cervix	☐☐☐☐
4. Technique	☐☐☐☐
5. Accuracy	☐☐☐☐
C. Amniotomy (with Allis Forceps) assisting Physician	☐☐☐☐
D. Timing Contractions	☐☐☐☐
E. Catheterization	☐☐☐☐
1. Urine Specimen	☐☐☐☐
F. Transfer to Delivery Room	☐☐☐☐
G. Positioning	☐☐☐☐
H. Preparation	☐☐☐☐
I. Draping	☐☐☐☐
J. Table Setup	☐☐☐☐

PRACTICAL APPLICATION	Initial of Supervisor
K. Administration of I.M. Medication	
1. Technique – Sterile	☐☐☐☐
2. Technique – Administration	☐☐☐☐
3. Knowledge of Drug	☐☐☐☐
L. Care of Newborn	
1. Identification	☐☐☐☐
2. Receiving	☐☐☐☐
3. Observation	☐☐☐☐
4. Suctioning	☐☐☐☐
5. Cord Blood	☐☐☐☐
M. Delivery Room Record	☐☐☐☐
N. Transfer of Patient to Room	
1. Chart	☐☐☐☐
2. Method	☐☐☐☐
O. Transfer of Baby to Nursery	
1. Chart	☐☐☐☐
2. Method	☐☐☐☐
P. Terminal Cleaning of Delivery Room	
1. Disposal of Placenta	☐☐☐☐
2. Instruments	☐☐☐☐
Q. Records (Book)	☐☐☐☐
R. Safety in Labor	
1. Siderails	☐☐☐☐
2. Bed Height	☐☐☐☐
S. Safety in Delivery	☐☐☐☐

GLOSSARY

abortion — expulsion of the product of conception before the fetus is viable (able to live; approximately 20 weeks)

acceleration — quickening; increase in speed

acidosis — depletion of the alkaline reserve in the blood and body tissues

acme — period of time when contractions increase

adolescence — period of time between puberty and maturity

afterbirth — lay term for the placenta and membranes

albuminuria — albumin in the urine

amenorrhea — a temporary or permanent absence of menstruation

amnesic — relating to impairment of memory

amniocentesis — a procedure whereby the amniotic sac is punctured with a needle and amniotic fluid is withdrawn

amnion — innermost of the two fetal membranes forming the amniotic sac or bag of waters that encloses the fetus

amnioscope — device for looking inside the amniotic cavity

amniotic fluid — slightly alkaline and about 98 percent water filling the amniotic sac and surrounding the fetus

amniotic sac — the amnion and chorion fuse forming a sac or bag in which the embryo is suspended

analgesia — absence of sensibility to pain

analgesic — relieving pain

android — malelike; refers to shape of pelvis meaning it is heavier, narrower and deeper

anemia — a decrease in the erythrocyte and/or hemoglobin content of the blood

anesthesia — partial or complete loss of sensation resulting from administration of drug

anomalies — deviations from normal

anovulatory menstruation — menses which occur when the ovary has failed to expel the ovum

anoxia — reduction of oxygen in body tissue

anteflexed — the bending of an organ so that its top is thrust forward

antigen — any substance which, when introduced into the blood or tissues, incites the formation of antibodies

anus — the opening of the rectum

apathy — lack of feeling of emotions

Apgar scoring system — guide for evaluation of infant's condition at birth

apnea — cessation of respiration

apneic — temporary loss of breath

areola — the darkened ring surrounding the nipple of the breast

asphyxia neonatorum — imperfect breathing in newborn infants

atony — lack of muscle tone

atrophy — decrease in size of an organ or tissue which is normally developed

attitude — state of flexion or extension of the fetus

auscultation — listening for sounds within the body

ballottement — literally means tossing. A term used in an examination when the fetus can be pushed about in the uterus

benign — tending not to progress or recur

bilirubin — a red bile pigment formed from the hemoglobin of erythrocytes

bladder — a storage receptacle for urine

blastocyst — the developing ovum during the second week after fertilization when it is a small hollow ball of cells

blastoderm — stage of development of the embryo in which it is a disc of cells from which the primary germ layers are derived

bradycardia — abnormal slowness of the pulse

Braxton-Hicks sign — painless uterine contractions occurring periodically throughout pregnancy, thereby enlarging the uterus to accommodate the growing fetus

breech — presentation in which the buttocks precedes the head

broad ligament — two structures which extend from the walls of the uterus to the pelvic wall and to which the ovaries and fallopian tubes are attached

bulbourethral glands — two small glands located below the prostate gland on either side of the urethra. They add secretions to the semen through ducts that open into the urethra.

canthus — the angle at the junction of the eyelids at either corner of the eye

caput — the head

carcinogen — a substance which causes cancer

carcinoma — malignant tumor

cataract — an opacity of the crystalline eye lens

caudal anesthesia — local anesthesia injected in the epidural space of the sacrococcygeal area

cephalic — pertaining to the head of the baby

cephalopelvic disproportion — the head of the baby is of such size, shape, or position that it cannot pass through the mother's pelvis

cervix — the narrow lower portion of the uterus

cesarean section — delivery of baby through abdominal surgery

Chadwick's sign — the violet color on the mucous membrane of the vagina just below the urethral orifice which is seen after the fourth week of pregnancy

chloasma gravidarum — various kinds of pigmentary discoloration of the skin during pregnancy

chorion — the outermost of fetal membranes

chorionic villi — fingerlike projections, developed from fetal tissue, which contain blood vessels communicating with the fetus and developing early in pregnancy

chromosome — the structure which carries the gene in the nucleus of a cell

cilia — hairlike projections which help carry the ovum along the fallopian tubes with their waving actions

circumcision — excision of the foreskin

cleavage — the early successful splitting of a fertilized ovum into smaller cells by mitosis

clitoris — a small elongated mass of tissue and muscle richly supplied with blood vessels — a female counterpart to the male penis

coccyx — small triangular bone made up of four vertebrae fused together which is found at the end of the spine

coitus — sexual union; intercourse

colostrum — the thin, yellowish fluid released by the breasts during the latter part of pregnancy and for the first few days after delivery, before milk is released.

conception — union of the sperm and ovum; see also fertilization

congenital — existing at birth as a result of heredity or some other factor occurring during intrauterine development

contraceptive — that which prevents conception

contraction — involuntary tightening of the uterine muscle

Coombs test — test done on Rh negative mothers to measure the presence of Rh antibodies

copulation — the sexual act whereby sperm is delivered to the female uterus by the erect penis

corpus — a body or mass formed in the follicle after discharge of the ovum

corpus luteum — yellowish mass formed in the graafian follicle after the egg has been released

creatinine — a basic substance in the urine

Crede treatment — instillation of 1 percent silver nitrate solution in the eyes of the newborn infant

crowning — stage at which the fetal head can be seen at the vaginal orifice

cyanosis — bluish discoloration of the skin due to insufficient oxygen in the blood

cystitis — infection of the bladder

dartos — involuntary muscle fibers which allow the scrotum to contract or relax with temperature changes

deceleration — decrease in speed

decidua basalis — a portion of the endometrium which lies directly beneath the embedded ovum in the uterus

deciduous — temporary or falling out

decrement — period of time when intensity of contractions diminishes

delivery — expulsion or extraction of a child at birth

dental caries — cavity; decay of the teeth

desquamated — peeled off; separated

Dick-Read method — a method of childbirth that uses specific exercises and relaxation techniques

differentiation — development into a more specialized or complex form

diffusion — the movement of a substance from an area of high concentration to one of lower concentration until both sides are equal

dilatation — stretching of an opening, as in the cervix during labor

DNA (deoxyribonucleic acid) — nucleic acid which contains the full genetic information needed for the formation of the human body

dominant — a trait or characteristic that appears in the offspring even though it is present in only one of the parents

Down's syndrome — congenital disorder characterized by brain and body damage

ductus arteriosus — a fetal blood vessel which joins the aorta and pulmonary artery

ductus venosus — a fetal vessel which connects the umbilical vein and the inferior vena cava

dysmenorrhea — painful menstruation

dyspnea — difficult breathing

dystocia — excessively painful, difficult or slow labor or delivery

eclampsia — an acute toxemia of pregnancy causing coma and convulsions, proteinuria, edema and hypertension

ectoderm — the outermost layer of the three primary germ layers of the embryo

ectopic — out of normal place; the fertilized ovum begins to develop outside the uterus

effacement — thinning and shortening of the cervix during labor

ejaculation — release of seminal fluid (semen) from the penis

electrode — an electric conductor through which current enters or leaves a cell, apparatus, or body

embolus — any material that is carried by the blood to another part of the body and obstructs a blood vessel

embryo — a new organism during the first eight weeks of development

endoderm — the innermost of the three primary germ layers of the embryo

endometrium —the mucous membrane lining of the uterus

engagement — presenting part decends and fully enters the pelvis

engorgement — excessive fullness of any organ or passage

epididymis — coiled tube located on the testes which is the principal storehouse for sperm. It also adds secretion to the semen which activates the spermatozoa.

episiotomy — surgical incision of the perineum toward the end of the second stage of labor to facilitate delivery

erectile — process of becoming turgid and upright

erection — the enlarging and stiffening of the penis caused by the cavernous bodies in the penis filling with blood; it generally occurs from sexual excitement.

erythroblastosis fetalis — a hemolytic disease of the newborn

estrogen — a female hormone responsible for causing female sexual changes

expiratory grunt — noisy expulsion of air from the lung

expulsion — expelling or pushing out

extension — fetal head becomes unflexed; pushes upward out of vaginal canal

external os — the opening from the cervix into the vagina

extrauterine — outside the uterus

fascia — bonds of connective tissue which help to support organs in the pelvis

fertilization — the union of the male and female reproductive cells leading to the creation of a new individual

fetal monitoring — a method used to gather data about fetal condition

fetone — an instrument which can detect fetal heart tones as early as the twelfth week

fetoscope — an obstetrical stethoscope worn on the examiner's head used to detect fetal heartbeat

fetus — the developing individual in the uterus after the eighth week of pregnancy

flaccid — limp

flatulence — excessive formation of gas in stomach or intestine

flexion — act of bending

follicle-stimulating hormone (FSH) — hormone in the female partly responsible for control of ovarian function

fontanel — unossified space or soft spot between two or more sutures of the fetal skull.

foramen ovale — opening between the auricles of the fetal heart

foreskin — see prepuce

fourchet — the posterior junction of the labia majora

fundus — the upper, rounded end of the uterus

funic souffle — a soft, flowing or whistling sound produced by the blood flowing through the umbilical cord; it synchronizes with the fetal heart sounds

gavage — feeding by means of a stomach tube

gene — one of the biologic units of heredity contained in the chromosome, each of which controls the inheritance of one or more characteristics

geneticist — a student of genetics (dealing with heredity)

gestation — the period of development of a new individual within the uterus from conception to birth

glans penis — the enlarged structure at the distal end of the penis which contains the orifice of the urethra

gonadotropic hormone — hormone secreted by the anterior lobe of the pituitary gland which helps to control ovarian function

Goodell's sign — softening of the cervix, a presumptive sign of pregnancy

graafian follicle — microscopic sac in which the ovum develops

gravida — pregnant woman

gynecoid — womanlike shape of pelvis; slightly heart-shaped and best for childbearing

heartburn — burning sensation in the epigastrium

Hegar's sign — softening of the lower uterine segment; a sign of pregnancy

hemoglobin — the oxygen-carrying pigment of human blood

hemolysis — disintegration of elements of red blood cells

hemophilia — a condition characterized by impaired co-agulability of the blood and a strong tendency to bleed

hemorrhoid — dilatation of the veins in the lower rectum and anus

heparinized — to render blood coagulable with heparin

heredity — transmission of characters from parent to offspring

heterozygote — a person having unlike genes in regard to a given characteristic

heterozygous — hybrid; having one or many pairs of unlike genes in regard to characteristics as a result of cross-breeding

histone — a simple protein found in cell nuclei which interferes with coagulation

Homans' sign — pain or discomfort behind the knee or in the calf due to an inflammation of a vein resulting from a blood clot

homozygote — a person having like genes in regard to a given character trait

homozygous — pure bred; like genes carry the dominant trait

hyaline membrane disease — respiratory distress syndrome. Condition in which alveoli of lungs fail to expand due to lack of surfactant (phospholipid)

hyaluronidase — enzyme that dissolves the layer of cells surrounding the ovum

hydramnios — amniotic fluid in amounts greater than 2000 milliliters at time of delivery

hymen — a fold of mucous membrane partly closing the vaginal opening

hyperbilirubinemia — excessive bilirubin in the blood

hyperemesis gravidarum — excessive vomiting

hyperglycemia — an excess of sugar in the blood

hypoglycemia — a deficiency of sugar in the blood

hypotension — diminished tension; low blood pressure

ilium — the lateral, flaring portion of the pelvis

impotent — term used when a man cannot have an erection or an ejaculation

increased titers — a rise in a substance required to react with another substance

increment — the amount by which a quantity is increased; increase in intensity of labor contraction

insomnia — inability to sleep

internal os — the inside opening from the uterus leading to the cervix

intrauterine — within the uterus

intrauterine transfusion — injection of Rh-negative erythrocytes into the peritoneal cavity of the fetus while it is still in the uterus

involution — return of the uterus to its normal size after childbirth

ischium — the posterior heavy portion of the pelvis

jaundice — yellowish discoloration of the skin and eyes from bile pigments

kernicterus — a severe form of icterus neonatorum with involvement of brain and spinal cord (jaundice)

labia majora — the two heavy outer lips which help make up the vulva

labia minora — the two smaller lips which lie inside the labia majora and help make up the vulva

labor — the function by which a new individual is expelled through the vagina to the outside world

lanugo — fine hair covering the body of the fetus

Leboyer method — a method of gentle, controlled childbirth with minimal trauma to the child and mother

let-down reflex — a release of milk from alveoli to the main milk sinuses under the nipple in the breast

leukorrhea — white viscid vaginal discharge

levator ani — a powerful muscle which helps support the organs in the pelvis

lie — the relationship of the long axis of the baby to that of the mother

lightening — dropping of the uterus due to the settling of the fetal head into the pelvis in the last weeks before delivery

linea nigra — a dark line appearing on the abdomen and extending from the pubis toward the umbilicus. Considered one of the signs of pregnancy

lingual — pertaining to the tongue

lipid — any one group of substances which include the fats and esters having analogous properties

lochia — vaginal discharge following delivery

lochial discharge — vaginal drainage during the six-week period following delivery

longitudinal presentation — When the long axis of the baby is parallel to the long axis of the mother

lunar month — a period of approximately 28 days; from one cycle of the moon to the next

luteinizing hormone (LH) — a hormone of the anterior pituitary gland which stimulates formation of the corpus luteum

maceration — the softening of a solid by soaking

mask of pregnancy — a pigmentary discoloration of the face during pregnancy

mastitis — inflammation or infection of the breasts

masturbation — stimulation of the sex organs by means other than sexual intercourse

maternal xiphoid — female breast bone or lowest segment of the sternum

meconium — dark green, tarlike substance in the intestines of a full-term fetus

meiosis — the process in the maturation of the germ cells by which the chromosome number is reduced from two sets to one set of chromosomes

menarche — the beginning of the menstrual function

menopause — cessation of menstruation

menorrhagia — prolonged or excessive bleeding during menstruation

menses — the periodic discharge of blood from the uterus, occurring at approximately four-week intervals

menstruation — cyclic, physiologic discharge of blood from a nonpregnant uterus occurring at about four-week intervals

mentum — chin

mesoderm — the middle layer of the three primary germ layers of the embryo

metrorrhagia — uterine bleeding which occurs at a time other than menstruation

microcephaly — condition in which the head is abnormally small

miscarriage — expulsion of fetus before the stage of viability

mitosis — indirect cell division

monilial vaginitis — vaginal infection caused by fungi

Montgomery tubercles — small nodular follicles or glands on the areolae around the nipple

Moro reflex — startle response of newborn

multipara — a woman who has borne more than one child

nullipara — a woman who has not produced a living child

Naegle's rule — a method used for calculating the expected delivery date by adding 7 days to the first day of the last menstrual period, subtracting 3 calendar months from the new date and adding 1 year.

narcosis — a stuporous, anesthetic condition

naris — nostril

neonate — a newborn in its first four weeks of life

nuchal cord — umbilical cord wrapped around neck of the fetus

nursing process — a systematic and logical framework for planning nursing care; it consists of four steps: assessment, planning, implementation, and evaluation

obstetrics — a branch of medicine which deals with childbirth and that which precedes and follows it

occiput — back part of skull

omentum — a double fold of the peritoneum attaching the stomach to adjacent organs

osmosis — the diffusion of solvent molecules through a semipermeable membrane, going from the side of lower concentration to that of higher concentration

ossification — formation of bone; conversion of other tissue into bone

ovary — the sex glands of the female which discharge and produce hormones necessary to the process of reproduction. The ovary also stores, matures, and expels ovum.

oviducts — the tubelike structures which carry the ovum from the ovary to the uterus

ovulation — the maturation and release of the ovum from the ovary

ovum — the female reproductive cell which is capable of becoming a new individual after being fertilized by sperm oxytocin — a posterior pituitary hormone which stimulates uterine contractions

Pap smear — a cervical smear (mucus from cervix placed on slide) for a cancer cytology test; short for Papanicolaou smear

para — refers to the number of previous pregnancies that have gone to the period of viability

parasympathetic — part of the autonomic nervous system which controls many internal functions of the body (heart, lungs, organs of the abdomen)

parenteral — administration of fluids, food, or drugs by means other than through the intestinal canal

parturition — expulsion or delivery of the fetus

penis — the male organ of copulation

perineal squeeze — tightening of the pelvic floor muscle

perineum — the area of skin tissue and muscle which lies between the vulva and anus

peritoneum — the membrane lining of the abdominal walls

permeable — able to be passed through

phagocytosis — the ingestion of solid particles by living cells

phenylketonuria (PKU) — rare metabolic abnormality in which phenylketones are excreted in the urine and can cause retardation

phocomelia — fetus with hands and feet but no legs or arms

phototherapy — treatment of disease by light rays; used to treat jaundice

pica — craving for nonfood substance

pigmentation — the deposit of a coloring matter in the skin

pituitary gland — a gland at the base of the brain divided into anterior and posterior lobes

placenta — a fleshy organ that develops from embryonic and maternal tissue; it serves as a respiratory, nutritive and excretory organ for the fetus

placenta abruptio — a premature separation of a normally implanted placenta

placenta previa — placenta is implanted in the lower segment of the uterus and either wholly or partially covers the cervix

placental souffle — a soft murmur produced by the blood flow in the placenta synchronized with the mother's pulse

position — pertaining to the presenting part of the child to the right or left side of the mother

postpartum — the period following childbirth

precocious dentition — early eruption of teeth

pre-eclampsia — a toxemia of pregnancy occurring in the last few months; the symptoms are elevated blood pressure, edema and albuminuria

pregnancy — the state of developing a fertilized ovum within the uterus

premature infant — infant born before 37 weeks gestation that weighs less than 5 1/2 pounds

prepuce — fold of skin over the glans penis; sometimes referred to as foreskin

presentation — the presenting part of the fetus, such as the head, face, buttocks, or shoulder, that first enters the pelvis

presenting part — that part of the fetus that lies nearest the internal opening of the cervix

previable fetus — a fetus that is not sufficiently developed to live outside of the uterus

primigravida — a woman who is pregnant for the first time

primipara — a woman who has given birth to her first child

progesterone — a hormone secreted by the corpus luteum which prepares the endometrium for the reception and development of the fertilized ovum and causes uterine secretions

projectile vomiting — vomitus ejected with force

prolactin — a hormone secreted by the anterior pituitary which stimulates milk production

prolapsed cord — presence of the umbilical cord beside or ahead of the presenting part

prostate gland — gland that surrounds the urethra at the base of the bladder; it adds an alkaline secretion to the semen which neutralizes the acidic fluid from the testes.

proteinuria — albumin in the urine

psychoprophylaxis — a method of childbirth in which the discomfort of labor and delivery is controlled by mental and physical means rather than chemical ones

puberty — period of time between the ages of nine and fourteen; an increased amount of sex hormones is usually released into the bloodstream at this time as secondary sex characteristics develop

pubis — the anterior portion of the pelvis

pudendal block anesthesia — anesthesia which affects the perineum and vulva

puerperal sepsis — postpartal infection of the pelvic organs

puerperium — period of time following delivery until complete involution of the organs (about six weeks)

pyelitis — inflammation of the kidney with special involvement of the renal pelvis

quickening — the mother's first perception of the movements of the fetus

recessive — the lesser strength of one of a pair or more of similar or contrasting factors

rectum — distal portion of the large intestine

regurgitation — abnormal backward progression of fluids or undigested food from the stomach; vomiting

renal — pertaining to the kidney

restitution — after the baby's head is delivered, it rotates back to resume its normal relationship with the shoulders

Rh factor — a term applied to an inherited antigen in the human blood

RhoGAM — Solution of gamma globulin containing Rh antibodies

ribonucleic acid (RNA) — a nucleic acid that is responsible for transferring genetic information within a cell

rickets — a deficiency disease of infancy and childhood that causes abnormalities in structure and shape of bones

rooting reflex — baby turns head to side and begins sucking response when cheek is touched

round ligament — a structure which helps support the pelvic organs and is attached to the side walls of the uterus and the mons veneris

rubella — German measles. An acute infectious disease that can cause serious anomalies in the developing fetus if the mother contracts the disease in the first two or three months of pregnancy

rugae — small folds or ridges within the mucous membrane lining the vagina

sacrum — lower back (triangular bone between lumbar and coccyx), formed of five unified vertebrae

scapula — shoulder

scrotum — pouch of loose skin and superficial fascia which contains the testes; it keeps the sperm at lower than body temperature

scurvy — a disease due to deficiency in ascorbic acid; characterized by bone deformities

sedative — a drug that allays activity and excitement

semen — fluid in which the sperm is carried; it consists of secretions from the epididymis, the prostate gland, the seminal vesicles, and the bulbourethral (Cowper's) gland.

seminal vesicle glands — two saclike structures located behind the prostate gland which secrete a fluid that makes up a part of the semen

sensorium — any sensory nerve center

sex-limited — traits that appear in one sex only

sex-linked — physical traits which are associated with the genes in the sex chromosomes

spectrophotometer — instrument used to measure the intensity of various wavelengths of light transmitted

spermatogenic — sperm-producing

spermatozoa — mature male sex cells which are formed in the testes; also called sperm

stasis — maintaining a constant level

station — degree of engagement above or below the ischial spines

sterility — the inability to bring about conception

sterilization — process of making conception impossible

stillbirth — a fetus that is born dead

striae gravidarum — streaks on the sides of the abdomen, breasts and thighs caused by stretching of the skin

subcutaneous — beneath the layers of the skin

surfactant — an agent that stabilizes the alveolar sacs by lowering surface tension; it is necessary for normal respiratory function

suture — junction between bones of the skull; also refers to sewing together an incision

symphysis pubis — line of fusion between the pubic bones

tachycardia — excessively rapid heart beat

talipes — clubfoot

teratogen — having the ability to cause abnormal development

testes — primary sex organs of the male; they produce sperm and testosterone

testosterone — primary male sex hormone contributing to the development of secondary sex characteristics such as hair distribution and growth, changes in body contour, and voice changes.

tetany — a nervous disorder characterized by sharp flexion of the wrist and ankle joints, muscle twitching, cramps, and convulsions

tetonic — prolonged uterine contractions lasting over ninety seconds

thrombus — blood clot that remains at the place it was formed

thrush — fungus infection in the mouth

titers — the quantity of a substance required to react with a given amount of another substance

tonus — tone or contraction of skeletal muscles

torturous — causing torture; cruelly painful

toxemia — a disorder encountered during gestation or early in the puerperium which is characterized by one or more of the following signs: hypertension, edema, albuminuria, and in severe cases, convulsion and coma

trait — a distinguishing quality or feature

transducer — a piece of equipment used to convert one form of energy into another form of energy

transverse presentation — shoulder is the presenting part

trichomonas vaginalis — parasitic flagellate protozoa found in acid secretion in the vagina

trimester — a three month period during gestation

tubal ligation — a form of sterilization for a woman whereby the fallopian tubes are cut and tied off

tubal pregnancy — fertilized ovum implanted within the fallopian tube

tyrosine — amino acid in the body

ultrasonography — a form of sound wave that views pelvic organs

umbilical cord — a structure, approximately twenty inches long containing two arteries and one vein which attaches the fetus to the placenta

umbilicus — navel

ureter — tube carrying urine from the kidneys to the bladder

urethra — tube leading from the bladder to an opening in the vulva

urinary meatus — the opening in the vulva through which urine is voided

uterine activity transducer — type of fetal monitoring unit

uterine dysfunction — a delay in any phase of labor

uterogestation — gestation (development of life) in the uterus

uterus — female organ which carries the fetus during pregnancy

vagina — a tubelike passage leading from the vulva to the uterus

varicose vein — a vein which has become abnormally painful and swollen as a result of prolonged increased pressure

vas deferens — slim, muscular tube about 18 inches long which carries semen to the urethra

vasectomy — surgical prevention of sperm traveling beyond the vas deferens resulting in permanent sterility for the male

venereal disease — an infection transmitted through sexual contact

vernix caseosa — cheeselike substance which covers the skin of the fetus and acts as a protection

version — altering of the fetal position in utero

vertex — the crown or top of the head

vulva — the external female genitalia

Wharton's jelly — a mucoid substance which surrounds the umbilical cord and protects the blood vessels inside the cord

zygote — a cell produced by genetic union. One cell with one nucleus containing all the necessary elements for future development of the offspring.

BIBLIOGRAPHY

BOOKS

Andre-Thomas, C.Y., Y. Chesni and S. Saint Anne Dargassies. *Neurological Examination of the Infant.* London: National Spastic Society Publication, 1960.

Baird, Dugald. *Combined Textbook of Obstetrics and Gynecology*, 9th ed. New York: Longman, Inc., 1976.

Bates, Barbara. *A Guide to Physical Examination*, 3rd ed. Philadelphia: J.B. Lippincott Co., 1983.

Benson, Ralph C. *Current Obstetric and Gynecologic Diagnosis and Treatment*, 5th ed. Los Altos, CA: Lange Medical Publications, 1984.

_____. *Handbook of Obstetrics and Gynecology*, 7th ed. Los Altos, CA: Lange Medical Publications, 1980.

Berkowitz, Richard, Donald Coustan, and Tara Mochizuke. *Handbook for Prescribing Medication During Pregnancy*, 2nd ed. Boston: Little, Brown and Co., 1986.

Brazelton, T.B., ed. *A Neonatal Behavioral Assessment Scale*, 2nd ed. (Clinics in Developmental Medicine Ser. Vol. 50.) New York: J.B. Lippincott Co., 1984.

Brenner, Erma A. *A New Baby! A New Life!* New York: McGraw-Hill, 1973.

Brigley, Catherine M. *Pediatrics for the Practical Nurse.* Albany, NY: Delmar Publishers Inc., 1973.

Burrow, Gerald N. and Thomas F. Ferris, *Medical Complications During Pregnancy*, 3rd ed. Philadelphia: W.B. Saunders Co., 1988.

Ibid, No. 287.

Childbirth Education Association of Seattle. *Becoming Parents.* Seattle: Ballard Printing and Publishing, 1976.

Cianfrani, Theodore. *A Short History of Obstetrics and Gynecology.* Springfield, IL: Charles C. Thomas Pubs., 1960.

Clausen, Joy, et al. *Maternity Nursing Today*, 2nd ed. New York: McGraw-Hill, 1977.

Crawford, J. Selwyn. *Principles and Practice of Obstetric Anaesthesia*, 5th ed. Philadelphia: J.B. Lippincott Co., 1984.

Crouch, James E. *Functional Human Anatomy*, 4th ed. Philadelphia: Lea and Febiger, 1985.

Danforth, David N. and James R. Scott. *Obstetrics and Gynecology*, 5th ed. Philadelphia: J.B. Lippincott, 1986.

Dickason, Jean and Martha Schult. *Maternal and Infant Care*, 2nd ed. New York: McGraw-Hill, 1979.

Fischbach, Frances T. *A Manual of Laboratory Diagnostic Tests*, 2nd ed. Philadelphia: J.B. Lippincott, 1984.

Gluck, Louis, ed. *Modern Perinatal Medicine.* Chicago: Year Book Medical Pubs., Inc., 1975.

Griffin, Joanne K., et al., eds. *Maternal and Child Health Nursing*, 3rd ed. Flushing, NY: Medical Examination Publishing Co., Inc. 1972.

Guyton, Arthur C. *Textbook of Medical Physiology*, 7th ed. Philadelphia: W.B. Saunders Co., 1986.

Hamilton, Persis Mary. *Basic Maternity Nursing*, 5th ed. St. Louis: The C.V. Mosby Co., 1984.

Hassid, Patricia. *A Textbook for Childbirth Educators.* New York: Harper & Row, 1978.

Hatcher, Robert. *Contraceptive Technology 1986–1987*, 13th ed. New York: Irvington Publishers, Inc., 1986.

Hawkins, Joellen Watson and Loretta Pierfedeici. *Maternity and Gynecological Nursing.* New York: J.B. Lippincott Co., 1981.

Helsing, Elizabet and T. Savage King. *Breast Feeding in Practice.* New York: Oxford University Press, 1982.

Hoerr, Normand L. and Arthur Osol, eds. *Blakiston's Illustrated Pocket Medical Dictionary* (1952), p. 110.

Iorio, Josephine. *Principles of Obstetrics and Gynecology for Nurses*, 3rd rev. ed. St. Louis: The C.V. Mosby Co., 1975.

Jenson, Margaret Duncan, Ralph Benson and Irene Bobsk. *Maternity Care: The Nurse and the Family*, 3rd ed. St. Louis: The C.V. Mosby Co., 1985.

Jornsay, Donna, Anne Duckles and Lois Jovanovic. *Gestational Diabetes*. Indianapolis, IN: Boehringer Mannheim, 1986.

Kay, Margarita A. *Anthropology of Human Birth*, Philadelphia: F.A. Davis (1982) p. 200.

Law, Barbara. *Family Planning in Nursing*. New York: Beedman Pubs., Inc., 1973.

Lerch, Constance. *Workbook for Maternity Nursing*, 3rd ed. St. Louis: The C.V. Mosby Co., 1978.

Lesner, Patricia. *Pediatric Nursing*, 2nd ed. Albany, New York: Delmar Publishers Inc., 1985.

Lorenze, Larry. *Fitness and Pregnancy*. New York: Drake Pubs., Inc., 1975.

McNall, Leota K. *Obstetric and Gynecologic Nursing*. St. Louis: The C.V. Mosby Co., 1980.

Martini, Arthur P. (unpub.).

Moore, Mary L. and Ora Strickland. *Realities in Childbearing*, 2nd ed. Philadelphia: W.B. Saunders Co., 1983.

Niswander, Kenneth R. *Manual of Obstetrics, Diagnosis and Therapy*, 2nd ed. Boston: Little, Brown and Company, 1983.

Olds, Sally W. and Marvin S. Eiger. *Maternal-Newborn*. Reading, MA: Addison-Wesley, 1984.

_____. *Maternal Newborn Nursing*, 2nd ed. Reading, MA: Addison-Wesley, 1984.

Oxorn, Harry. *Oxorn-Foote Human Labor and Birth*, 5th ed. East Norwalk, CT: Appleton-Century-Crofts, 1986.

Page, Ernest W., Claude A. Villee and Dorothy B. Villee. *Human Reproduction*, 3rd ed. Philadelphia: W.B. Saunders Co., 1981.

Pillitteri, Adele. *Maternal-Newborn Nursing: Care of the Growing Family*, 2nd ed. Boston: Little, Brown and Co., 1981.

Pritchard, Jack A., Paul C. MacDonald and Norman F. Grant. *Williams Obstetrics*, 17th ed. E. Norwalk, CT: Appleton-Century-Crofts, 1985.

Reeder, Sharon R., et al. *Maternity Nursing*, 14th ed. Philadelphia: J.B. Lippincott Co., 1980.

Reeder, Sharon, Luigi Mastroianni, Jr., and Leonide Martin. *Maternity Nursing*, 16th ed. New York: J.B. Lippincott Co., 1987.

Romney S., et al. *Gynecology and Obstetrics: The Health Care of Women*, 2nd ed. New York: McGraw-Hill, 1980.

Sabbagha, Ruby E. *Diagnostic Ultrasound Applied to Obstetrics and Gynecology*, 2nd ed. Philadelphia: J.B. Lippincott, 1987.

Sagebeer, Josephine. *Maternal Health Nursing Review*, 2nd ed. New York: Arco Publishing Co., Inc., 1979.

Sasmor, Jeannette. *Childbirth Education: A Nursing Perspective*. New York: John Wiley & Sons, 1979.

Sherman, Alfred I., ed. *Pathways to Conception: The Role of the Cervix and the Oviduct in Reproduction*. Springfield, IL: Charles C. Thomas, Pubs., 1971.

Simkin, Penny, Janet Whalley and Ann Keppler. *Pregnancy, Childbirth and the Newborn*. Deephaven, MN: Meadowbrook Books, 1984.

Smith, Clement A. *The Critically Ill Child*, 3rd ed. Philadelphia: W.B. Saunders, 1985.

_____. *Physiology of the Newborn Infant*, 4th ed. Springfield, IL: Charles C. Thomas, Pubs., 1975.

Spector, Rachel E. *The Utilization of Parteras as a Source of Maternal/Child Health Care Along the U.S./Mexico Border*. UT Austin, (1983), p 5.

Speert, Harold. *A Pictorial History of Gynecology and Obstetrics*. Philadelphia: F.A. Davis Co., 1973.

_____. *Obstetrics and Gynecology in America—A History*. Baltimore, MD: Waverly Press, 1980.

Stevenson, Roger E. *The Fetus and the Newly Born Infant: Influences of the Prenatal Environment*, 2nd ed. St. Louis: The C.V. Mosby Co., 1977.

Time-Life Education Materials. *Life Before Birth*. 1965.

Tucker, Susan Martin and Sandra L. Bryant. *Fetal Monitoring and Fetal Assessment in High-Risk Pregnancy*. St. Louis: The C.V. Mosby Co., 1978.

_____. *Patient Care Standards*, 3rd ed. St. Louis: The C.V. Mosby Co., 1984.

Van Bergen, William S., ed. *Obstetric Ultrasound: Applications and Principles*. Reading, MA: Addison-Wesley Pub. Co., 1980.

Wason, Candace and Boyd Metzger. *Diabetes Management for the Mother-to-be*. Chicago: Abelson-Taylor-Frizsimmons, Inc., 1986.

Williams, *Italian Folkways*, p. 88.

Worthington-Roberts, Bonnie S., Joyce Vermeesch and Sue. R. Williams. *Nutrition in Pregnancy and Lactation*, 3rd ed. St. Louis: Times Mirror-Mobsy, 1985.

Ziegel, Erna and Mecca S. Cranley. *Obstetric Nursing*, 7th ed. New York: Macmillan, 1978.

PERIODICALS

Affonso, D. "The Newborn's Potential for Interaction." *Journal of Obstetric, Gynecological and Neonatal Nursing* 5(6):9–14, November–December 1976.

Apgar, V.A. "A Proposal for a New Method of Evaluation of the Newborn Infant." *Current Researches in Anesthesia and Analgesia* 32:260, 1960.

Brazelton, T.B. "Does the Neonate Shape His Environment?" *Birth Defects* 10(2):131–40, 1974.

_____. "Psychophysiological Reactions in the Neonate, No. I: The Value of Observation of the Newborn." *Journal of Pediatrics* 48:508, 1961.

Brazelton, T.B., et al. "Early Mother-Infant Reciprocity." *Ciba Foundation Symposium* (33):137–54, 1975.

Brazelton, T.B., W.B. Parker, and B. Zuckerman. "Importance of Behavioral Assessment of the Neonate." *Current Problems in Pediatrics* 7(2):1–82, December 1976.

Brazelton, T.B. and J.S. Robey. "Observations of Neonatal Behavior, the Effect of Perinatal Variables in Particular that of Maternal Medication." *Journal of Child Psychiatry* 4:613, 1965.

Cannon, *Utah*, No. 289.

Clark, A.L. and D.D. Affonso. "Mother-Child Relationships. Infant Behavior and Maternal Attachment: Two Sides to the Coin." *Maternal-Child Nursing Journal* 1(2):94–9, March–April 1976.

Cook, Nancy and Paulina Periz. "The Brazelton Scale." *Childbirth Educator*, 4(4):31–35, 1985.

Cohen, S.N. and S.K. Ganapathy. "Drugs in the Fetus and Newborn Infant." *Clinical Endocrinology and Metabology* 5(1):176–90, March 1976.

Cox, B.S. "Rooming-in." *Nursing Times* 70(32):1246–7, 8 August 1974.

Done, A.K. "Perinatal Pharmacology." *Annual Review of Pharmacology* 6:189–208, 1966.

Gelber, *Colorado*, No. 57.

Gombel, J. and J. Nocon. "The Physiological Basis for the Leboyer Approach to Childbirth. *Journal of Obstetric, Gynecological, and Neonatal Nursing* 6:11–15, January–February 1977.

Grausz, J.P. "The Fetus and the Newborn." *Medical Clinics of North America* 53(5):1051–62, September 1969.

Green, H.G. "Infants of Alcoholic Mothers." *American Journal of Obstetrics and Gynecology* 118(5):713–6, 1 March 1974.

Griepp, E. and D. Baum. "Circulatory Adjustments at Birth." *Obstetrics and Gynecology Annual* 4:99–118, 1975.

Hoffeld, D.R., J. McNew, and R.L. Webster. "Effect of Tranquilizing Drugs During Pregnancy on Activity of Offspring." *Nature* 218:357, 1968.

Klein, R.E., J.P. Habicht, and C. Yarbrough. "Effect of Protein-Calorie Malnutrition on Mental Development." (Advances of Pediatrics, Incap publication No. 1-571), 1971.

Lavery, J. Patrick. "Nonstress Fetal Heart Rate Testing." *Clinical Obstetrics and Gynecology* 25(4):689, December 1982.

Mirkin, B.L. "Perinatal Pharmacology: Placental Transfer, Fetal Localization, and Neonatal Disposition of Drugs." *Anesthesiology* 43(2):156–70, August 1975.

Parkin, J.M., E.N. Hey, and J.S. Clowes. "Rapid Assessment of Gestational Age at Birth." *Archives of Diseases of Childhood* 51(4):259–63, April 1976.

Plante, Dawn and Bonnie Stiles. "Expanding the Nurse's Role Through Formal Assessment of the Neonate." *JOGN Nursing* 13(1):25–29, January–February, 1984.

Prechtl, H.F. "The Behavioral States of the Newborn Infant (A Review)." *Brain Research* 76(2):185–212, 16 August 1974.

Reiber, V.D. "Is the Nurturing Role Natural to Fathers?" *Maternal-Child Nursing Journal* 1(6):366–71, November–December 1976.

Richman, N. "Individual Differences at Birth." *Developmental Medicine and Child Neurology* 14(3):400–1, June 1972.

Scanlon, J.W., et al. "Neurobehavioral Responses and Drug Concentrations in Newborns After Maternal Epidural Anesthesia with Bupicacaine." *Anesthesiology* 45(4):400–5, October 1976.

Scanlon, J.W. "Obstetric Anesthesia as a Neonatal Risk Factor in Normal Labor and Delivery." *Clinical Perinatology* 1(2):465–82, September 1974.

Smith, Pamela C. "Diabetes in Pregnancy." *Childbirth Educator* 1(2):8–12, 1982.

Snapper, Isadore. "Midwifery, Past and Present." *Bulletin of the New York Academy of Medicine* 39:503–32.

Sorimshaw, N.S., C.E. Taylor, and J.E. Gordon. "Interactions of Nutrition and Infection." *American Journal of Medical Sciences* 237:367, 1959.

Standley, K., et al. "Local-Regional Anesthesia During Childbirth: Effect on Newborn Behaviors." *Science* 186(4164):634–5, 15 November 1974.

Stringer, Marilyn. "Chorionic Villi Sampling: A Nursing Perspective." *JOGNN* 17(1):19–22, January–February, 1988.

Stone, F.H. "Psychological Aspects of Early Mother-Infant Relationships." *British Medical Journal* 4(781):224–6, 23 October 1971.

Thomas, E.B., et al. "Feeding Behaviors of Newborn Infants as a Function of Parity of the Mother." *Child Development* 42(5):1471–83, November 1971.

Wingate, M.B., et al. "The Effect of Epidural Analgesia Upon Fetal and Neonatal Status." *American Journal of Obstetrics and Gynecology* 119(8):1011–6, 15 August 1974.

Yaffee, S.J. and C.S. Catz. "Pharmacology of the Perinatal Period." *Clinical Obstetrics and Gynecology* 14(3):722–44, September 1971.

Yao, A.C. and J. Lind. "Placental Transfusion." *American Journal of Diseases of Children* 127(1):128–41, January 1974.

Zigrossi, Suzanne and S. Riga-Ziegler. "The Stress of Medical Management on Pregnant Diabetics." *MCN* 11:320–323, September–October, 1986.

ACKNOWLEDGMENTS

The authors wish to express their appreciation to the following individuals and organizations for permission to use information, tabular data, and illustrations:

Advanced Technology Laboratories, Bothell, WA, figures 11-8 and 11-9
Air-Shields, Inc., Hatboro, PA, figure 19-9
Virginia Apgar, M.D., figure 16-7
Astra Pharmaceutical Products, Inc., Worcester, MA, figures 15-1 and 15-3
Baby Talk Magazine, New York, NY, figure 19-1
Robert J. Brady Company, Washington, DC, figures 11-3, 11-5, 12-4, 12-5
Carnation Company, Buffalo, NY, figures 12-10, 12-11, 12-14, 18-1
Century Manufacturing Company, Aurora, NE, figure 13-8
Childbirth Education Association of Seattle, figure 10-5
Corometrics Medical Systems, Inc., and Dr. Edward Hon, figure 14-7
Doubleday & Company, New York, NY
Evergreen General Medical Center, Kirkland, WA, figures 1-1, 1-2 and 1-3
Hill-Rom Corp., Batesville, IN, figures 13-6 and 19-8
Johns Hopkins Press, Baltimore, MD
Patricia Lesner, R.N., Elyria, Ohio, figures 20-4, 20-5, and 20-6
Littlefield, Adams & Co., Totowa, NJ, figures 11-6, 13-7, 13-8, 16-2
Maternity Center Association, New York, NY, figures 8-1, 10-2, 18-3
New York Academy of Medicine, New York, NY
Ross Laboratories, Columbus, OH, figures 2-4, 7-1, 7-2, 11-2, 11-4, 12-3, 12-8, 12-9, 12-13, 16-7, 19-2, 19-4, 19-10, 20-2
W.B. Saunders Co., Philadelphia, PA, figures 3-1, 5-1, 5-4, 5-5, 12-12, 13-9, 16-1
Jack M. Schneider, M.D., figure 14-8
Shering Corp., Bloomfield, NJ, figures 6-1, 6-2, 6-3
Sherwood Medical Industries, Inc., St. Louis, MO, figure 15-6
Tampax, Inc., Palmer, MA, figures 2-2, 2-3, 3-4
Charles C. Thomas, Evanston, IL
Winthrop Laboratories, Division of Sterling Drug Corp., Inc., figure 19-3
Wyeth Laboratories, Philadelphia, PA, figure 2-4
W.A. Silverman, M.D. and D.H. Anderson, M.D., figure 20-1

The authors also wish to acknowledge their indebtedness to:

Kenneth C. Welch M.D. for his professional expertise.
Michael, David, and Jeffrey Shapiro for their understanding, love, and encouragement to Mom and Tutu in the preparation of this book.

INDEX

Drugs
    dependency on, prenatal development and, 44
    effect on fetus, 74
Ductus
    arteriosus, 50
    deferens, 26
    venosus, 50
Dysmenorrhea, 21

E

Eclampsia, 112, 117
Ectoderm, 34
Ectopic pregnancy, 115, 118, 119
Effacement in labor, 138–39, 142–44
Ejaculation, 27
Ejaculatory, ducts, 26
EKG electrode, 170
Elimination
    during pregnancy, 84
    newborn, 259
    postpartum period and, 241, 245
Embryo, 34
Embryonic development, 40
Emerson Birtheez method, 193
Endocrine system, pregnancy and, 63
Endoderm, 34
Endometrium, 12
Enema, during labor, 154
Engagement, fetus, 137, 142, 144
Engorgement, 267–68
    postpartum period, 237
Enzymes, hyaluronidase, 28–29
Epididymis, 25, 26
Episiotomy, 146, 235
Epithelial cells, desquamated, 43
Epithelium, 19
Erb's palsy, 294
Erythroblastosis fetalis, 128, 287–88
Erythromycin, effect on fetus, 74
Estrogen, 17, 18
    effect on fetus, 74
Exercise
    during pregnancy, 89–91
        pelvic floor contraction, 90
    postpartum period and, 244, 245
Expulsion
    fetus, 146
    labor and, 144–46
Extension, fetus, 146
External os, 12

F

Face presentations, 219
Facial paralysis, 293
Fallopian tubes, 12, 18–19

False labor, 138
Family planning, 301–9
    father's role in, 301–2
    methods of, 302–8
        cervical cap, 305
        coitus interruptus, 306
        condoms, 206–7
        diaphragm, 305
        effectiveness of, *307*
        intrauterine devices, 304–5
        oral contraceptives, 302, 304
        rhythm, 305
        spermicidals, 307
        sterilization, 307–8
Fascias, 14
Fertilization, 9, *32*
Fetal
    alcohol syndrome, 78
    blood sampling, 183–85
        test, 126
    bradycardia, 171–72, 173–74
    circulation, 50–52
    development, 41–43
    diseases effect on, 74
    distress, *174*
        acute, 172, 173
        assessing, 122–30
    drugs effect on, 74
    flexion, 144
    heart beat, 64
    heart rate
        internal monitor, 182–83
        monitor tracing, *172*
        patterns, 171, 173–76
    heart tones, during labor, 153, *154*
    membrane, 34
    monitoring 166–87
        direct method, 170
        indirect method, 168–70
        interpretations, 170–73
        intrauterine catheter insertion, 181–82
        nonstress test, 178–80
        oxytocin challenge test, 175, 177–78
        selecting patients for, 167
    movements, 65
    positions, 140, 141–42
        abnormal, 218–20
        tachycardia, 172, 173
Fetone, 41–42, 64
Fetoscope, 42
Fetus, 34
    diseases effect on, 74
    drugs effect on, 74
    flexion, 144